THIRD EDITION

JOINT MOBILIZATION/ MANIPULATION

EXTREMITY AND SPINAL TECHNIQUES

Susan L. Edmond, P.T., D.Sc., O.C.S.

Professor

School of Health Related Professions

Rehabilitation and Movement Sciences

Rutgers, The State University of New Jersey

New Brunswick, New Jersey

ELSEVIER

ELSEVIER

3251 Riverport Lane
St. Louis, Missouri 63043

JOINT MOBILISATION/MANIPULATION:
EXTREMITY AND SPINAL TECHNIQUES, 10TH EDITION

ISBN: 978-0-323-29469-0

Notices

Previous editions copyrighted 1993 and 2006.

Library of Congress Cataloging-in-Publication Data

Names: Edmond, Susan L., author.
Title: Joint mobilization/manipulation : extremity and spinal techniques/
    Susan L. Edmond.
Other titles: Joint mobilization manipulation
Description: Third edition. | St. Louis, Missouri : Elsevier, [2017] |
    Includes bibliographical references and index.
Identifiers: LCCN 2015050577| ISBN 9780323294690 (paper back : alk. paper) |
    ISBN 0323027261 (paper back : alk. paper)
Subjects: | MESH: Manipulation, Orthopedic | Manipulation, Spinal | Range of
    Motion, Articular–physiology
Classification: LCC RD736.M25 | NLM WB 535 | DDC 615.8/2–dc23 LC record available at
http://lccn.loc.gov/2015050577

Executive Content Strategist: Kathy Falk
Content Development Manager: Jolynn Gower
Senior Content Development Specialist: Brian S. Loehr
Project Manager: Srividhya Vidhyashankar
Designer: Ryan Cook

Printed in United States of America

Last digit is the print number: 9 8 7 6 5 4 3

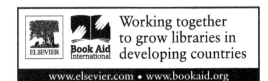

To
Derek,
my son

Reviewers of the Second Edition

Katherine L. Beissner, Ph.D., P.T.
Ithaca College
Ithaca, New York

Lee C. Grinonneau, M.S., P.T.
Owens State Community College
Toledo, Ohio

Peter M. Leininger, M.S., P.T., O.C.S., C.S.C.S.
The University of Scranton
Scranton, Pennsylvania

L. Vince Lepak III, P.T., M.P.H., C.W.S.
University of Oklahoma Health Sciences Center
Tulsa, Oklahoma

Becky J. Rodda, P.T., M.H.S., O.C.S., O.M.P.T.
University of Michigan–Flint
Flint, Michigan

Richard Biff Williams, Ph.D., A.T.C., L.A.T.
University of Northern Iowa
Cedar Falls, Iowa

Preface

The motivation for writing the first edition of this book was to provide entry-level students and practicing clinicians with a practical guide for learning the art and science of joint mobilization/manipulation. Since the publication of the first edition in 1993, much has changed in the discipline of manual therapeutic techniques. One notable change is the increased emphasis on evidence-based practice. Implicit in the use of evidence-based practice is the critical appraisal of theories and techniques that are commonly used to evaluate and treat patients using the best available research.

I firmly believe that we serve our patients most effectively when we consistently apply results from clinical research to our decisions regarding patient care. In this third edition, I have incorporated information from available research regarding evaluation and intervention techniques associated with joint mobilization/manipulation. There is much we have yet to learn about this discipline, especially in relation to linking effective interventions to examination findings. I trust that with the changes and additions to this third edition, I have provided the reader with an important resource for advancing the understanding and implementation of effective evaluation and treatment procedures involving mobilization/manipulation of the extremities and spine.

Susan L. Edmond, P.T., D.Sc., O.C.S.

Contributor

Richard Crowell, PT, MS, GDMT, MCTA, FAAOMPT
Center for Fitness and Therapy
Essentia Health
Duluth, Minnesota

Acknowledgments

To my students and colleagues, who continually educate and inspire me.

To the folks at Elsevier, who made this book happen.

To my colleagues, Allison M Brown, PT, PhD and Robyn Lieberman, PT DPT, whose editing, advice, and support were invaluable, and who contributed their time and energy to model for videos and stills.

Susan L. Edmond, P.T., D.Sc., O.C.S.

Contents

INTRODUCTION

1 General Concepts, 3
2 Principles of Examination, Evaluation, and Intervention, 11

THE APPENDICULAR SKELETAL SYSTEM

3 The Shoulder, 28
4 The Elbow and Forearm, 60
5 The Wrist and Hand, 82
6 The Hip Joint, 138
7 The Knee, 150
8 The Lower Leg, Ankle, and Foot, 170

THE AXILLARY SKELETAL SYSTEM

9 Introduction to the Axillary Skeletal System, 219
10 The Temporomandibular Joint, 222
11 Cervical Spine, 230
12 The Thoracic Spine and Ribs, 260
13 The Lumbar Spine, 290
14 Pelvic Joints, 314

Index, 327

Introduction

CHAPTER 1

General Concepts

DEFINITION

Joint mobilization has been defined by Maitland[1] as an externally imposed, small-amplitude passive motion that is intended to produce gliding or traction at a joint. Joint manipulation traditionally has been defined as a specific technique in which the articular capsule is passively stretched by delivering a quick thrust maneuver to the joint and has been considered by many clinicians to be a specific type of joint mobilization technique as defined by Maitland. In an attempt to consolidate these definitions, the American Physical Therapy Association[2] provided the following definition of mobilization/manipulation: manual therapy techniques comprising a continuum of skilled passive movements to the joints and/or related soft tissues that are applied at varying speeds and amplitudes, including a small-amplitude/high-velocity therapeutic movement. This definition encompasses multiple techniques, including those referred to by Maitland in the aforementioned definition, passive joint movement techniques in which the mobilization/manipulation force is created by active contraction of the patient's own muscles (called muscle energy), and passive joint movements that occur simultaneously with active range or passive range of motion (called mobilization with movement). As a general rule, muscle energy and mobilization with movement are only performed using slower maneuvers, whereas the traditional method of joint mobilization/manipulation as defined by Maitland can generally be performed using either a quick thrust or slower-amplitude force. Manual therapy encompasses a broader array of hands-on techniques including joint mobilization/manipulation and soft tissue mobilization techniques.

HISTORY

Joint mobilization/manipulation has been a part of medicine throughout recorded history. There is some evidence that manual techniques were used in Thailand around 2000 B.C. as well as in ancient Egypt. Hippocrates used manual traction in the treatment of spinal deformities. In Europe during the 1600s, bonesetters developed an entire practice consisting of joint mobilization/manipulation techniques. This discipline persisted throughout the 1800s. Although ignorant of much of the anatomic and physiologic basis for mobilization/manipulation, bonesetters used a series of techniques that were often successful in reducing pain and deformity.

The practices of osteopathic and chiropractic medicine were conceived of in the late nineteenth to early twentieth century. Osteopathic and chiropractic medicine are based on the theory that diseases, including spinal conditions, are due to vertebral joint impairment. Some of the techniques practiced by osteopaths and chiropractors resemble those of bonesetters.

Osteopathy is based on the premise that disease processes frequently manifest themselves in the neuromusculoskeletal system, resulting in somatic dysfunction. Somatic dysfunction is defined as impairment in the skeletal, arthrodial, and myofascial systems with resultant alteration in vascular, lymphatic, and neural tissue. Manual therapy is believed to normalize the somatic system.

The osteopathic neuromusculoskeletal examination includes a determination of the presence of joint asymmetry, joint movement restrictions, and soft tissue texture changes. Treatment includes thrust joint manipulation, slower-amplitude mobilization, and muscle energy, among other techniques.

Chiropractors also believe that disease processes can manifest themselves in the neuromusculoskeletal system, causing somatic dysfunction, although they place greater emphasis on the role of spinal nerves. The chiropractic examination also focuses primarily on joint asymmetry and restrictions, and treatment most often consists of thrust joint manipulation.

Osteopaths continue to use mobilization/manipulation as an adjunct to medical intervention but have expanded their education to a level comparable to that of medical physicians, with additional training in mobilization/manipulation. Most chiropractors now believe that diseases cannot be cured by spinal manipulation and focus their treatments to specifically address spinal impairments. Both of these disciplines have contributed to the knowledge base of mobilization/manipulation as currently practiced by physical therapists.

PRACTITIONERS CONTRIBUTING TO THE KNOWLEDGE BASE OF JOINT MOBILIZATION/MANIPULATION

Numerous practitioners, including medical physicians and physical therapists, have contributed to the current knowledge base of joint mobilization/manipulation evaluation and intervention techniques.

Mennell

Mennell was an early proponent of using joint mobilization/manipulation techniques to treat joint pain. He developed the concept that joint adhesions are a common cause of joint impairments, as they alter movement between two joint surfaces. Furthermore, he advocated that clinicians evaluate patients for loss of joint motion and promoted the concept that this loss of joint motion could be treated effectively with mobilization techniques.

Cyriax

Cyriax was an orthopedic physician who contributed to the development of a system of examining patients with musculoskeletal impairments, components of which are commonly used by physical therapists. This system focuses on using different examination procedures involving active, passive, and resisted movements to selectively isolate one soft tissue from another to determine which soft tissue is responsible for the patient's symptoms, a concept he termed *selective tissue tension testing*. As part of the examination process, Cyriax proposed identifying the presence of a capsular pattern, which is a specific pattern of osteokinematic (angular or physiologic) range-of-motion restrictions that he believed accompanies conditions in which the whole joint is involved. Cyriax advocated including joint mobilization as part of the examination and subsequent treatment. He also brought into common use some of the thrust joint manipulation treatment techniques practiced today, many of which were developed to address spinal disc disorders.

Kaltenborn

Kaltenborn proposed that the clinician should evaluate patients for joint mobility impairments and soft tissue changes. Joint mobility impairments are evaluated by performing gliding and traction joint mobilization procedures, and joint restrictions are treated with these same techniques. Kaltenborn advocates that glide mobilization interventions should be performed in a specific direction, based on the evaluation of the restriction in range of motion and the shape of the articular surface. He also developed the concepts of loose-packed and close-packed joint positions, joint positions in which the joint capsule is most and least lax, respectively.

Mulligan

Mulligan built on the approach established by Kaltenborn. He advocated combining pain free joint mobilization glide techniques with concomitant active or passive osteokinematic (angular or physiologic) range of movement, a technique he calls mobilization with movement. Mulligan proposed evaluating joint impairments by performing the treatment technique being considered, taking care not to reproduce pain, with and without the mobilization force. If pain and/or range of motion is improved with the mobilization force compared with performing the technique without the mobilization force, then the technique is indicated. Techniques are chosen for evaluation purposes based on a strategy that Mulligan calls the Client Specific Impairment Measure (CSIM), a painful movement that is associated with a specific disorder.

Maitland

Maitland was a strong advocate of performing a thorough examination of each patient to determine the position, movement, or test that reproduces the patient's symptoms. This examination includes testing osteokinematic (angular or physiologic movement) and accessory (joint) movements. Maitland also developed a system of determining the irritability, or ease in which a patient's pain is exacerbated, based on the intensity of symptoms as they relate to the physical examination and to functional activities, and an intervention strategy in which the aggressiveness of treatment is based on this determination. He also proposed using the concept of identifying a comparable sign: an easily reproduced position, movement, or activity that reproduces the patient's symptoms. The comparable sign is repeated after treatment to determine whether a change has occurred in the symptoms that were present when the comparable sign was originally identified. A reduction in symptoms indicates that the treatment was beneficial, whereas an increase in symptoms indicates that the treatment was not appropriate. Intervention often includes joint mobilization/manipulation. The direction of the intervention mobilization/manipulation is determined primarily by the direction of the examination technique that reproduced symptoms; however, the aggressiveness of the intervention, determined by tissue irritability, should not reproduce symptoms. Maitland also developed the five-grade (I, II, III, IV, and V) categorization system of mobilization/manipulation intervention techniques that is in common use today.

SUMMARY

The role of joint mobilization/manipulation in the evaluation and intervention of movement impairments is strongly influenced by the experiences, insight, and charisma of numerous clinicians. In some cases these different philosophies and strategies of mobilization/manipulation evaluation and intervention conflict with one another. There is a paucity of research comparing the specific tenets of these various philosophies with one another. It remains unclear whether, or under what circumstances, choosing one discipline or practitioner's approach over another would result in better outcomes and, if so, which approach is optimal.

EVIDENCE-BASED/EVIDENCE-INFORMED PRACTICE

Traditionally, much of the practice of physical therapy, including joint mobilization/manipulation, has evolved because of the influence of practitioners who were able to organize their clinical experience into a cohesive framework and disseminate this information to other clinicians. These clinicians are to be commended for their insight and effort. Nevertheless, as Rothstein[3] eloquently stated, "we do a disservice to the pioneers of manual therapy when we worship their words and fail to advance the scientific basis on which they first developed."

Evidence-based practice is a process of health care decision making that has evolved since the 1970s and is increasingly influencing physical therapy practice. One consequence of the movement toward evidence-based practice is a greater emphasis on the critical evaluation of health care theories and techniques using the best available research.

Adhering to evidence-based practice principles involves not only applying the best research evidence to a patient scenario but also integrating clinical expertise and patient values into the decision-making process.[4] Using the best research evidence entails the conscientious, explicit, and judicious use of clinically relevant research in making decisions about the care of individual patients.[4,5] The integration of clinical expertise involves the ability to use clinical skills and past experience to identify a patient's unique health status and the risks and benefits of potential interventions. Finally, each patient has unique preferences, concerns, and expectations that have an impact on the outcome of the therapeutic intervention. Patient-care decisions should entail the identification and consideration of patient values.[4] The term *evidence-informed practice* has evolved from the tenets of evidence-based practice to reflect the component of evidence-based practice that addresses the value of incorporating clinical expertise and patient values in the decision-making process.

Take the example of a patient who reports experiencing a recent exacerbation of low back pain accompanied by radicular symptoms of lower leg pain and numbness and weakness in the L4 nerve root distribution that had been treated successfully in the past with lumbar spine thrust joint manipulation. A review of the literature on the efficacy of lumbar spine manipulation interventions for acute lumbar radiculopathy suggests that it might not be effective for these patients. The decision whether to intervene with spinal manipulation would involve a process of weighing the evidence, which does not strongly support the intervention, with the patient's expectations, which do support the intervention, and the clinician's own experience with using spinal manipulation on similar patients. One of several solutions to this clinical dilemma might be to use the least aggressive manipulation procedure known to the clinician, perform it only once during that treatment session, and monitor the result of that intervention carefully for the purpose of determining future actions. By adhering to the tenets of evidence-based (evidence-informed) practice, we are recognizing the importance of all three of the aforementioned components and not just information gleaned from research studies.

The objective of this book is to describe the strategies and techniques commonly used by physical therapists to examine, evaluate, and treat musculoskeletal impairments with joint mobilization/manipulation techniques and to evaluate them in relation to the best evidence. The articles referenced in this book were chosen based on research evidence principles, relative to the specific issue being addressed. Clinical expertise and patient values are determined and weighted into the treatment decision making process on a case by case basis.

There are numerous concerns with determining the validity of studies addressing the efficacy of manual techniques in the treatment of patients with musculoskeletal conditions. Foremost is the issue with the strong placebo effects that accompany interventions involving the laying on of hands: patients respond positively to interventions that they believe will work and many patients believe that manual techniques will improve their disorder. Although placebo effects produce positive clinical outcomes, clinicians should not choose a technique based on that criterion alone, because greater effects occur when placebo effects are combined with a positive physiologic response. One additional concern with manual therapy intervention studies is that some musculoskeletal conditions are self-limiting: many patients improve with time regardless of the intervention. For these reasons, in this book priority was given to reporting efficacy studies that used a placebo or comparison group.

One other major concern with study validity involves the difficulty in blinding clinicians and subjects to the intervention the subjects are receiving. Especially in relation to clinician blinding, most intervention studies investigating mobilization/manipulation techniques were unsuccessful in avoiding this pitfall, adversely affecting the validity of these study results.

An evolving issue related to spine research, but applicable to all musculoskeletal impairments, is the manner in which disorders are classified. For example, if joint mobilization/manipulation is extremely effective with one category of back pain, but relatively ineffective with other categories, studies that do not correctly classify patients in such a way as to identify this relation would be less likely to show positive effects from the mobilization/manipulation intervention than studies in which the characteristics of the subjects matched the intervention being studied. Many studies do not make an attempt to classify subjects beyond identifying them as having pain in a particular location. At best, subjects also are classified based on symptom acuity. An alternative explanation for results of studies indicating that joint mobilization/manipulation is not efficacious would be that the inclusion criteria were not suitable for finding an effect. This is evidenced by the conclusion of one systematic review, published in 2012, in which the authors concluded that there is preliminary evidence demonstrating the efficacy of categorizing subjects into meaningful subgroups to inform better clinical outcomes.[6] These findings suggest that the choice of mobilization/manipulation technique is less important than characteristics of the patient receiving the intervention. Inroads are currently being made to subclassify patients to identify effective interventions; however, this research approach is still in its infancy.

One advance in applying evidence-based practice to clinical decision making is the proliferation of systematic reviews, published papers addressing a research question with the objective of identifying, appraising, selecting, and synthesizing research evidence relevant to that question. Systematic reviews are believed to represent the highest level of evidence[7] and are therefore used extensively in this book.

EFFECTS OF JOINT MOBILIZATION AND MANIPULATION

Despite the wide use of mobilization/manipulation in clinical practice and the volumes of research addressing the processes by which mobilization/manipulation might alter musculoskeletal disorders, the mechanisms behind the efficacy of mobilization/manipulation remains unknown. Furthermore, research suggests that the effects of joint mobilization/manipulation might differ depending on whether the technique is administered to spinal or peripheral joints or whether a nonthrust or thrust procedure is performed. The most commonly cited effects of joint mobilization/manipulation can be categorized as those producing mechanical effects and those producing neurophysiological effects. It is likely that these two mechanisms interact because changes in the mechanics of the musculoskeletal system are accompanied by neurophysiologic changes and changes in neural states are accompanied by changes in the musculoskeletal system, each in turn producing changes in function, movement, and pain.

Mechanical Effects

All joints are capable of osteokinematic movement. This movement occurs when muscles contract concentrically or eccentrically or when gravity causes the position of one bone of a joint to change in relation to the other bone. The different directions of movement that each joint is capable of are called its osteokinematic degrees of freedom, defined as the number of components within a movement system that specify position in space. Osteokinematic degrees of freedom are usually referenced by movements in cardinal planes. A maximum of six

different degrees of freedom are possible in each joint: four degrees of freedom occur as the bone moves in both directions in two planes of motion perpendicular to one another, and two degrees of freedom occur as the bone rotates around an axis perpendicular to the joint surfaces. In most cases, the joint motion accompanying functional activities is the result of a combination of more than one osteokinematic motion.

Joints also undergo arthrokinematic motion, which is defined as movement between two articulating surfaces without reference to any of the external forces being applied to that joint. The number of arthrokinematic movements that occur at each joint is determined by the number of accessory motions. Accessory motion has been defined as movement occurring between two joint surfaces that is produced by forces applied by the examiner[8] and, as with osteokinematic motion, usually refers only to movement in cardinal planes.

Normal accessory motion is believed to be necessary for full, pain-free osteokinematic movement to occur. Joint mobilization/manipulation entails moving a joint through its accessory motion, thereby maintaining or increasing the extensibility of articular structures. Joint mobilization/manipulation is therefore the recommended treatment for restoring normal accessory motion, which is one criterion for the restoration of normal osteokinematic motion. Although theoretically the joint capsule is the structure affected by joint mobilization/manipulation intervention techniques, most likely other periarticular tissues, such as tendons, muscles, and fascia, also are targeted when joint mobilization/manipulation is performed.

Articular and periarticular restrictions have been shown to result from immobilization of joints. Early studies have identified many of the biomechanical and biochemical effects of immobilization on joint capsules. With immobilization, there is a decrease in water content, resulting in a reduction in the distance between the fibers constituting the joint capsule. This causes an increase in fiber cross-link formation, which produces adhesions. In the absence of movement, as new collagen tissue is produced, additional cross-linking occurs. Immobilization also produces adhesions between synovial folds. Additionally, fibrofatty connective tissue proliferates within the joint and adheres to cartilaginous structures. Finally, the strength of collagen tissue decreases, resulting in a decrease in the load-to-failure rate.[9-11]

Joint mobilization/manipulation is thought to reverse these changes by promoting movement between capsular fibers. This movement is believed to stretch synovial tissue in a selective manner, causing a gradual rearrangement of collagen tissue, a reduction of cross-link formation, and the development of parallel fiber configuration in newly forming collagen tissue. More aggressive manipulation techniques are thought to break adhesion in the joint capsule and synovial folds, and increase the length of capsular fibers. These responses to mobilization/manipulation are believed to have the mechanical effect of increasing the amount of arthrokinematic motion and consequently osteokinematic motion at a joint.

These assumptions regarding lengthening of capsular tissue with joint mobilization/manipulation interventions are being evaluated. In a 2012 systematic review of nine studies addressing the mechanical effects of spinal manipulation, the investigators concluded that, although there is very little evidence to support these conclusions, the best evidence suggests that in relation to symptomatic individuals, there are no long-term changes in spinal stiffness, although there might be a decrease in spinal stiffness short term.[12] These findings were congruent with a 2009 systematic review of manual therapy, which suggested that only transient biomechanical effects occur.[13]

Nevertheless, increasing joint mobility is the most common reason cited by clinicians for performing joint mobilization/manipulation techniques. It is possible that to obtain a more permanent effect on joint mobility following mobilization/manipulation techniques, it might be necessary to ensure that the patient performs range-of-motion and/or strengthening exercises and functional activities that bring the treated joint through its newly gained range of motion. It stands to reason that by doing so, the gains in arthrokinematic movement obtained during a treatment session would more likely be retained.

One other commonly cited effect of joint mobilization/manipulation is the correction of positional faults. A positional fault is defined as a minor displacement of two joint articulating surfaces in relation to one another. If the displacement is moderate or severe, the joint would be labeled *subluxed*. Positional faults are believed to cause pain and neuromuscular dysfunction.

Mobilization/manipulation of one of the joint surfaces in the direction consistent with realigning it into its correct position is thought by some clinicians to normalize the static positioning of one joint surface in relation to the other, thereby reducing pain. For example, if the lunate was positioned in a posterior direction in relation to the radius, treatment would be directed toward mobilizing/manipulating the lunate in an anterior direction in relation to the radius; this could result in the restoration of normal alignment of the two articular surfaces.

The existence and clinical relevance of spinal positional faults, called *subluxations* in the chiropractic literature, have caused a great deal of controversy because they provide a justification for chiropractic manipulation interventions. Current evidence suggests that the identification and treatment of spinal subluxations/positional faults are not based on sound science.[14] In relation to positional faults in peripheral joints, most of the clinical literature has focused on the tibiofibular joints. In several studies, the investigators concluded that positional faults exist in the distal tibiofibular joint in patients with chronic ankle instability[15-17]; however, treatment of positional faults with joint mobilization/manipulation for these patients does not affect outcome.[18] In summary, in relation to spinal as well as peripheral joints, there is currently insufficient evidence to support the treatment of positional faults with joint mobilization/manipulation techniques.

Neurophysiological Effects

A number of studies have identified changes in the nervous system that occur as a result of the application of joint mobilization/manipulation interventions. These changes have been shown to occur throughout the nervous system, via peripheral, spinal, and supraspinal mechanisms.[13] Examples of these nervous system effects include such diverse alterations as increases in blood composition of b-endorphin and serotonin,[19] changes in alpha motor neuron activity,[20] and changes in the autonomic response systems.[21] To date, no unifying theory has evolved to explain the mechanism or mechanisms behind these neurophysiological effects. It is likely that joint mobilization/manipulation produces multiple neurophysiological responses that in some cases interact with one another and sometimes operate alone, making it difficult to identify the physiologic mechanisms behind specific effects.

The most commonly reported therapeutic outcome arising from these neurophysiological effects is a reduction in pain. In a 2012 systematic review of 20 articles, the authors evaluated whether and to what extent this effect on pain occurs. They concluded that spinal manipulation increases pain pressure threshold immediately after the intervention is administered. Furthermore, they stated that this effect was greater than those of other commonly used conservative interventions.[22] One implication of these findings is that joint mobilization/manipulation interventions, via pain-reduction mechanisms, can provide the patient with an opportunity to perform more aggressive exercises, normalize movement patterns, and increase functional activities, thereby promoting long-term improvement in symptoms. Adding exercise and education regarding movement patterns and activity level would thereby be a necessary addition to any mobilization/manipulation intervention.

Some investigators have reported that mobilization/manipulation produces changes in muscle activity through its effects on the nervous system via changes in alpha motor neuron activity. In some cases, the result is an increase in the ability of muscles to generate force, for example, in shoulder lateral rotators[23] and in the lower trapezius muscle,[24] whereas in other cases joint mobilization/manipulation interventions decrease muscle tone, as was shown to be the case in relation to the hamstring muscles.[25,26] To date, no cohesive theory has been proposed to explain these apparent contradictory effects or to describe under what conditions an increase in strength or a decrease in muscle tone can be expected from a joint mobilization/manipulation intervention technique.

Perhaps for these reasons, changing muscle activity is not a commonly cited indication for joint mobilization/manipulation interventions.

Because the relation between joint mobilization/manipulation interventions and neurophysiological effects is not entirely clear, patients might request an explanation regarding why joint mobilization/manipulation procedures are being performed. The following justification has been recommended: mobilization/manipulation forces produce a barrage of impulses within the nervous system, which has the effect of "resetting" nervous activity.[27] This alteration in nervous activity likely results in less pain and muscle activity that is more consistent with normal movement patterns.

REGIONAL INTERDEPENDENCE

Regional interdependence, formally introduced into the rehabilitation literature by Wainner et al.[28] in 2007, refers to the phenomenon that "seemingly unrelated impairments in a remote anatomic region may contribute to, or be associated with, a client's primary complaint." This concept provides structure to diverse clinical observations involving multiple anatomic locations, such as the effect that correcting foot mechanics can have on patellofemoral pain. In relation to joint mobilization/manipulation, this concept provided a framework for understanding observations such as why a thoracic spine manipulation intervention might reduce neck pain or why a cervical spine mobilization intervention might be an effective treatment for lateral epicondylalgia.

In 2013, Sueki et al.[29] redefined regional interdependence to state "the concept that a patient's primary musculoskeletal symptom(s) may be directly or indirectly related or influenced by impairments from various body regions and systems regardless of proximity to the primary symptom(s)", explicitly stating that the mechanism behind regional interdependence is likely multifactorial and regional interdependence can occur irrespective of the proximity of the structures to one another.

Regional interdependence involving joint mobilization/manipulation techniques likely occurs via a combination of mechanical and neurophysiological effects; however, the specifics of how these effects occur remain unknown. Identifying patterns related to interventions that produce specific outcomes at specific remote areas also needs further exploration. Several patterns have been established, for example, the effect of thoracic manipulation on neck pain, whereas other proposed patterns require additional investigation. Nevertheless, the concept of regional interdependence provides a rationale for treatment with joint mobilization/manipulation in one area to effect a change in a different area. One strategy recommended in several systematic reviews for addressing regional interdependence effects is to simply treat all hypomobile joints along the kinematic chain associated with the symptomatic joint.[30,31]

INTERVENTION STRATEGIES

Current best evidence suggests that the choice of technique performed does not appear to have much effect on outcomes. This conclusion has given rise to the expression, "move it and move on."[32] Nevertheless, several different strategies are recommended for determining which mobilization/manipulation interventions are indicated, based in part on the clinical experience and opinions of the individual promoting the specific approach.

The most common strategy involves identifying joint hypomobility using accessory motion testing procedures, correlating these hypomobile accessory motions to decreases in osteokinematic motion, and treating with mobilization/manipulation techniques that move the joint in the same direction as the hypomobility. This strategy is consistent with that which is taught by Kaltenborn.

Another strategy is based on Maitland and involves identifying the painful accessory motion using accessory motion testing. The disorder is then treated with mobilization/manipulation techniques that move the joint in the same direction as the painful accessory motion but never with a technique that is aggressive enough to reproduce pain.

A third approach is based on recognizing patterns of signs and symptoms and treating with a specific technique or one of several techniques based on the presence of these signs and symptoms. Clinicians basing interventions on patterns of regional interdependence, treatment-based classifications, or Mulligan's CSIM would be using methods of determining joint mobilization/manipulation interventions consistent with this approach.

REFERENCES

1. Maitland GD. *Vertebral Manipulation*. 5th ed. London: Butterworth; 1986.
2. <WWW.APTA.org>; Accessed 10/2015.
3. Rothstein JM. Editor's note: manual therapy—a special issue and a special topic. *Phys Ther.* 1992;72:839-842.
4. Sackett DL, Straus SE, Richardson WS, Rosenberg W, Haynes RB. *Evidence-Based Medicine: How to Practice and Teach EBM.* 2nd ed. Philadelphia: Churchill Livingstone; 2000.
5. Sackett DL, Rosenberg WM, Gray JA, Haynes RB, Richardson WS. Evidence based medicine:

what it is and what it isn't. *BMJ.* 1996;312: 71-72.

6. Slater SL, Ford JJ, Richards MC, et al. The effectiveness of sub-group specific manual therapy for low back pain: a systematic review. *Man Ther.* 2012;17:201-212.

7. Oxford Centre for Evidence-based Medicine. Levels of evidence. <http://www.cebm.net/oxford-centre-evidence-based-medicine-levels-evidence-march-2009>; Accessed 5/2015.

8. Riddle DL. Measurement of accessory motion: critical issues and related concepts. *Phys Ther.* 1992;72:865-874.

9. Woo SL-Y, Matthews JV, Akeson WH, et al. Connective tissue response to immobility: correlative study of biomechanical and biochemical measurements of normal and immobilized rabbit knees. *Arthritis Rheum.* 1975;18:257-264.

10. Akeson WH. Immobilization effects on synovial joints. *Biorheology.* 1980;17:95-110.

11. Akeson WH, Amiel D, Abel JF, et al. Effects of immobilization on joints. *Clin Orthop.* 1987;219:28-37.

12. Snodgrass SJ, Haskins R, Rivett DA. A structured review of spinal stiffness as a kinesiological outcome of manipulation: its measurement and utility in diagnosis, prognosis and treatment decision-making. *J Electromyogr Kinesiol.* 2012;22:708-723.

13. Bialosky JE, Bishop MD, Price DD, Robinson ME, George SZ. The mechanisms of manual therapy in the treatment of musculoskeletal pain: a comprehensive model. *Man Ther.* 2009;14:531-538.

14. Ernst E. Chiropractic: a critical evaluation. *J Pain Symptom Manage.* 2008;35:544-562.

15. Hubbard TJ, Hertel J. Anterior positional fault of the fibula after sub-acute lateral ankle sprains. *Man Ther.* 2008;13:63-67.

16. Hubbard TH, Hertel J, Sherbondy P. Fibular position in individuals with self-reported chronic ankle instability. *J Orthop Sports Phys Ther.* 2006;36:3-9.

17. Wikstrom EA, Hubbard TJ. Talar positional fault in persons with chronic ankle instability. *Arch Phys Med Rehabil.* 2010;91:1267-1271.

18. Beazell JR, Grindstaff TL, Sauer LD, et al. Effects of a proximal or distal tibiofibular joint manipulation on ankle range of motion and functional outcomes in individuals with chronic ankle instability. *J Orthop Sports Phys Ther.* 2012;42:125-134.

19. Degenhardt BF, Darmani NA, Johnson JC, et al. Role of osteopathic manipulative treatment in altering pain biomarkers: a pilot study. *J Am Osteopath Assoc.* 2007;107:387-400.

20. Dishman JD, Greco DS, Burke JR. Motor-evoked potentials recorded from lumbar erector spinae muscles: a study of corticospinal excitability changes associated with spinal manipulation. *J Manipulative Physiol Ther.* 2008;31:258-270.

21. Perry J, Green A. An investigation into the effects of a unilaterally applied lumbar mobilisation technique on peripheral sympathetic nervous system activity in the lower limbs. *Man Ther.* 2008;13:492-499.

22. Coronado RA, Gay CW, Bialosky JE, et al. Changes in pain sensitivity following spinal manipulation: a systematic review and meta-analysis. *J Electromyogr Kinesiol.* 2012;22:752-767.

23. Wang SS, Meadows J. Immediate and carryover changes of C5-6 joint mobilization on shoulder external rotation muscle strength. *J Manipulative Physiol Ther.* 2010;33:102-108.

24. Cleland JA, Selleck B, Stowell T, et al. Short-term effects of thoracic manipulation on lower trapezius muscle strength. *J Man Manip Ther.* 2004;12:82-90.

25. Szlezak AM, Georgilopoulos P, Bullock-Saxton JE, Steele MC. The immediate effect of unilateral lumbar Z-joint mobilization on posterior chain neurodynamics: a randomized controlled study. *Man Ther.* 2011;16:609-613.

26. Ganesh GS, Mohanty P, Pattnaik SS. The immediate and 24-hour follow-up effect of unilateral lumbar Z-joint mobilisation on posterior chain neurodynamics. *J Bodyw Mov Ther.* 2015;19:226-231.

27. Bialosky JE, George SZ, Bishop MD. How spinal manipulative therapy works: why ask why? *J Orthop Sports Phys Ther.* 2008;38:293-295.

28. Wainner RS, Whitman JM, Cleland JA, Flynn TW. Regional interdependence: a musculoskeletal examination model whose time has come. *J Orthop Sports Phys Ther.* 2007;37:658-660.

29. Sueki DG, Cleland JA, Wainner RS. A regional interdependence model of musculoskeletal dysfunction: research, mechanisms, and clinical implications. *J Man Manip Ther.* 2013;21:90-102.

30. Brantingham JW, Cassa TK, Bonnefin D, et al. Manipulative and multimodal therapy for upper extremity and temporomandibular disorders: a systematic review. *J Manipulative Physiol Ther.* 2013;36:143-201.

31. Brantingham JW, Bonnefin D, Perle SM, et al. Manipulative therapy for lower extremity conditions: update of a literature review. *J Manipulative Physiol Ther.* 2012;35:127-166.

32. Flynn TW. Move it and move on (guest editorial). *J Orthop Sports Phys Ther.* 2002;32:192-193.

CHAPTER 2

Principles of Examination, Evaluation, and Intervention

EXAMINATION AND EVALUATION

All patients should undergo an evaluation before any physical therapy intervention is performed, including treatment with joint mobilization/manipulation. The evaluation should consist of a history and a thorough physical examination, which includes an inspection of posture, positioning, gait, and body type; palpation of relevant soft and bony tissue; assessment of range of motion; examination of accessory movements; muscle strength testing; neurologic testing; and special tests designed to rule in or out specific conditions. Radiographs should be examined whenever possible. Signs and symptoms should be consistent with the diagnosis, and a plan of care should be generated from the diagnosis and clinical findings, taking into consideration the acuity of the injury and any medical, surgical, psychosocial, cultural, or financial concerns.

Examination of accessory movements is a prerequisite to the performance of most joint mobilization/manipulation techniques. Testing is generally initiated by positioning the joint to be examined in the *resting*, or *loose-packed*, *position*. Kaltenborn[1] defined the resting position as the joint position in which the periarticular tissues are most lax. Joints are tested in the resting position because this is the position with the greatest amount of accessory movement. The resting position also is often the position that is most comfortable for patients with joint pain. If limitations in range of motion or pain prevent the clinician from placing the joint in the resting position, the position that is most comfortable for the patient and in which there is the least amount of soft tissue tension should be used to examine accessory movements. Kaltenborn used the term *actual resting position* to describe this position.[1]

In a study addressing hip biomechanics, hip joint separation was greater when the joint was placed in the resting position compared with the position believed to have the least joint laxity,[2] thereby providing validation for the resting position of the hip. Investigators evaluating the resting position of the glenohumeral joint, however, concluded that the position varies depending on whether arthrokinematic (joint) or osteokinematic (angular or physiologic) motion is being evaluated.[3] For most other joints, the resting position has not been determined using research methodology. Nevertheless, Kaltenborn has described resting positions for most of the joints that are treated with mobilization/manipulation techniques, presumably based on clinical experience. These positions are described in their respective chapters.

Accessory motions are generally examined by moving one of the articular surfaces of the joint in a direction that is perpendicular or parallel to the joint. These directions are determined by identifying the concave joint surface and visualizing the plane in which that joint surface would exist in if it were flattened out. This plane is called the *treatment plane*.

Moving either bone in a direction perpendicular to the treatment plane such that the bones separate constitutes a traction or a distraction technique, and moving either bone in a direction perpendicular to the treatment plane such that the two bones approximate one another constitutes a compression technique (Figure 2-1). If the bones are moved in a direction parallel to the treatment plane, a glide accessory motion is being performed (Figure 2-2). In many joints, glides can be performed in several directions. An oscillation motion often accompanies the glide mobilization. Less often, but occasionally, tractions are accompanied by this oscillation movement.

Because the treatment plane is identified in reference to the concave joint surface, it moves if the concave joint surface is part of the moving bone and remains stationary if the convex joint surface moves. The direction of the mobilization/manipulation force would thereby remain unchanged with changes in joint position when the moving bone is convex but would change with the osteokinematic joint motion when the moving bone is concave.

A mobilization/manipulation administered to a long bone is not always performed parallel or perpendicular to the long axis of that bone. For example, because of the anteriorly directed angulation of the forearm in relation to the treatment plane of the ulna, humeroulnar traction mobilizations/manipulations are performed in a direction of 45 degrees less flexion than the angle of the forearm (Figure 2-3) because this is the direction perpendicular to the treatment plane. Based on the definition of a traction mobilization/manipulation, techniques that are directed along the axis of the long bone are not always

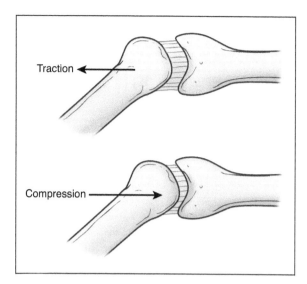

Figure 2-1 Traction and compression.

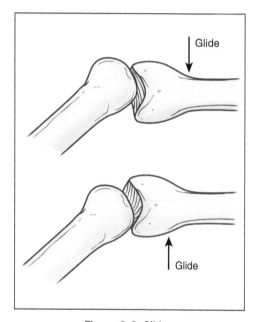

Figure 2-2 Glides.

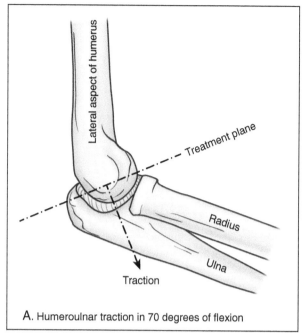

A. Humeroulnar traction in 70 degrees of flexion

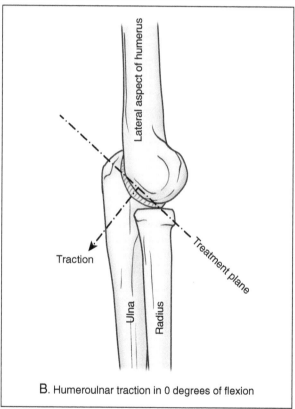

B. Humeroulnar traction in 0 degrees of flexion

Figure 2-3 Humeroulnar traction.

true traction techniques. These techniques are called long-axis tractions to distinguish them from tractions administered perpendicular to the treatment plane.

The examination procedure is performed such that the motion is taken up to and slightly through tissue resistance and is usually performed in the same direction as the intended treatment mobilization/manipulation technique. In this text, in cases in which the examination technique differs from the corresponding treatment technique, the examination technique is also described in the section with the description of the intervention mobilization/manipulation.

As a rule, the clinician evaluates all possible accessory motions for each joint being evaluated. An accessory

motion examination entails an evaluation of the amount of excursion or mobility present in a particular joint when moved in a particular direction, an evaluation of the presence of pain, and a determination of the type of tissue resistance felt at the end of the range for each accessory motion. The clinician evaluating the patient also should consider whether, and if so, how these accessory motion findings corroborate with other components of the physical examination. The implication for most joint mobilization/manipulation interventions is that if an accessory motion is hypomobile, then treatment with the technique that constituted the examination procedure should be considered.

Excursion

To understand more clearly the nature of soft tissue extensibility and its relationship to joint mobilization/ manipulation, it is important to become familiar with the characteristics of the stress-strain curve (Figure 2-4). Rules of stress-strain, or load deformation, are applicable to all solid tissue. As an external tensile force is applied to a tissue (stress or, in this case, a mobilization/ manipulation force), the tissue undergoes several transitions (strain). The first stage is the elastic phase, in which the stretched tissue returns to its original configuration when the external force is removed. The second stage is the plastic phase, in which permanent elongation of the stretched tissue occurs when the external force is removed.

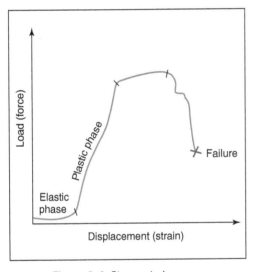

Figure 2-4 Stress-strain curve.

The third stage is the failure or breaking point, in which separation of the elongated tissue occurs. Within the plastic phase, there is a point at which a decrease in load is accompanied by an increase in deformation. This is called the necking point and is an indication that the breaking point is about to be reached.

Joint mobility is evaluated by performing either a glide or a traction mobilization and by moving the bone up to and slightly through the limit of the available motion into tissue resistance. The clinician is evaluating the amount of motion that occurs up to the point where an increase in tissue resistance is felt. This point theoretically corresponds to the end of the elastic phase and the beginning of the plastic phase on the stress-strain curve.

The amount of motion from the starting position for the two joint surfaces to the point where tissue resistance is felt is graded according to the amount of excursion the bone undergoes. Most clinicians grade the amount of excursion, or joint accessory motion, by comparing the joint being tested with the same joint on the opposite side, assuming the joint being used for comparison is not impaired. Despite this recommendation, there is no evidence to show that, in normal joints, excursion at one joint is the same as excursion into the same direction at the same joint on the opposite side. One alternative to this approach, especially useful if both of the patient's joints are affected, is to compare the joint excursion with the clinician's perceived experience with evaluating the same joint on other patients of similar age, sex, and body type, although this approach is not likely to be highly reliable. Both of these concerns affect the reliability and internal validity of joint mobilization/manipulation examination procedures.

The amount of joint excursion can be graded according to the scale shown in Figure 2-5, with the following implications for determining a plan of care:

Grade 0: There is no motion between the two articulating surfaces. Mobilization/manipulation is not indicated because the joint is ankylosed.

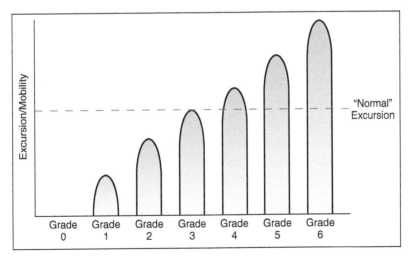

Figure 2-5 Grades of joint excursion.

Grade 1: There is considerable limitation in the excursion between the two joint surfaces. Mobilization/manipulation into this accessory motion is indicated to increase joint mobility.

Grade 2: There is a slight limitation in the excursion between the two joint surfaces. Mobilization/manipulation into this accessory motion is indicated to increase joint mobility.

Grade 3: The amount of movement between the joint surfaces is normal. Mobilization/manipulation into this accessory motion is not indicated to increase joint mobility.

Grade 4: There is a slight increase in the excursion between the two joint surfaces. Mobilization/manipulation into this accessory motion is not indicated to increase joint mobility. The patient should be treated with stabilization exercises and should be educated regarding correct posture and positions to avoid. Taping and/or bracing are also treatment options.

Grade 5: There is a considerable increase in the excursion between the two joint surfaces. Mobilization/manipulation into this accessory motion is not indicated to increase joint mobility. The patient should be treated with stabilization exercises and should be educated regarding correct posture and positions to avoid. Taping and/or bracing are also treatment options.

Grade 6: The joint is unstable. Mobilization/manipulation into this accessory motion is not indicated to increase joint mobility. The patient can be treated with stabilization exercises, patient education, and taping/bracing, but this intervention is less likely to be successful than if the joint was less hypermobile.

An alternative grading scale consists of three categories: hypomobile, normal, and hypermobile, with the same plan-of-care implications as the aforementioned seven-category scale. This alternative scale is likely to be more reliable, because there are fewer categories.

Pain

It is important to examine whether pain is produced or increased when evaluating accessory motion and to interpret this finding in conjunction with the results of the accessory motion examination. Pain in conjunction with hypomobility usually indicates a need for joint mobilization/manipulation intervention theoretically because treating the hypomobility would eliminate the joint impairment that might be causing the pain. Conversely, it might be a sign that there is an acute sprain with guarding or an inflamed joint. In these latter circumstances, it is important to consider whether what appears to be hypomobility is in fact muscle guarding and whether the muscle guarding is masking a hypermobile condition. If so, joint mobilization/manipulation might be detrimental. This condition can be determined by evaluating for periarticular muscle spasm and, if present, ensuring that these muscles are relaxed during the examination procedure.

In the absence of these concerns, the examination of joint excursion, combined with a determination of the presence or absence of pain, has the following implications for determining whether treatment consisting of joint mobilization/manipulation procedures that correspond to the evaluation procedure are indicated as part of the plan of care:

- Hypomobility with pain is believed to indicate an adhesion or contracture that is causing the patient to have pain. Mobilization/manipulation techniques that bring the joint through tissue resistance are indicated in this situation, although any techniques that produce or increase the patient's pain should only be performed if the benefits outweigh the potential to aggravate the painful condition.
- Hypomobility without pain is believed to indicate a chronic adhesion or contracture. Mobilization/manipulation techniques that bring the joint through tissue resistance might be indicated in this situation, although in the absence of pain the possibility that hypomobility is a normal state for that patient also should be considered.
- Normal mobility with pain indicates a mild sprain without disruption of capsular fibers. Joint mobilization/manipulation for stretching of periarticular structures is not indicated in the presence of normal mobility, but the patient might benefit from more gentle mobilization techniques to decrease pain and promote normal alignment of newly forming collagen fibers.
- Normal mobility without pain indicates an absence of joint capsular impairment. Joint mobilization/manipulation is not indicated.
- Hypermobility with pain indicates a partial sprain of capsular tissue. Joint mobilization/manipulation techniques that bring the joint through tissue resistance are not indicated. Rather, stabilization techniques are recommended. When pain accompanies hypermobility, gentle mobilizations carefully administered so as not to take the joint up to tissue resistance can be used to decrease pain and promote normal alignment of newly forming collagen tissue.
- Hypermobility without pain, or with far less pain than would be expected given other examination findings such as swelling and guarding, indicates a complete sprain of capsular tissue. Joint mobilization/manipulation techniques are not indicated. Rather, stabilization techniques are recommended.

End Feel

End feels also are examined during the evaluation of accessory motion. Accessory motion end feels are either bony or firm. With bony end feels, the joint-tissue resistance is felt as an abrupt change in joint extensibility,

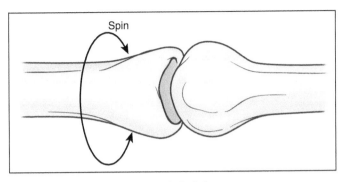

Figure 2-6 Spin.

whereas firm end feels are less abrupt. A bony end feel indicates that either there is bony hypertrophy in the joint blocking additional motion or the restrictions in the joint capsule are causing the two joint surfaces to jam together. If bony hypertrophy is blocking joint motion, performing joint mobilization/manipulation techniques might be harmful to the patient. A firm end feel indicates that capsular tissue is limiting further motion. If the firm end feel is accompanied by no pain and normal excursion, there is no joint capsular impairment involving that accessory motion. A firm end feel accompanied by an abnormal amount of excursion is considered an abnormal end feel. If the firm end feel is accompanied by hypomobility, joint mobilization/manipulation interventions should be considered. A hypermobile joint should be treated with stabilization interventions, regardless of end feel.

In the situation in which a firm end feel is present, most experienced clinicians make an additional determination regarding the quality of the firm end feel, based on the relative "give" or "play" in the tissue. Firm end feels that have relatively more play are more likely to be judged hypermobile, even if the amount of joint excursion is not judged to be excessive.

Accessory motion testing is a complex task to perform. Maitland[4] provided the following description of the skills required to evaluate accessory motion: The clinician must

> "... apply a force to a joint and ... evaluate the joint's response to that force. The student (clinician) is supposed to appreciate the amount of force applied to the joint, the speed and direction at which it is applied, the amount of movement produced at the joint, the way in which the joint moves or resists movement in response to that force, the pain produced by that movement, the presence of muscle activity evoked during the movement, and the comparison of this reaction to the expected normal response and to that of adjacent joints when palpated in a presumably similar way."

For most joints, these components of accessory motion examination have not been clearly defined or studied. As

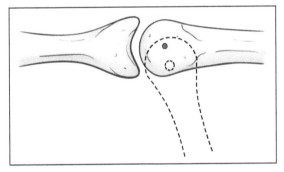

Figure 2-7 Roll.

a general rule, testing procedures involving the palpation of position and movement are associated with poor reliability. Pain provocation tests show greater reliability. The implication of these findings for joint accessory motion testing is that clinicians are more accurate in identifying pain than excursion or end feel when evaluating accessory motion.

INTEGRATING ACCESSORY MOTION EXAMINATION RESULTS WITH OTHER EXAMINATION FINDINGS

Convex-Concave Rules

Joints are capable of several types of joint motion. Spinning is one type (Figure 2-6) and consists of movement of one bone on the other such that one point on both bones remains in contact with the other and the rest of the articular surface of one bone rotates in relation to the other. The radius spins on the humerus during forearm pronation and supination. Rolling is another type of motion (Figure 2-7) and occurs when one point on one bone comes into contact with a point on the other bone that is equidistant from the original contact point. Much of the motion associated with knee flexion and extension occurs by way of rolling motion. Gliding is the third type of motion (Figure 2-8) and occurs when one point on one bone stays in contact with the articulating surface of the other bone, but at a new point. Talocrural joint motion occurs primarily by gliding.

Kaltenborn[1] proposed that restrictions in range of motion are associated most often with a decrease in the gliding component. He further stated that the direction of the glide corresponds to a specific osteokinematic movement, which depends on the shape of the articular surface.

Most joints are composed of a convex surface articulating with a reciprocally shaped concave surface. If the concave surface is the moving surface, the direction of the glide is the same as the osteokinematic movement. If

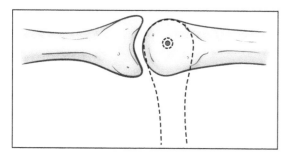

Figure 2-8 Glide.

the convex surface is the moving surface, the direction of the glide is opposite that of the osteokinematic movement (Figure 2-9). The direction of force imparted with an examination glide should therefore theoretically correspond to a specific osteokinematic movement based on the convex-concave relationship of the joint surfaces, and the grade of joint mobility (grade 1 to 6) given to that examination glide should correlate with the corresponding range-of-motion examination results.[1] If a concave tibia moves on a convex femur, as in open kinematic chain knee flexion activities, the tibia glides in the same direction as the osteokinematic motion. If knee flexion occurs in a closed kinematic chain situation, the femur moves on the tibia, and the femur glides in a direction opposite that of the osteokinematic motion. Assuming range-of-motion limitations correspond to the limitation in accessory motion based on these convex-concave rules, a decrease in accessory motion of the tibia gliding in a posterior direction on the femur or of the femur gliding in an anterior direction on the tibia should be present when there is a decrease in knee flexion range of motion (Figure 2-10). To restore knee flexion, the direction of the mobilization/manipulation glide should therefore be such that the tibia is glided in a posterior direction on the

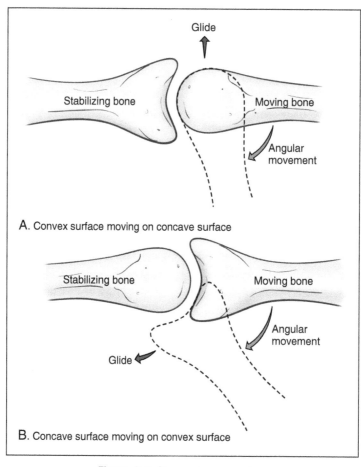

A. Convex surface moving on concave surface

B. Concave surface moving on convex surface

Figure 2-9 Convex-concave rules.

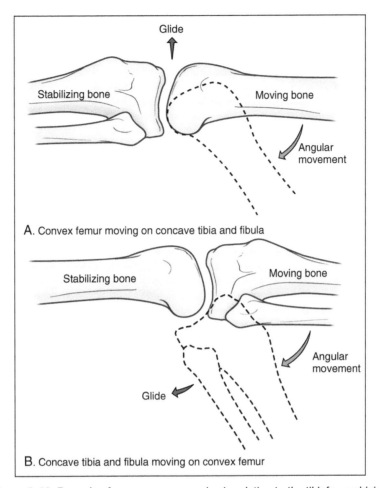

Figure 2-10 Example of convex-concave rules in relation to the tibiofemoral joint.

femur or the femur is glided in an anterior direction on the tibia.

Ovoid joints are shaped such that one joint surface is concave in its entirety. This joint surface articulates with a joint surface that is convex in its entirety (Figure 2-11). Sellar joints are shaped such that one joint surface is convex in one direction and concave in the direction perpendicular to the convex surface, similar to the shape of a saddle. The articulating joint surface is reciprocally concave to match the convex surface of its adjoining articulation and convex in the direction perpendicular to the concave surface (Figure 2-12). The two articulating surfaces are therefore congruent. The moving bone glides in the same direction as the osteokinematic movement in one plane of motion and opposite the direction of the osteokinematic movement occurring in the perpendicular plane.

Convex-concave rules are conceptualized more easily when the moving joint surface is perpendicular to the axis of a long bone, as is the case with the tibia and the femur. The patellofemoral joint is an example of a joint for which the convex-concave rules are less easy to visualize.

The validity of this strategy for determining the direction of the glide intervention to evaluate and treat a range-of-motion restriction in a particular direction has been evaluated in relation to several joints, most notably the glenohumeral joint. The studies involving the glenohumeral joint were summarized in a 2007 systematic review, in which the authors noted that the humeral head moved opposite the direction predicted by the convex-concave rules for glenohumeral lateral rotation and abduction.[5] In relation to the proximal radioulnar joint, investigators studying joint arthrokinematics similarly reported that the direction of radial head migration occurred in a direction opposite expectation with forearm pronation and supination.[6]

As a follow-up to the aforementioned findings regarding the glenohumeral joint, in a study of patients with shoulder adhesive capsulitis, the investigators reported that changes in lateral rotation range of motion were greater after performing a posterior glide, which theoretically should increase medial rotation, compared with an anterior glide, which theoretically should increase lateral rotation.[7]

These discrepancies highlight several issues related to applying the convex-concave rules to determining the direction of intervention mobilization/manipulation glides. Early theories of convex-concave rules were

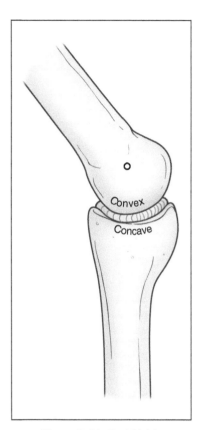

Figure 2-11 Ovoid joint.

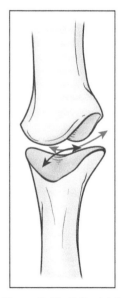

Figure 2-12 Sellar joint.

conceptualized based on movement in healthy individuals, and might not apply to those with painful, restricted or weak joints. For example, in relation to the glenohumeral joint, it is possible that the joint disorder might cause the humeral head to be positioned more anterior in the glenoid, thereby requiring a different direction of glide to treat the disorder than that which

would be recommended based on convex-concave rules. Additionally, kinematic studies likely measure combinations of rolling and gliding motions. The role of joint mobilization/manipulation techniques to restore rolling have not been addressed in the clinical literature. Nevertheless, rolling is likely a necessary component of normal arthrokinematic motion that is addressed with joint mobilization/manipulation intervention techniques and that does not necessarily follow the convex-concave rules, because these rules theoretically apply exclusively to gliding.

Determining the direction of mobilization/manipulation glides clearly is more complicated than simply applying convex-concave rules. To summarize, there is evidence refuting the use of Kaltenborn's convex-concave rules when treating patients with glenohumeral joint mobilization/manipulation for the purpose of increasing range of motion into lateral rotation and insufficient evidence to support or refute the validity of these convex-concave rules in relation to other glenohumeral motions and other joints. Nevertheless, it is possible that the clinician would be relatively more effective with mobilization/manipulation interventions for the purpose of increasing motion in a particular direction if he or she considered Kaltenborn's convex-concave rules in the determination of glide direction for most joints. The information that is required to apply these convex-concave rules is therefore provided in Table 2-1 and in the description of the relevant joint mobilization/manipulation procedures in subsequent chapters.

Capsular Patterns

Numerous components of the physical examination, used in conjunction with the results of an accessory motion examination, can aid in determining the patient's diagnosis. One of these components often entails an evaluation of the presence of a capsular pattern. According to Cyriax,[8] when the joint impairment affects the entire joint, the capsule of each joint undergoes a characteristic pattern of restriction in passive range of motion. This pattern of restriction is called the capsular pattern. Cyriax[8] proposed that there is a specific pattern of restriction for each joint, in which the proportional limitation in one motion is greater than one or more other motions. For example, the capsular pattern for the shoulder joint is described as lateral rotation being proportionally more limited than abduction, which is proportionally more limited than medial rotation. If a capsular pattern is present, there is a limitation in lateral rotation that is, in relation to the normal range of motion for lateral rotation, more limited than abduction, which is more limited than medial rotation. Movements not listed are irrelevant to the identification of the capsular pattern. As an example, a patient with 10 degrees of shoulder lateral rotation (10 degrees out of a possible 90 degrees of motion), 90 degrees of abduction (90 degrees out of a possible 180 degrees of motion), and

TABLE 2-1	Articular Anatomy as per Kaltenborn and Interpretation Based on Kaltenborn's Concave-Convex Rules	

Name of Joint	Articulation Anatomy	Osteokinematic Motion and Arthrokinematic Glide
Sternoclavicular joint	For elevation/depression: the sternum is concave; the clavicle is convex	Opposite direction
	For protraction/retraction: the sternum is convex; the clavicle is concave	Same direction
Acromioclavicular joint	The acromion is concave; the clavicle is convex	Opposite direction
Glenohumeral joint	The glenoid is concave; the humerus is convex	Opposite direction
Humeroulnar joint	The humerus is convex; the ulna is concave	Same direction
Humeroradial joint	The humerus is convex; the radius is concave	Same direction
Proximal radioulnar joint	The ulna is concave; the radius is convex	Opposite direction
Distal radioulnar joint	The ulna is convex; the radius is concave	Same direction
Radiocarpal joints	The radius is concave; the carpals are convex	Opposite direction
Intercarpal joints	The scaphoid is convex; the trapezium and trapezoid are concave	Same direction
	Otherwise: the proximal bones are concave; the distal bones are convex	Opposite direction
Carpometacarpal joint of the thumb	For flexion/extension: the carpal is convex; the metacarpal is concave	Same direction
	For abduction/adduction: the carpal is concave; the metacarpal is convex	Opposite direction
Intermetacarpal joints	In relation to metacarpal III: the more medial metacarpals are convex; the more lateral metacarpals are concave	Same direction
Metacarpophalangeal joint of the thumb	The metacarpal is convex; the phalanx is concave	Same direction
Metacarpophalangeal joints of digits 2-5	The metacarpals are convex; the phalanges are concave	Same direction
Proximal and distal interphalangeal joints of the hand	The proximal phalanges are convex; the distal phalanges are concave	Same direction
Hip joint	The acetabulum is concave; the femur is convex	Opposite direction
Tibiofemoral joint	The femur is convex; the tibia is concave	Same direction
Patellofemoral joint	The femur is concave; the patella is convex	Opposite direction
Proximal tibiofibular joint	The tibia is convex; the fibula is concave	Same direction
Distal tibiofibular joint	The tibia is concave; the fibula is convex	Opposite direction
Talocrural joint	The tibia and fibula are concave; the talus is convex	Opposite direction
Subtalar joint	The anterior and middle talus are convex; the anterior and middle calcaneus are concave	Same direction
	The posterior talus is concave; the posterior calcaneus is convex	Opposite direction
Talonavicular joint	The talus is convex; the navicular is concave	Same direction
Calcaneocuboid joint	For flexion/extension: the calcaneus is convex; the cuboid is concave	Same direction
	For abduction/adduction: the calcaneus is concave; the cuboid is convex	Opposite direction
Intermetatarsal joints	In relation to metatarsal II: the more medial metatarsals are convex; the more lateral metatarsals are concave	Same direction
Metatarsophalangeal joints	The metatarsals are convex; the phalanges are concave	Same direction
Interphalangeal joints of the toes	The proximal phalanges are convex; the distal phalanges are concave	Same direction
Temporomandibular joint	The temporalis is concave; the mandible is convex	Opposite direction

Adapted from Kaltenborn FM. Manual Mobilization of the Joints: The Kaltenborn Method of Joint Examination and Treatment, Vol I: The Extremities, 6th ed. OPTP, Oslo, Norway, Norli, 2002.

60 degrees of medial rotation (60 degrees out of a possible 90 degrees) would have a capsular pattern.

According to Cyriax,[8] if passive range of motion of a joint is limited in this characteristic pattern of restriction, this indicates that the impairment involves the entire joint capsule. Determining the presence of capsular patterns is helpful in diagnosing articular lesions because the presence of a capsular pattern would indicate that the diagnosis is therefore one in which the entire joint capsule is involved, suggesting that mobilization/manipulation interventions in all directions would be indicated. Examples of impairments involving the entire joint capsule are osteoarthritis and conditions involving trauma to the entire joint capsule. Joint conditions that would not cause a capsular pattern of restriction include knee meniscus tears, ligamentous injuries, and extraarticular lesions. Capsular patterns of restriction for all of the joints are listed in the introduction section of the respective chapter for each joint.

The determination of the motion limitations that constitute a capsular pattern is not evidence based, but rather is based on Cyriax's descriptions. In several studies, the validity of the concept of capsular patterns was addressed. In relation to subjects with adhesive capsulitis of the shoulder[9,10] and osteoarthritis of the hip,[11,12] there was no evidence of a capsular pattern, whereas the question of whether there is a capsular pattern in patients with knee osteoarthritis remains unanswered.[11,13,14]

Positional Faults

The clinician might choose to identify positional faults as part of the examination procedure, in which case he or she should determine during the palpation component of the evaluation process whether the joint surfaces appear to be aligned correctly in relation to one another by comparing the position of bony landmarks with the same landmarks on the opposite side. When a suspected positional fault is identified, the clinician should examine whether the perceived alignment impairment is a positional fault or simply a bony abnormality by palpating adjacent bony landmarks. For example, if a clinician suspects, by palpating the position of a spinous process, that a thoracic vertebra has a rotational positional fault, the transverse processes corresponding to that vertebra should also be asymmetric consistent with the direction of rotation. A T5 vertebral body that is rotated right should be accompanied by a spinous process that is positioned left of midline and a right T5 transverse process that is positioned more posterior than the left T5 transverse process. If the transverse processes are aligned symmetrically, any alignment asymmetry of the spinous process is more likely due to a bony anomaly of that spinous process. There are additional criteria for identifying the presence of a symptomatic positional fault: the joint should be hypomobile and painful with accessory motion testing.

PRECAUTIONS AND CONTRAINDICATIONS

Many of the conditions that have been identified as precautions or contraindications have been identified as such simply because they appeal to common sense: they are not evidence based.

Most of the conditions listed here are therefore precautions and not contraindications. The clinician should weigh the risks and benefits carefully before choosing whether or not to administer a particular joint mobilization/manipulation intervention.

When considering whether to perform a particular technique, it is important to take into account the amount of force produced and the duration of treatment. In general, it is a good strategy to use the least aggressive technique that would accomplish the goal of treatment. In the case of determining whether to intervene with mobilization/manipulation for all patients, especially patients with the precautions listed here, it is therefore important to consider whether less aggressive techniques (joint mobilization/manipulation or some other intervention) would produce the desired outcome with less risk of an adverse reaction than more aggressive techniques or whether the best course of action is no intervention whatsoever.

Numerous precautions and contraindications relate specifically to spine mobilization/manipulation interventions. These are described in Chapter 9. Precautions and contraindications relating to all joints are as follows:

1. Any condition that has not been fully evaluated
2. Joint ankylosis
3. Joint hypermobility, if techniques that take the joint through its end range are being considered, unless a positional fault is being treated
4. An infection in the area being treated
5. A malignancy in the area being treated
6. An unhealed fracture in the area being treated
7. Inflammatory arthritis in the area being treated, especially if it is in a state of exacerbation
8. Metabolic bone diseases, such as osteoporosis, Paget's disease, and tuberculosis
9. Any debilitating disease that compromises the integrity of periarticular tissue (e.g., advanced diabetes)
10. Long-term use of corticosteroids
11. When there is considerable joint effusion in the area being treated (because it is difficult to evaluate joint mobility accurately, as swelling takes up some of the slack in the joint capsule)
12. Considerable joint irritability or pain in the area being treated
13. Protective muscle spasm to the extent that the clinician is unable to evaluate mobility in the area being treated
14. Pain in adjacent segments that is aggravated by the placement of the clinician's hands when attempting to perform mobilization/manipulation techniques
15. Coagulation disorders
16. Skin rashes or open or healing skin lesions in the area being treated

INTERVENTION

Numerous treatment parameters must be determined when designing an intervention that includes joint mobilization/manipulation, including joint position, direction of force, amount and speed of force, timing of the intervention, and pain considerations.

Joint Position

Treatment should be initiated with the joint in the resting position. This is the safest position in which to treat, because compressive forces are minimal and the patient's response can be observed before proceeding to techniques involving more aggressive positions. Most of the techniques discussed in this book are described in the resting position for these reasons. Nevertheless, research has shown that if the goal is to increase joint mobility, positions approximating the restricted range of motion yield greater increases in joint range of motion.[15]

It is generally recommended that mobilizations/manipulations should not be performed in the *close-packed position*. Kaltenborn[1] described the *close-packed position* as the position in which the joint capsule and ligaments are maximally tensed, and there is maximal contact between the two articular surfaces. Kaltenborn proposed that mobilization/manipulation performed in the *close-packed position* produces too much compressive force on the articulating surfaces. As is the case with the resting position, few studies have been performed to determine the *close-packed position* for specific joints, making it difficult to accurately identify the true *close-packed position*. To complicate this issue further, in one study investigating glenohumeral joint stiffness, the investigators concluded that close-packed positioning is most likely different for different mobilization/manipulation glides.[16] The *close-packed positions* are listed in the introductory section of each chapter. They are based on Kaltenborn's work, as Kaltenborn was the first clinician to introduce this concept in relation to joint mobilization/manipulation.

Direction of Force

When the goal of the mobilization/manipulation technique is to increase joint mobility, the direction of the mobilization/manipulation force is usually performed in the same direction as the hypomobile accessory motion. In most cases, the actual technique used to identify a decrease in accessory motion is also the technique used to treat that impairment. An exception to this statement involves performing some of the spinal techniques, in which case the examination technique can differ from the treatment technique.

Positional faults are most often treated with mobilization/manipulation interventions that realign the two bones in the correct position, although some clinicians advocate gliding in the direction of the greatest hypomobility. The direction of the intervention mobilization/manipulation is less relevant when considering the other indications for treatment, such as pain reduction.

Amount and Speed of Force

Intervention mobilizations/manipulations are graded according to the amount and speed of motion imparted to the joint and numbered in order from least to most aggressive. Although several descriptions of mobilization/manipulation grades have been proposed, the system described by Maitland[4] (Figure 2-13) is most commonly used and is described as follows:

Grade I: A slow, small-amplitude movement that does not take the joint capsule to the limit of available joint motion

Grade II: A slow, large-amplitude movement that does not take the joint capsule to the limit of available joint motion

Grade III: A slow, large-amplitude movement that takes the joint up to and slightly through the limit of available joint motion and into tissue resistance

Grade IV: A slow, small-amplitude movement that is performed through the limit of available joint motion and into tissue resistance

Grade V movements are used to describe thrust joint manipulations and can be defined as follows:

Grade V/thrust joint manipulation: A high-velocity, small-amplitude, nonoscillatory movement that begins at the limit of available joint motion and takes the joint into tissue resistance

The grade of movement used to evaluate joint motion corresponds to a grade III mobilization.

Research suggests that joint mobilization/manipulation treatment techniques used to increase the mobility of joint and periarticular tissue should be forceful enough to bring the tissue into the plastic phase of the stress-strain curve (grade III or higher),[17] but not so forceful as to reach the failure point, unless the goal is to break adhesions. The research suggests that mobilizations/manipulations also should be at least a grade III to optimally decrease pain.

Maitland[4] described one method of determining how aggressively a patient can be safely treated with mobilization/manipulation techniques. This method involves examining the pattern of pain to tissue resistance with the passive range of motion corresponding to the particular mobilization/manipulation technique being considered and determining the severity of the patient's condition through history taking. If pain occurs before the end range is met with passive range of motion, and if the patient has symptoms that are easily provoked and persist for a long time, grade I and II techniques are indicated to treat the pain. If pain occurs after the end range is met with passive range of motion or if passive range of motion is pain-free, and if symptoms increase only after a moderate amount of activity and last for a short time, the patient should be able to tolerate grade III or higher mobilizations/manipulations. The aim of this approach is to avoid reproducing the patient's pain with mobilization/manipulation interventions.

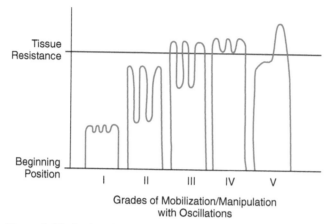

Figure 2-13 Grades of mobilization/manipulation with oscillations.

Timing of Mobilization and Manipulation Intervention

Recommendations for the length of time a single mobilization maneuver should last range from two to three maneuvers a second to one maneuver every 10 seconds. There is also wide variability in the recommended total amount of time to spend mobilizing/manipulating a patient with a musculoskeletal impairment, ranging from treatments lasting seconds to treatments lasting up to 60 minutes. Other treatment parameters likely to influence outcomes from the application of a mobilization/manipulation technique include whether the technique is accompanied by an oscillatory movement and the number of repetitions per technique.

Mobilization/manipulation interventions that take the joint through tissue resistance could cause irritation to stretched periarticular structures. As a general rule, mobilization/manipulation interventions should be curtailed if they aggravate the patient's symptoms. The patient might also experience soreness after treatment. If the patient experiences an increase in symptoms for more than 12 hours after treatment or experiences swelling or muscle guarding in the area of the joint being treated, either the wrong technique was performed or the treatment was too aggressive. In such cases, a reevaluation is indicated. Finally, treatment sessions should be spaced at least 48 hours apart to allow the patient to recover from any joint irritation from the previous treatment.

Pain with Accessory Motion Testing

There is currently no consensus regarding determining the direction of joint mobilization/manipulation interventions based on whether pain occurred during accessory motion testing. Maitland recommends mobilizing/manipulating into the direction of pain, with the caveat that the amount of force should be determined based on the severity of the condition and should not cause symptoms to commence or increase. Other clinicians advocate using different strategies that result in mobilizing/manipulating in a pain-free direction. Other clinicians advocate using different strategies, such as identifying hypomobility with accessory motion testing to determine the direction of joint mobilization/manipulation force.

TECHNIQUE

When performing most joint mobilization/manipulation techniques, either as examination or as treatment procedures, the clinician should keep the following principles in mind:

1. The patient should exhibit no muscle guarding and should be as relaxed as possible.
2. The clinician should be efficient with body mechanics. The mobilizing/manipulating force should be as close to the clinician's center of gravity as possible. The force ideally should be directed downward. If a downward force is not feasible, a horizontally directed force can be performed. This is especially important when evaluating and treating larger joints. When performing joint mobilization/manipulation techniques on the smaller joints of the hand and the foot, the role of gravity in executing the technique is relatively unimportant.
3. The stabilizing force and the mobilizing/manipulating force should be as close to the joint surfaces as possible.
4. When mobilizing/manipulating proximal joints, the mobilization/manipulation technique should be timed with the patient's breathing such that the patient exhales while the mobilization/manipulation is being performed.

5. Pain should be monitored during the mobilization/manipulation procedure, and appropriate modifications to the technique being performed should be made to minimize patient discomfort.

6. Each technique is an evaluative technique and an intervention technique; the clinician continually evaluates during treatment.

7. For reasons related to patient safety and comfort, when feasible, glides are performed with a grade I traction to decrease compression forces on the joint surfaces.

Joint Cavitation

Manipulation procedures applied to joint structures are sometimes accompanied by a cracking noise, or cavitation. Evidence suggests that this noise occurs because the manipulation procedure causes the volume of the joint to expand rapidly, resulting in the formation of an air cavity accompanied by a cracking sound.[18]

Some clinicians believe that producing an audible crack during a manipulation procedure maximizes the therapeutic effect of the intervention. Several studies have indicated that this is not the case. In relation to grade V lumbar manipulations in subjects with low back pain when range of motion, pain, and disability outcomes were assessed, there were no differences between subjects whose manipulations did and did not result in an audible crack.[19] Similarly, in patients with neck pain who received thoracic manipulations,[20] and in asymptomatic subjects who received lumbar manipulations,[21] there was no difference in pain sensitivity or reduction in perceived pain, respectively, between subjects who did and those who did not experience joint cavitation.

Common folklore suggests that habitual self-cracking might result in osteoarthritic changes. In several studies in which investigators compared the prevalence of osteoarthritis among subjects with and without a history of habitual joint cracking, no such relationship was found.[22-24] In one of these studies, however, habitual knuckle cracking was associated with hand swelling and a decrease in hand strength.[23]

VARIATIONS IN JOINT MOBILIZATION/MANIPULATION APPROACHES

Mobilization with Movement

Mobilization with movement techniques, conceived and disseminated by Brian Mulligan, entails a pain-free joint mobilization force that is applied to a joint while simultaneously either an active or passive joint osteokinematic motion is performed. The mobilization force is maintained throughout pain free movement toward to end range and during the return movement to the start position. If pain free, the joint osteokinematic motion is taken to the end range and overpressure into that end-range position is applied momentarily, before the joint is brought back to its start position. This sustained end-range positioning and overpressure is believed to be necessary for long-term improvement.

The evaluation procedure to determine whether a specific mobilization with movement technique is indicated is to first identify a painful and/or restricted joint osteokinematic motion and then repeat that motion while performing the mobilization with movement procedure. If the patient demonstrates a decrease in pain and/or an increase in pain-free range of motion while the mobilization with movement technique is being performed compared with that same motion without the mobilization with movement technique, then that technique is deemed to be an appropriate intervention. Mobilization with movement intervention techniques, therefore, should never reproduce the patient's symptoms.

Mulligan initially proposed that these techniques are effective because they correct positional faults.[25] Recently, this premise has been called into question.[26] Several other models, including biomechanical and neurophysiological explanations, have been proposed; however, the underlying rationale for the efficacy of mobilization with movement interventions remains unclear.[26] More in-depth discussion on clinical reasoning mechanisms and dosage can be found in *Mobilisation with Movement: The Art and the Science.*[27]

Muscle Energy

Muscle energy is a specific type of mobilization intervention that uses a voluntary contraction of the patient's muscles to move one bone on another. To perform this technique, the joint first is placed in a specific position that facilitates optimal contraction of a particular muscle or muscle group. The patient is asked to contract that muscle or muscle group isometrically against the clinician's counter pressure. This contraction causes the muscle to pull on the bony attachment of one of the bones that composes the joint to be mobilized, moving one bone in relation to its articulating counterpart. The articulating counterpart must be stabilized for this accessory movement to occur. The contraction occurs in a precisely controlled direction with a precisely controlled joint position in all three planes and requires a precisely executed counterforce. After holding the contraction for 3 to 7 seconds, the patient is instructed to relax, and the muscle is passively stretched. The clinician repeats the sequence from this new position. The technique is commonly performed three times before reexamination.

Muscle energy techniques have the advantage of allowing the patient to control the mobilization; if too much pain is reproduced during the maneuver, the patient can terminate the procedure. In some situations, muscle-energy techniques can also alleviate joint impairment by stretching and/or strengthening muscles that influence joint mechanics.

PLAN OF CARE

There is evidence to support the premise that combining treatment with joint mobilization/manipulation with other physical therapy interventions enhances outcomes. These interventions should minimally include therapeutic exercises for improving strength, range of motion, and/or motor control, as well as patient education regarding body mechanics, activity level, and prognosis, but could also include other interventions such as bracing, taping, and/or therapeutic agents.

REFERENCES

1. Kaltenborn FM. *Manual Mobilization of the Joints: The Kaltenborn Method of Joint Examination and Treatment*. Vol. I. The Extremities. 6th ed. Oslo, Norway: Norli; 2002.
2. Arvidsson I. The hip joint: forces needed for distraction and appearance of the vacuum phenomenon. *Scand J Rehabil Med*. 1990;22:157-162.
3. Lin HT, Hsu AT, Chang GL, et al. Determining the resting position of the glenohumeral joint in subjects who are healthy. *Phys Ther*. 2007;87:1669-1682.
4. Maitland GD. *Vertebral Manipulation*. 5th ed. London: Butterworth; 1986.
5. Brandt C, Sole G, Krause MW, Nel M. An evidence-based review on the validity of the Kaltenborn rule as applied to the glenohumeral joint. *Man Ther*. 2007;12:3-11.
6. Baeyens J-P, van Glabbeek F, Goossens M, et al. In vivo 3D arthrokinematics of the proximal and distal radioulnar joints during active pronation and supination. *Clin Biomech*. 2006;21:S9-S12.
7. Johnson AJ, Godges JJ, Zimmerman GJ, Ounanian LL. The effect of anterior versus posterior glide joint mobilization on external rotation range of motion in patients with shoulder adhesive capsulitis. *J Orthop Sports Phys Ther*. 2007;37:88-99.
8. Cyriax J. *Textbook of Orthopaedic Medicine*. Vol. 1. Diagnosis of Soft Tissue Lesions. 8th ed. London: Bailliere Tindall; 1982.
9. Rundquist PJ, Anderson DD, Guanche CA, Ludewig PM. Shoulder kinematics in subjects with frozen shoulder. *Arch Phys Med Rehabil*. 2003;84: 1473-1479.
10. Rundquist PJ, Ludewig PM. Patterns of motion loss in subjects with idiopathic loss of shoulder range of motion. *Clin Biomech*. 2004;19:810-818.
11. Biji D, Dekker J, van Baar ME, et al. Validity of Cyriax's concept capsular pattern for the diagnosis of osteoarthritis of hip and/or knee. *Scan J Rheum*. 1998; 27:347-351.
12. Klassbo M, Harms-Ringdahl K, Larsson G. Examination of passive ROM and capsular patterns in the hip. *Physiother Res Int*. 2003;8:1-12.
13. Fritz JM, Delitto A, Erhard RE, Roman M. An examination of the selective tissue tension scheme, with evidence for the concept of a capsular pattern of the knee. *Phys Ther*. 1998;78:1046-1061.
14. Hayes KW, Petersen C, Falconer J. An examination of Cyriax's passive motion tests with patients having osteoarthritis of the knee. *Phys Ther*. 1994;74: 697-709.
15. Hsu A-T, Ho L, Ho S, Hedman T. Joint position during anterior-posterior glide mobilization: its effect on glenohumeral abduction range of motion. *Arch Phys Med Rehabil*. 2000;81:210-214.
16. McQuade KJ, Shelley I, Cvitkovic J. Patterns of stiffness during clinical examination of the glenohumeral joint. *Clin Biomech*. 1999;14:620-627.
17. Vermeulen HM, Rozing PM, Obermann WR, le Cessie S, Vliet Vlieland TP. Comparison of high-grade and low-grade mobilization techniques in the management of adhesive capsulitis of the shoulder: randomized controlled trial. *Phys Ther*. 2006;86: 355-368.
18. Kawchuk GN, Fryer J, Jaremko JL, et al. Real-time visualization of joint cavitation. *PLoS ONE*. 2015; 10(4):e0119470.
19. Flynn TW, Fritz JM, Wainner RS, et al. The audible pop is not necessary for successful spinal high-velocity thrust manipulation in individuals with low back pain. *Arch Phys Med Rehab*. 2003;84: 1057-1060.
20. Sillevis R, Cleland J. Immediate effects of the audible pop from a thoracic spine thrust manipulation on the autonomic nervous system and pain: a secondary analysis of a randomized clinical trial. *J Manipulative Physiol Ther*. 2011;34:37-45.
21. Bialosky JE, Bishop MD, Robinson ME, George SZ. The relationship of the audible pop to hypoalgesia associated with high-velocity, low-amplitude thrust manipulation: a secondary analysis of an experimental study in pain-free participants. *J Manipulative Physiol Ther*. 2010;33:117-124.
22. Swezey RL, Swezey SE. The consequences of habitual knuckle cracking. *West J Med*. 1975;122: 377-379.
23. Castellanos J, Axelrod D. Effect of habitual knuckle cracking on hand function. *Ann Rheum Dis*. 1990;49:308-309.

24. deWeber K, Olszewski M, Ortolano R. Knuckle cracking and hand osteoarthritis. *J Am Board Fam Med.* 2011;24:169-174.

25. Mulligan B. Mobilisation with movement (MWM's). *J Man Manip Ther.* 1993;1:154-156.

26. Vicenzino B, Paungmali A, Teys P. Mulligan's mobilization-with-movement, positional faults and pain relief: Current concepts from a critical review of literature. *Man Ther.* 2007;12:98-108.

27. Vicenzino B, Hing W, Rivett D, Hall T. *Mobilisation with movement: the art and the science.* Elsevier; 2010.

The Appendicular Skeletal System

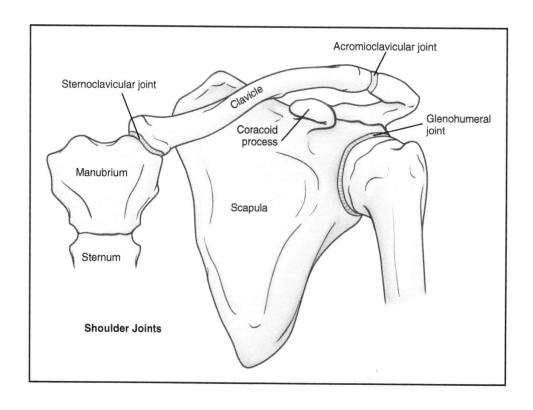

Sternoclavicular joint

Acromioclavicular joint

Clavicle

Coracoid process

Glenohumeral joint

Manubrium

Scapula

Sternum

Shoulder Joints

CHAPTER 3

The Shoulder

BASICS

The shoulder complex comprises four joints, all of which contribute to attaining full range of motion at the shoulder: the glenohumeral joint, scapulothoracic joint, sternoclavicular joint, and acromioclavicular joint. Approximately 120 degrees of motion into flexion and abduction must occur at the shoulder complex for most basic activities of daily living to occur.

Glenohumeral Joint

The glenohumeral articulation is the most mobile joint in the human body. This mobility is achieved in part because the humeral head is much larger than its articulating counterpart, the glenoid cavity. The sole bony attachment of the shoulder complex to the axial skeletal system at the sternoclavicular joint also contributes to its mobility. Many conditions affecting the shoulder can be attributable to its large arc of motion.

Scapulothoracic Joint

Scapular lateral rotation occurs with shoulder elevation. During the first 30 degrees of elevation, the scapula attempts to stabilize itself against the thorax. In this phase a greater proportion of the motion occurs at the glenohumeral joint. After this phase there is variability as to the relative amount of glenohumeral versus scapulothoracic motion.

Sternoclavicular and Acromioclavicular Joints

Movement at the sternoclavicular and acromioclavicular joints accompanies shoulder elevation. As the scapula elevates and laterally rotates, the clavicle rotates on its longitudinal axis, contributing to full shoulder elevation range of motion.

SPECIFIC PATHOLOGY AND SHOULDER JOINT MOBILIZATION/ MANIPULATION

Adhesive Capsulitis

In a 2014 systematic review, the authors reported on the efficacy of conservative interventions for the management of adhesive capsulitis. They concluded that, in relation to short-term outcomes, a combination of manual therapy and exercise was not as effective as a glucocorticoid injection. The authors were unable to draw firm conclusions regarding long-term outcomes.[1] These conclusions were consistent with clinical practice guidelines addressing physical therapy interventions for patients with adhesive capsulitis, in which the authors could only base their recommendations that mobilization interventions were indicated to decrease pain and improve function and range of motion on weak evidence.[2] These findings contradict a 2011 systematic review, however, in which the authors reported that there was fair evidence that manual therapy, which included manipulation, mobilization, and mobilization with movement, along with proprioceptive training was an effective intervention for adhesive capsulitis.[3]

Impingement Syndrome

In a 2014 systematic review of two different studies, investigators reported that mobilization in addition to exercises resulted in greater improvements in pain at 3 weeks compared with exercises alone. In one of these studies, however, the exercise alone group had greater improvements in function than the exercise plus mobilization group.[4]

Rotator Cuff Injuries

In a 2011 systematic review, the authors concluded that there was fair evidence supporting interventions consisting of manipulation, soft tissue mobilization, and/or exercise for treatment of rotator cuff injuries.[3]

Nonspecific Shoulder Pain

Two different systematic reviews addressed nonspecific shoulder pain. In one review, published in 2011, the authors reported that there was fair evidence supporting multi-modal interventions including manipulation,[3] whereas in the other review, also published in 2011, investigators stated that studies were inconclusive regarding whether mobilization in addition to exercise interventions was more effective than exercise alone.[5] This latter conclusion was corroborated in a study, published concurrently, in which the investigators reported no difference in function or pain outcomes when joint mobilization was added to advice and exercises. This was the case at 1-, 3-, and 6-month follow-ups.[6]

GLENOHUMERAL JOINT

Osteokinematic motions:
  Flexion/extension
  Abduction/adduction
  Medial/lateral rotation
  Horizontal abduction/adduction
Ligaments:
  Superior glenohumeral ligament
  Middle glenohumeral ligament
  Inferior glenohumeral ligament
  Coracohumeral ligament
  Coracoacromial ligament
Joint orientation:
  Glenoid: lateral, anterior, inferior
  Humerus: medial, posterior, superior
Concave joint surface:
  Glenoid
Type of joint:
  Synovial
Resting position:
  55 degrees of abduction and 30 degrees of horizontal adduction (55 degrees of scaption), slight lateral rotation[7]
  30 to 40 degrees of abduction, no flexion, neutral rotation[8]
Close-packed position:
  Full elevation[7]
Capsular pattern of restriction:
  Lateral rotation more limited than abduction, which is more limited than medial rotation[9]

Distraction (Figure 3-1, Video 3-1)

Purpose
- To examine for glenohumeral joint impairment
- To increase accessory motion into glenohumeral joint distraction
- To increase range of motion at the glenohumeral joint
- To decrease pain

Positioning
1. The patient is supine.
2. The glenohumeral joint is positioned in the resting position if conservative techniques are indicated or approximating restricted range of motion if more aggressive techniques are indicated.
3. The clinician can use a belt to hold the patient's scapula against the trunk, especially in the presence of scapulothoracic hypermobility or excessive movement at the scapulothoracic joint with shoulder elevation.
4. The clinician is at the patient's side, facing the glenohumeral joint.
5. The clinician can support the patient's forearm and hand by positioning them between the clinician's upper arm and trunk.
6. Both hands grip the proximal humerus as close to the axilla as possible from the medial and lateral side.

Procedure
1. Both hands move the humeral head lateral, anterior, and inferior, perpendicular to the glenoid joint surface (see Figure 3-1).

Particulars
- When the glenohumeral joint is positioned such that the long axis of the humerus is perpendicular to the flattened-out concave surface of the glenoid, this technique can be performed by pulling on the upper arm.

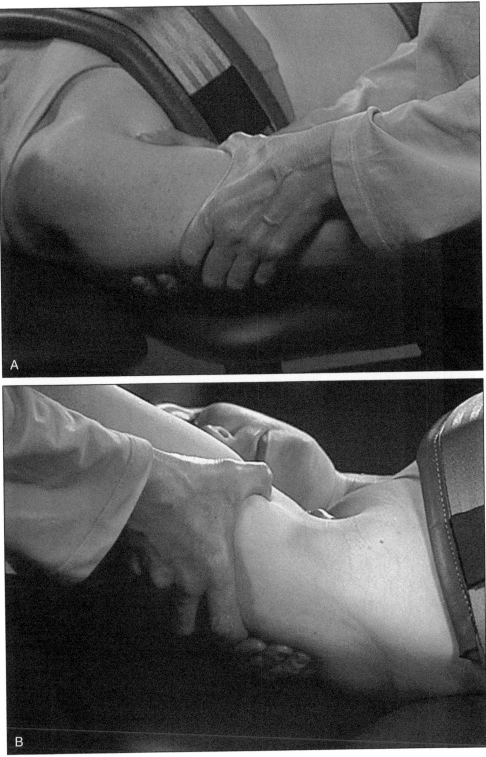

Figure 3-1 Distraction. **A,** Distraction performed in the resting position. **B,** Distraction performed approximating the restricted range of motion into flexion.

Inferior Glide (Figure 3-2, Video 3-2)

Purpose

- To examine for glenohumeral joint impairment
- To increase accessory motion into glenohumeral joint inferior glide
- To increase range of motion at the glenohumeral joint
- To decrease pain

Positioning

1. The patient is supine.
2. The glenohumeral joint is positioned in the resting position if conservative techniques are indicated or approximating restricted range of motion if more aggressive techniques are indicated.
3. The clinician can use a belt to hold the patient's scapula against the trunk.
4. The clinician is at the patient's head, facing the glenohumeral joint.
5. The clinician can support the patient's forearm and hand by positioning them between the clinician's upper arm and trunk.
6. The mobilizing/manipulating hand is positioned with the web space over the superior surface of the proximal humerus.
7. The guiding hand supports the upper limb from the medial side of the distal humerus.

Procedure

1. The clinician applies a grade I traction to the joint.
2. The mobilizing/manipulating hand glides the humerus in an inferior direction.
3. The guiding hand controls the position of the humerus (see Figure 3-2).

Particulars

- This technique might be especially effective for increasing range of motion into glenohumeral joint abduction.

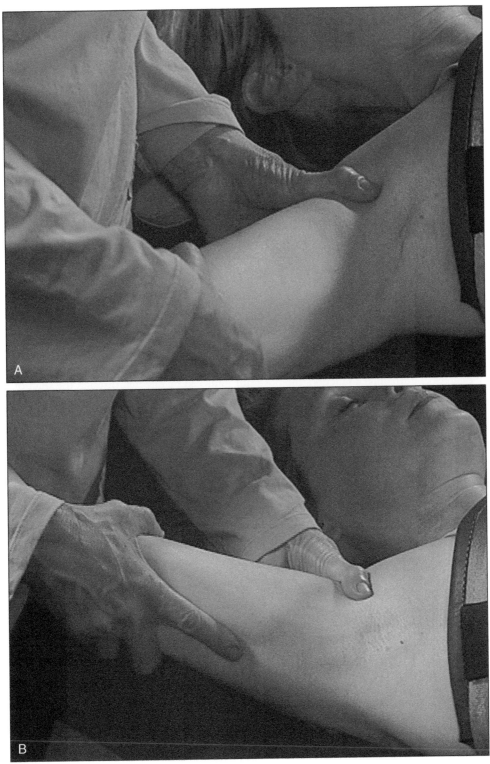

Figure 3-2 Inferior glide. **A,** Inferior glide performed in the resting position. **B,** Inferior glide performed approximating the restricted range of motion into abduction.

Posterior Glide (Figure 3-3, Video 3-3)

Purpose

- To examine for glenohumeral joint impairment
- To increase accessory motion into glenohumeral joint posterior glide
- To increase range of motion at the glenohumeral joint
- To decrease pain

Positioning

1. The patient is supine, with the humerus positioned off the edge of the treatment table.
2. The glenohumeral joint is positioned in the resting position if conservative techniques are indicated or approximating restricted range of motion if more aggressive techniques are indicated.
3. The clinician is at the patient's side, facing the patient.
4. The clinician can support the patient's forearm and hand by positioning them between the clinician's upper arm and trunk.
5. The mobilizing/manipulating hand is positioned over the anterior surface of the proximal humerus.
6. The guiding hand supports the upper limb from the posterior side of the distal humerus.

Procedure

1. The clinician applies a grade I traction to the joint.
2. The mobilizing/manipulating hand glides the humerus in a posterior direction.
3. The guiding hand controls the position of the humerus (see Figure 3-3).
4. When approximating the restricted range of motion for horizontal adduction, if the shoulder joint can be positioned in at least 90 degrees of horizontal adduction, the posterior glide can be directed through the shaft of the humerus.

Particulars

- This technique might be especially effective for increasing range of motion into glenohumeral joint medial rotation, flexion, and horizontal adduction. Nevertheless, it has been shown in a study to increase range of motion into lateral rotation to a greater extent than an anterior glide mobilization technique.[10]

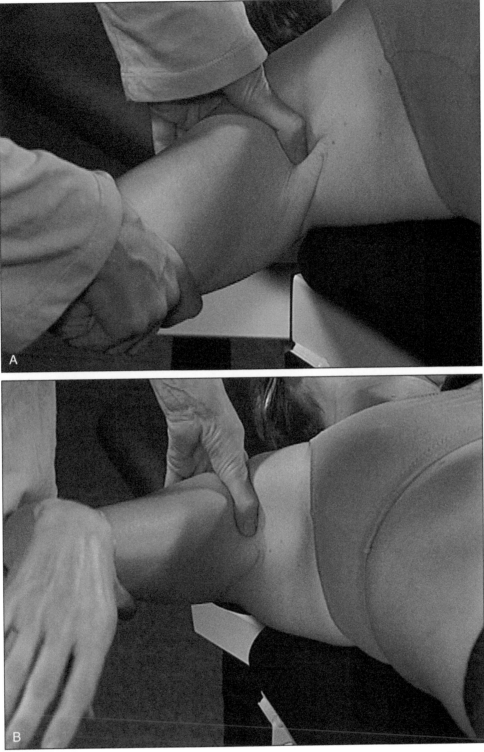

Figure 3-3 Posterior glide. **A,** Posterior glide performed in the resting position. **B,** Posterior glide performed approximating the restricted range of motion into medial rotation.

Anterior Glide: First Technique (Figure 3-4, Video 3-4)

Purpose

- To examine for glenohumeral joint impairment
- To increase accessory motion into glenohumeral joint anterior glide
- To increase range of motion at the glenohumeral joint
- To decrease pain

Positioning

1. The patient is supine.
2. The glenohumeral joint is positioned in the resting position if conservative techniques are indicated or approximating restricted range of motion if more aggressive techniques are indicated.
3. The clinician can use a belt to hold the patient's scapula against the trunk.
4. The clinician is at the patient's side, facing the glenohumeral joint.
5. The clinician can support the patient's forearm and hand by positioning them between the clinician's upper arm and trunk.
6. The mobilizing/manipulating hand is positioned over the posterior surface of the proximal humerus.
7. The guiding hand supports the upper limb from the anterior and posterior sides of the distal humerus.

Procedure

1. The clinician applies a grade I traction to the joint.
2. The mobilizing/manipulating hand glides the humerus in an anterior direction.
3. The guiding hand controls the position of the humerus (see Figure 3-4).

Particulars

- The clinician should use caution in performing this technique because this motion might be hypermobile. If it is, performing an anterior glide mobilization/manipulation technique might cause the glenohumeral joint to be more unstable.
- This position requires that the clinician move the humerus against gravity and should be used only when the mobilization/manipulation technique is to be performed for a short amount of time.
- This technique might be effective for increasing range of motion into glenohumeral joint lateral rotation, extension, and horizontal abduction. Nevertheless, it has been shown in a study that posterior gliding mobilization increases range of motion into lateral rotation to a greater extent than an anterior glide mobilization technique in subjects with adhesive capsulitis.[10]

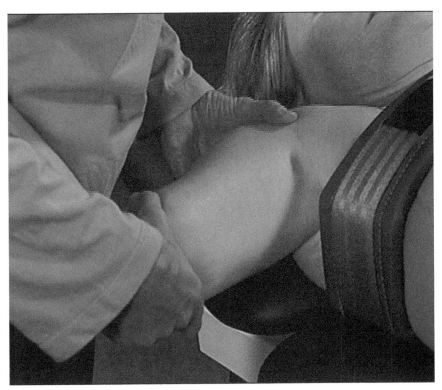

Figure 3-4 Anterior glide: first technique.

Anterior Glide: Second Technique (Figure 3-5, Video 3-5)

Purpose

- To examine for glenohumeral joint impairment
- To increase accessory motion into glenohumeral joint anterior glide
- To increase range of motion at the glenohumeral joint
- To decrease pain

Positioning

1. The patient is prone with the humerus positioned off the edge of the treatment table and a pillow supporting the coracoid process.
2. The glenohumeral joint is positioned in the resting position if conservative techniques are indicated or approximating restricted range of motion if more aggressive techniques are indicated.
3. The clinician can use a belt to hold the patient's scapula against the trunk.
4. The clinician is at the patient's side, facing the glenohumeral joint.
5. The mobilizing/manipulating hand is positioned over the posterior surface of the proximal humerus.
6. The guiding hand supports the upper limb from the anterior side of the distal humerus.

Procedure

1. The clinician applies a grade I traction to the joint.
2. The mobilizing/manipulating hand glides the humerus in an anterior direction.
3. The guiding hand controls the position of the humerus (see Figure 3-5).

Particulars

- The clinician should use caution in performing this technique because this motion might be hypermobile. If it is, performing an anterior glide mobilization/manipulation technique might cause the glenohumeral joint to be more unstable.
- This technique might be effective for increasing range of motion into glenohumeral joint lateral rotation, extension, and horizontal abduction. Nevertheless, it has been shown in a study that posterior gliding mobilization increases range of motion into lateral rotation to a greater extent than an anterior glide mobilization technique in subjects with adhesive capsulitis.[10]

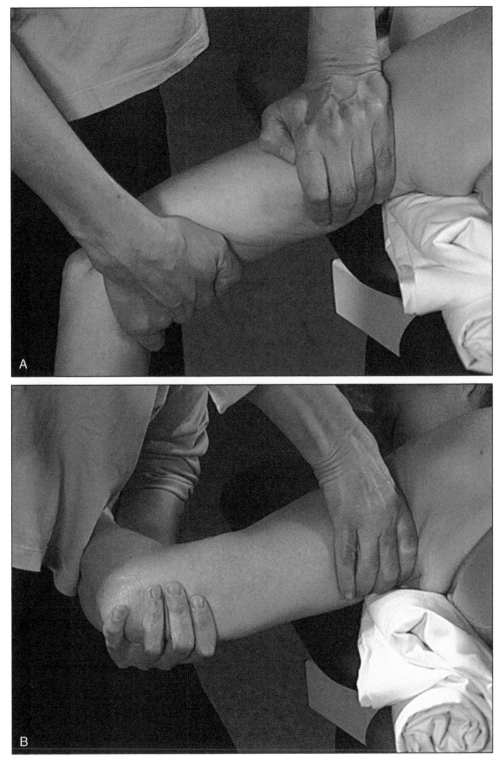

Figure 3-5 Anterior glide: second technique. **A,** Anterior glide performed in the resting position. **B,** Anterior glide performed approximating the restricted range of motion into lateral rotation.

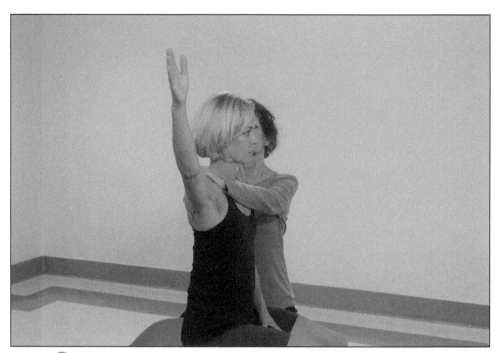

▶ **Figure 3-6** Posterolateral glide of the humerus mobilization with movement.

Posterolateral Glide of the Humerus Mobilization with Movement (Figure 3-6, Video 3-6)

Purpose
- To decrease pain
- To increase pain-free range of motion into shoulder flexion
- To increase pain-free range of motion into shoulder scaption/abduction

Positioning
1. The patient is sitting with the arm at the patient's side.
2. The clinician is standing on the side opposite the side being treated.
3. The stabilizing hand is positioned on the patient' scapula.
4. The mobilizing hand is positioned with the thenar eminence on the patient's anteromedial humeral head, and the distal forearm in contact with the chest wall inferior to the coracoid process.

Procedure

1. The clinician imparts a posterolateral glide to the humeral head.
2. While maintaining the posterolateral glide, the patient raises the arm through the pain-free range of motion into elevation in the scapular plane.
3. While providing stability to the scapula, the clinician also allows the scapula to upwardly rotate.
4. The clinician maintains the posterolateral glide while the patient moves the shoulder joint back to the starting position.
5. Due to the dynamic changes in the position of the glenoid fossa with shoulder elevation. Clinician continually adjusts his or her own position in relation to the patient's position to maintain the joint mobilization force during joint movement (see Figure 3-6).

Particulars

- This technique are indicated only if they can be performed without reproducing the patient's pain/symptoms.
- This technique should result in an immediate increase in range of motion and/or a decrease in pain.
- If effective (the technique results in an immediate increase in range of motion and/or decrease in pain), this technique should be repeated (~3 sets of 10).
- This technique was studied in a trial in which subjects with painful shoulders served as their own controls. When compared with placebo and control conditions, subjects receiving this technique demonstrated an increase in range of motion in the scapular plane and pain pressure threshold immediately following treatment.[11] A subsequent study, also performed on subjects with shoulder pain and using a repeated-measures design, compared this mobilization with movement technique with a combination of mobilization with movement and rigid sports tape. The group receiving both mobilization with movement and tape showed greater improvements in range of motion into elevation in the scapular plane, but no difference in pain pressure threshold at 1-week follow-up.[12] A third study randomly assigned subjects with shoulder pain to the mobilization with movement technique and kinesiology tape or a supervised exercise program. At 10 days follow-up, the group receiving mobilization with movement and taping demonstrated greater improvements in pain-free shoulder abduction and flexion range of motion.[13]

SCAPULOTHORACIC JOINT

Osteokinematic motions:
  Protraction/retraction
  Elevation/depression (these two motions are accompanied by upward and downward rotation)
Ligaments:
  None
Joint orientation:
  Thorax: posterior, lateral, superior
  Scapula: anterior, medial, inferior
Concave joint surface:
  Scapula
Type of joint:
  Functional articulation
Resting position:
  Not described by Kaltenborn
Close-packed position:
  None; not a synovial joint
Capsular pattern of restriction:
  None; not a synovial joint

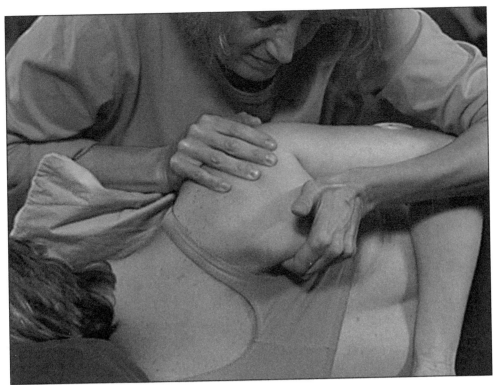

▶ **Figure 3-7** Distraction.

Distraction (Figure 3-7, Video 3-7)

Purpose
- To examine for scapulothoracic joint impairment
- To increase accessory motion into scapulothoracic joint distraction
- To increase range of motion at the shoulder complex
- To decrease pain

Positioning
1. The patient is lying on the unaffected side with the posterior surface of the hand positioned on the sacrum if shoulder range of motion allows.
2. The clinician is either in front or behind the patient, facing the patient's shoulder.
3. If the clinician is positioned in front of the patient, a pillow can be used to separate the patient's chest from the clinician.
4. The mobilizing hand is positioned over the acromion.
5. The guiding hand is positioned adjacent to the inferior angle of the scapula.

Procedure
1. The mobilizing hand moves the scapula medially and inferiorly over the guiding hand.
2. The guiding hand lifts the scapula away from the ribs (see Figure 3-7).

Particulars
- This joint can be difficult to mobilize, as it might take a great deal of effort on the part of the clinician to maneuver the hand between the scapula and thorax.
- This is not a grade V manipulation technique.

Superior Glide (Figure 3-8, Video 3-8)

Purpose
- To examine for scapulothoracic joint impairment
- To increase accessory motion into scapulothoracic superior glide
- To increase range of motion at the shoulder complex
- To decrease pain

Positioning
1. The patient is lying on the unaffected side with the arm in a neutral position.
2. The clinician is in front of the patient, facing the patient's shoulder.
3. A pillow can be used to separate the patient's chest from the clinician.
4. The mobilizing hand is positioned adjacent to the inferior angle of the scapula.
5. The guiding hand is positioned over the acromion.

Procedure
1. The clinician applies a grade I traction to the joint.
2. The mobilizing hand glides the scapula in a superior direction.
3. The guiding hand controls the position of the scapula (see Figure 3-8).

Particulars
- This is not a grade V manipulation technique.
- This technique might be especially effective for increasing range of motion into scapulothoracic joint elevation.

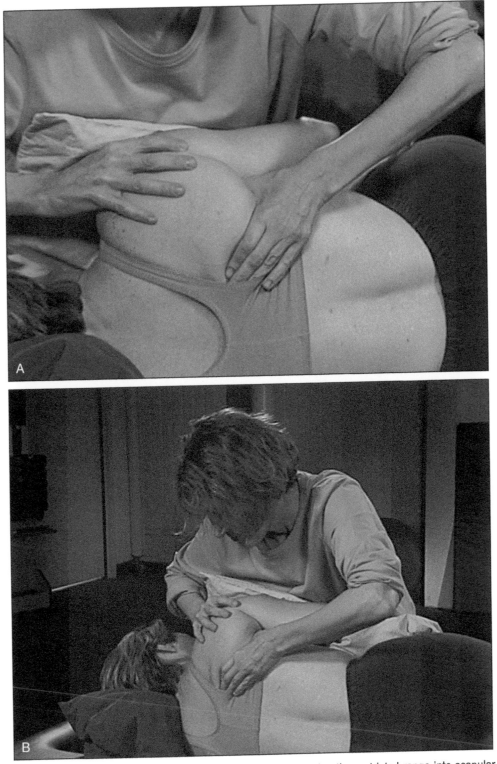

Figure 3-8 Superior glide. **A,** Initial hand placement. **B,** Approximating the restricted range into scapular elevation.

Inferior Glide (Figure 3-9, Video 3-9)

Purpose

- To examine for scapulothoracic joint impairment
- To increase accessory motion into scapulothoracic inferior glide
- To increase range of motion at the shoulder complex
- To decrease pain

Positioning

1. The patient is lying on the unaffected side with the arm in a neutral position.
2. The clinician is in front of the patient, facing the patient's shoulder.
3. A pillow can be used to separate the patient's chest from the clinician.
4. The mobilizing hand is positioned over the acromion.
5. The guiding hand is positioned over the inferior angle of the scapula.

Procedure

1. The clinician applies a grade I traction to the joint.
2. The mobilizing hand glides the acromion in an inferior direction.
3. The guiding hand controls the position of the scapula (see Figure 3-9).

Particulars

- This is not a grade V manipulation technique.
- This technique might be especially effective for increasing range of motion into scapulothoracic joint depression.

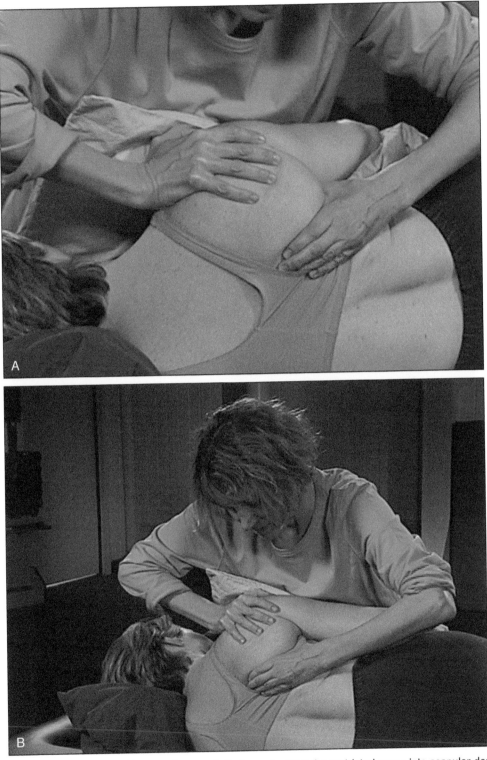

Figure 3-9 Inferior glide. **A,** Initial hand placement. **B,** Approximating the restricted range into scapular depression.

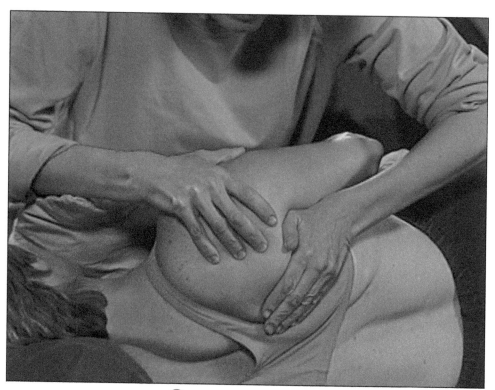

▶ **Figure 3-10** Medial glide.

Medial Glide (Figure 3-10, Video 3-10)

Purpose
- To examine for scapulothoracic joint impairment
- To increase accessory motion into scapulothoracic medial glide
- To increase range of motion at the shoulder complex
- To decrease pain

Positioning
1. The patient is lying on the unaffected side with the arm in a neutral position.
2. The clinician is in front of the patient, facing the patient's shoulder.
3. A pillow can be used to separate the patient's chest from the clinician.
4. Both hands are positioned over the lateral surface of the scapula, one hand over the axillary border and the other hand over the acromion.

Procedure
1. Both hands glide the scapula in a medial direction (see Figure 3-10).

Particulars
- This is not a grade V manipulation technique.
- This technique might be especially effective for increasing range of motion into scapulothoracic joint retraction.

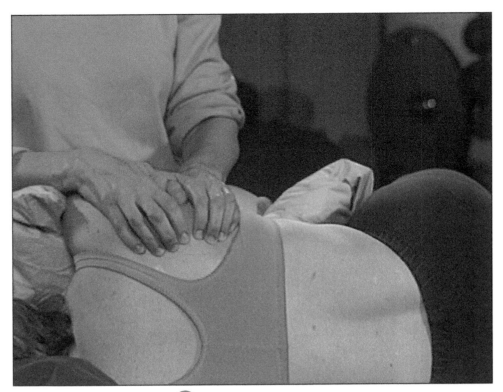

▶ **Figure 3-11** Lateral glide.

Lateral Glide (Figure 3-11, Video 3-11)

Purpose
- To examine for scapulothoracic joint impairment
- To increase accessory motion into scapulothoracic lateral glide
- To increase range of motion at the shoulder complex
- To decrease pain

Positioning
1. The patient is lying on the unaffected side with the arm in a neutral position.
2. The clinician is in front of the patient, facing the patient's shoulder.
3. A pillow can be used to separate the patient's chest from the clinician.
4. Both hands are positioned with the fingertips over the vertebral border of the scapula.

Procedure
1. Both hands glide the scapula in a lateral direction (see Figure 3-11).

Particulars
- This is not a grade V manipulation technique.
- The clinician should use caution in performing this technique because this motion might be hypermobile, especially among patients with posture impairments involving the shoulder.
- This technique might be especially effective for increasing range of motion into scapulothoracic joint protraction.

STERNOCLAVICULAR JOINT

Osteokinematic motions:
  Elevation/depression
  Protraction/retraction
Ligaments:
  Costoclavicular ligament
  Interclavicular ligament
  Posterior sternoclavicular ligament
  Anterior sternoclavicular ligament
Joint orientation:
  Manubrium: lateral, superior
  Clavicle: medial, inferior
Concave joint surface:
  Sternum concave superior to inferior
  Clavicle concave anterior to posterior
Type of joint:
  Synovial
Resting position:
  Not described by Kaltenborn
Close-packed position:
  Arm fully elevated[7]
Capsular pattern of restriction:
  Pain at the end of range of shoulder motion[9]

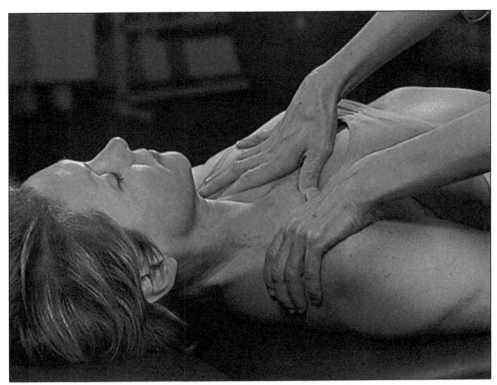

▶ **Figure 3-12** Superior glide.

Superior Glide (Figure 3-12, Video 3-12)

Purpose
- To examine for sternoclavicular joint impairment
- To increase accessory motion into sternoclavicular superior glide
- To increase range of motion at the shoulder complex
- To decrease pain

Positioning
1. The patient is supine with the arm resting at the side.
2. The clinician is at the patient's side, facing the sternoclavicular joint.
3. The mobilizing/manipulating hand is positioned with the thumb over the thumb of the guiding hand.
4. The guiding hand is positioned with the thumb over the inferior surface of the clavicle about 3 cm lateral to the most medial surface.

Procedure
1. The mobilizing/manipulating hand glides the clavicle in a superior direction.
2. The guiding hand controls the position of the mobilizing/manipulating hand (see Figure 3-12).

Particulars
- The clinician should use caution in performing this technique because this motion might be hypermobile.

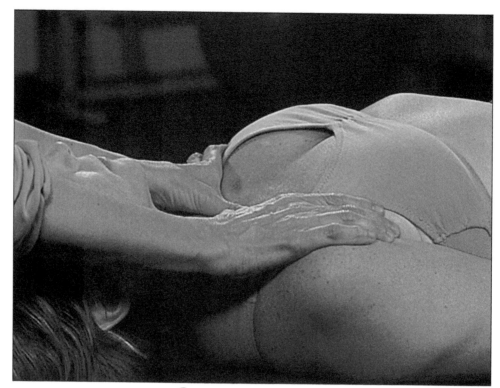

▶ **Figure 3-13** Inferior glide.

Inferior Glide (Figure 3-13, Video 3-13)

Purpose
- To examine for sternoclavicular joint impairment
- To increase accessory motion into sternoclavicular inferior glide
- To increase range of motion at the shoulder complex
- To decrease pain

Positioning
1. The patient is supine with the arm resting at the side.
2. The clinician is at the patient's head, facing the sternoclavicular joint.
3. The mobilizing/manipulating hand is positioned with the thumb over the thumb of the guiding hand.
4. The guiding hand is positioned with the thumb over the superior surface of the clavicle, about 3 cm lateral to the most medial surface.

Procedure
1. The mobilizing/manipulating hand glides the clavicle in an inferior direction.
2. The guiding hand controls the position of the mobilizing/manipulating hand (see Figure 3-13).

Particulars
- The clinician should use caution in performing this technique because this motion might be hypermobile.

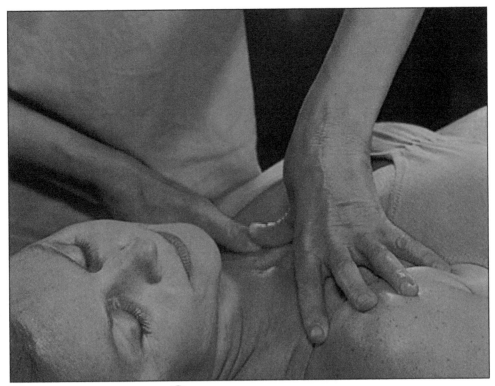

Figure 3-14 Posterior glide.

Posterior Glide (Figure 3-14, Video 3-14)

Purpose
- To examine for sternoclavicular joint impairment
- To increase accessory motion into sternoclavicular posterior glide
- To increase range of motion at the shoulder complex
- To decrease pain

Positioning
1. The patient is supine with the arm resting at the side.
2. The clinician is at the patient's head, facing the sternoclavicular joint.
3. The mobilizing/manipulating hand is positioned with the thumb over the thumb of the guiding hand.
4. The guiding hand is positioned with the thumb over the anterior surface of the clavicle.

Procedure
1. The mobilizing/manipulating hand glides the clavicle in a posterior direction.
2. The guiding hand controls the position of the mobilizing/manipulating hand (see Figure 3-14).

Particulars
- The clinician should use caution in performing this technique because this motion might be hypermobile.

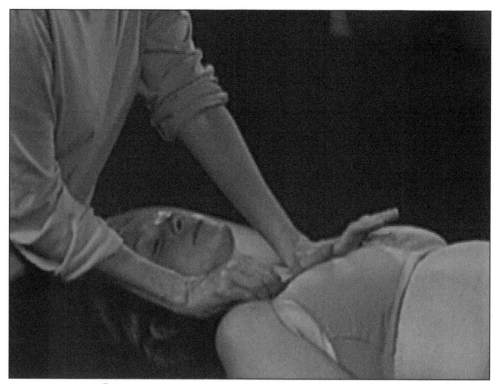

▶ **Figure 3-15** Anterior glide of the clavicle on the sternum.

Anterior Glide of the Clavicle on the Sternum (Figure 3-15, Video 3-15)

Purpose
- To examine for sternoclavicular joint impairment
- To increase accessory motion into sternoclavicular anterior glide
- To increase range of motion at the shoulder complex
- To decrease pain

Positioning
1. The patient is supine with the arm resting at the side.
2. The clinician is at the patient's head, facing the sternoclavicular joint.
3. The stabilizing hand grips around the clavicle superiorly and inferiorly as close to the posterior surface as possible with the fingers.
4. The mobilizing/manipulating hand is positioned over the patient's sternum.

Procedure
1. The stabilizing hand holds the clavicle in position.
2. The mobilizing/manipulating hand glides the sternum in a posterior direction, thereby imparting an anterior force to the clavicle on the sternum (see Figure 3-15).

Particulars
- The clinician should use caution in performing this technique because this motion might be hypermobile.
- The clinician should be aware that the grip on the clavicle might be uncomfortable for the patient.

ACROMIOCLAVICULAR JOINT

Osteokinematic motions:
  Elevation/depression
  Protraction/retraction
Ligaments:
  Superior acromioclavicular ligament
  Inferior acromioclavicular ligament
  Coracoclavicular ligaments (conoid and trapezoid)
Joint orientation:
  Acromion: superior, medial, anterior
  Clavicle: inferior, lateral, posterior
Concave joint surface:
  Acromion
Type of joint:
  Synovial
Resting position:
  Not described by Kaltenborn
Close-packed position:
  90 degrees of abduction[7]
Capsular pattern of restriction:
  Pain at the end of range of shoulder motion[9]

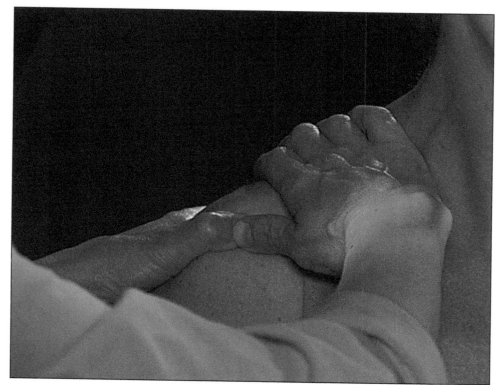

▶ **Figure 3-16** Posterior glide.

Posterior Glide (Figure 3-16, Video 3-16)
Purpose
- To examine for acromioclavicular joint impairment
- To increase accessory motion into acromioclavicular posterior glide
- To increase range of motion at the shoulder complex
- To decrease pain

Positioning
1. The patient is sitting with the arm resting at the side.
2. The clinician is in front of the patient, facing the anterior surface of the acromioclavicular joint.
3. The stabilizing hand is positioned over the posterior surface of the scapula.
4. The mobilizing/manipulating hand is positioned with the thumb over the thumb of the guiding hand.
5. The guiding hand, which is the same hand as the stabilizing hand, is positioned with the thumb over the anterolateral surface of the clavicle.

Procedure
1. The stabilizing hand holds the scapula in position.
2. The mobilizing/manipulating hand glides the clavicle in a posterior direction.
3. The guiding hand controls the position of the mobilizing/manipulating hand (see Figure 3-16).

Particulars
- The clinician should use caution in performing this technique because this motion might be hypermobile.

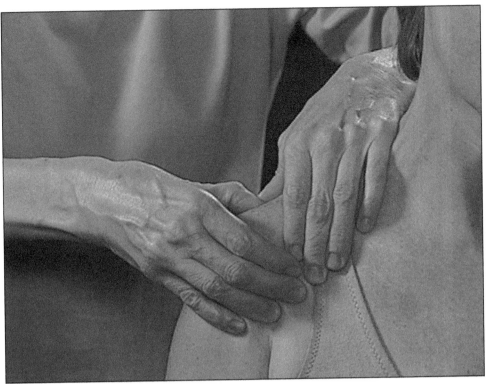

▶ **Figure 3-17** Anterior glide.

Anterior Glide (Figure 3-17, Video 3-17)

Purpose
- To examine for acromioclavicular joint impairment
- To increase accessory motion into acromioclavicular anterior glide
- To increase range of motion at the shoulder complex
- To decrease pain

Positioning
1. The patient is sitting with the arm resting at the side.
2. The clinician is behind the patient, facing the posterior surface of the acromioclavicular joint.
3. The stabilizing hand is positioned over the anterior acromion and over the anterior surface of the proximal humerus.
4. The mobilizing/manipulating hand is positioned with the thumb over the thumb of the guiding hand.
5. The guiding hand, which is the same hand as the stabilizing hand, is positioned with the thumb over the posterolateral surface of the clavicle.

Procedure
1. The stabilizing hand holds the acromion in position.
2. The mobilizing/manipulating hand glides the clavicle in an anterior direction.
3. The guiding hand controls the position of the mobilizing/manipulating hand (see Figure 3-17).

Particulars
- The clinician should use caution in performing this technique because this motion might be hypermobile.

REFERENCES

1. Page MJ, Green S, Kramer S, et al. Manual therapy and exercise for adhesive capsulitis (frozen shoulder). *Cochrane Database Syst Rev.* 2014;(8):CD011275.

2. Kelley MJ, Shaffer MA, Kuhn JE, et al. Shoulder pain and mobility deficits: adhesive capsulitis clinical practice guidelines linked to the International Classification of Functioning, Disability, and Health from the Orthopaedic Section of the American Physical Therapy Association. *J Orthop Sports Phys Ther.* 2013;43:A1-A31.

3. Brantingham JW, Cassa TK, Bonnefin D, et al. Manipulative therapy for shoulder pain and disorders: expansion of a systematic review. *J Manipulative Physiol Ther.* 2011;34:314-346.

4. Gebremariam L, Hay EM, van der Sande R, et al. Subacromial impingement syndrome—effectiveness of physiotherapy and manual therapy. *Br J Sports Med.* 2014;48:1202-1208.

5. Brudvig TJ, Kulkarni H, Shah S. The effect of therapeutic exercise and mobilization on patients with shoulder dysfunction: a systematic review with meta-analysis. *J Orthop Sports Phys Ther.* 2011;41:734-748.

6. Yiasemides R, Halaki M, Cathers I, Ginn KA. Does passive mobilization of shoulder region joints provide additional benefit over advice and exercise alone for people who have shoulder pain and minimal movement restriction? A randomized controlled trial 2011. *Phys Ther.* 2011;91:178-190.

7. Kaltenborn FM. *Manual Mobilization of the Joints: The Kaltenborn Method of Joint Examination and Treatment.* Vol 1. 6th ed. The Extremities. OPTP, Oslo, Norway: Norli; 2002.

8. Lind T, Blyme PJH, Strange-Vognsen HH, et al. Pressure-position relations in the glenohumeral joint. *Acta Orthop Belg.* 1992;58:81-83.

9. Cyriax J. *Textbook of Orthopaedic Medicine.* Vol 1. 8th ed. Diagnosis of Soft Tissue Lesions. London: Bailliere Tindall; 1982.

10. Johnson AJ, Godges JJ, Zimmerman GJ, Ounanian LL. The effect of anterior versus posterior glide joint mobilization on external rotation range of motion in patients with shoulder adhesive capsulitis. *J Orthop Sports Phys Ther.* 2007;37:88-99.

11. Teys P, Bisset L, Vicenzino B. The initial effects of a Mulligan's mobilization with movement technique on range of movement and pressure pain threshold in pain-limited shoulders. *Man Ther.* 2008;13:37-42.

12. Teys P, Bisset L, Collins N, Coombes B, Vicenzino B. One-week time course of the effects of Mulligan's Mobilisation with Movement and taping in painful shoulders. *Man Ther.* 2013;18:372-377.

13. Djordjevic OC, Vukicevic D, Katunac L, Jovic S. Mobilization with Movement and Kinesiotape compared with a supervised exercise program for painful shoulder: results of a clinical trial. *J Manipulative Physiol Ther.* 2012;35:454-463.

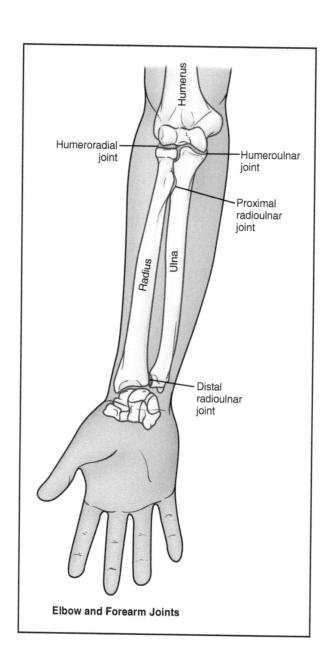

Elbow and Forearm Joints

CHAPTER 4

The Elbow and Forearm

BASICS

The elbow complex comprises three articulations: the humeroulnar and humeroradial joints and the proximal radioulnar joint. Flexion and extension occur at the humeroulnar and humeroradial joints. Pronation and supination are considered motions of the forearm and occur at the humeroradial joint, the proximal and distal radioulnar joints, and the ulnomeniscotriquetral joint of the wrist. Most basic activities of daily living occur between 30 and 130 degrees of elbow flexion and between 50 degrees of pronation and 50 degrees of supination.

Humeroulnar Joint

The humeroulnar joint is classified as a hinge joint. The ulnar concave articular surface has a larger curvature than most joint surfaces. Posterior and anterior glides might therefore be ineffective at this joint because the two joint surfaces are likely to jam together when these glide techniques are attempted. Assuming this is the case, humeroulnar joint techniques are limited to distraction and medial and lateral techniques.

Distraction techniques for all joints are performed such that the bone being mobilized/manipulated is moved in a direction perpendicular to the treatment plane. Because the proximal ulna is angulated 45 degrees anterior to the shaft of the ulna, the shaft of the ulna is not perpendicular to the treatment plane and humeroulnar distraction mobilization/manipulation occurs at an angle that is 45 degrees less flexion than the position of the shaft of the ulna (see Figure 2-3).

Humeroradial Joint

Positional faults are believed to occur at the humeroradial joint. Compression positional faults can be caused by a fall on an outstretched arm, causing the humerus to move closer to the radius, whereas distraction positional faults can occur when the arm is pulled, which causes the opposite alignment impairment to occur. Distraction positional faults are especially common in young children as a result of being pulled or spun by the arms. This condition is called a pulled elbow.

Proximal and Distal Radioulnar Joints

Motion into pronation and supination occurs simultaneously at the proximal and distal radioulnar joints. When the ulna is stationary, the radius rotates anteriorly and medially with pronation and posteriorly and laterally with supination. The radius also spins on the humerus during these two motions.

SPECIFIC PATHOLOGY AND ELBOW AND FOREARM JOINT MOBILIZATION/ MANIPULATION

Lateral Epicondylalgia

In a 2013 systemic review addressing conservative interventions for patients with lateral epicondylalgia,[1] the authors concluded that there is limited evidence to support the use of elbow lateral glide mobilization with movement interventions to decrease pain and increase pain-free grip strength immediately after treatment compared with placebo or control interventions and as an add-on to ultrasound and exercise to decrease pain and increase pain-free grip strength at 3-month follow-up. These conclusions were based on a review of two separate studies.

In a second systematic review published in the same year, the authors concluded that there was moderate evidence to support joint mobilization interventions for lateral epicondylalgia. They specifically recommended mobilization with movement techniques.[7]

HUMEROULNAR JOINT

Osteokinematic motion:
  Flexion/extension
Ligaments:
  Ulnar collateral ligament
Joint orientation:
  Humerus: inferior, posterior
  Ulna: superior, anterior
  Note: The flattened-out concave joint surface (the treatment plane) of the ulna forms a 45-degree angle with the shaft of the ulna
Concave joint surface:
  Ulna
Type of joint:
  Synovial
Resting position:
  70 degrees flexion, 10 degrees supination[2]
Close-packed position:
  Full extension and supination[2]
Capsular pattern of restriction:
  Flexion is more limited than extension[3]

Distraction (Figure 4-1, Video 4-1)

Purpose

- To examine for humeroulnar joint impairment
- To increase accessory motion into humeroulnar joint distraction
- To increase range of motion at the elbow joint
- To decrease pain

Positioning

1. The patient is supine.
2. The humeroulnar joint is positioned in the resting position if conservative techniques are indicated or approximating restricted range of motion if more aggressive techniques are indicated.
3. The clinician is at the patient's hip, facing the humeroulnar joint, with the patient's upper arm resting on the treatment table, the elbow joint positioned off the edge of the table, and the distal forearm resting on the clinician's shoulder.
4. The stabilizing hand grips the distal humerus from the anterior side.
5. Instead of or in addition to the stabilizing hand, the clinician can use a belt to hold the patient's humerus to the treatment table.
6. The mobilizing/manipulating hand grips the proximal ulna from the anterior side, avoiding contact with the radius.

Procedure

1. The stabilizing hand holds the distal humerus against the treatment table.
2. The mobilizing/manipulating hand moves the proximal ulna in a direction perpendicular to the ulnar joint surface, which is at an angle that is in 45 degrees less flexion than the position of the ulnar shaft (see Figure 2-3 and Figure 4-1).

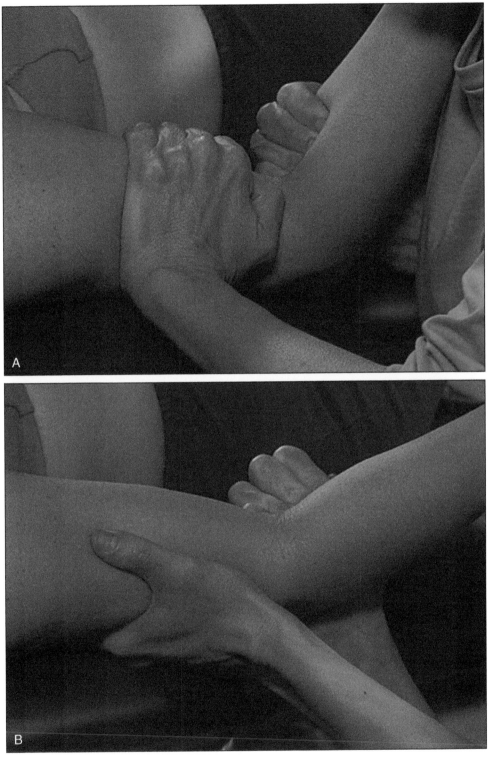

Figure 4-1 Distraction. **A,** Distraction performed in the resting position. **B,** Distraction performed approximating the restricted range of motion into extension.

Medial Glide (Figure 4-2, Video 4-2)

Purpose

- To examine for humeroulnar joint impairment
- To increase accessory motion into humeroulnar medial glide
- To increase range of motion at the elbow joint
- To decrease pain

Positioning

1. The patient is supine.
2. The humeroulnar joint is positioned in the resting position if conservative techniques are indicated or approximating restricted range of motion if more aggressive techniques are indicated.
3. The clinician is facing the patient, between the patient's arm and trunk, with the patient's forearm between the clinician's upper arm and trunk.
4. The stabilizing hand grips the distal humerus from the medial side.
5. The mobilizing/manipulating hand grips the proximal radius from the lateral side.

Procedure

1. The clinician applies a grade I traction to the joint.
2. The stabilizing hand holds the humerus in position.
3. The mobilizing/manipulating hand glides the proximal ulna in a medial direction indirectly through the radius while the clinician's trunk guides the motion (see Figure 4-2).

Particulars

- This technique is commonly performed with the elbow in slight flexion using a grade V manipulation.

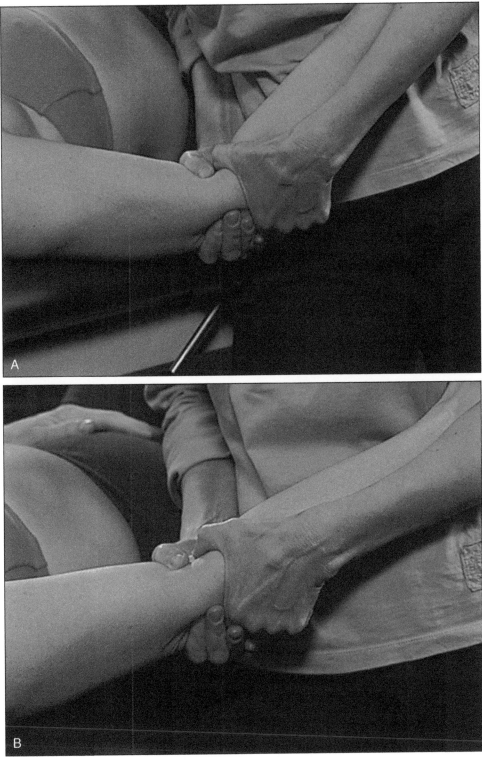

Figure 4-2 Medial glide. **A,** Medial glide performed in the resting position. **B,** Medial glide performed approximating the restricted range of motion into extension.

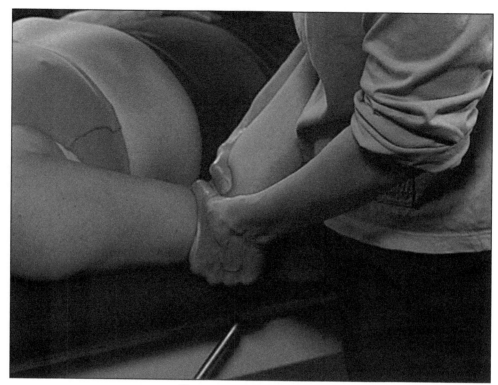

▶ **Figure 4-3** Lateral glide.

Lateral Glide (Figure 4-3, Video 4-3)

Purpose
- To examine for humeroulnar joint impairment
- To increase accessory motion into humeroulnar lateral glide
- To increase range of motion at the elbow joint
- To decrease pain

Positioning
1. The patient is supine.
2. The humeroulnar joint is positioned in the resting position if conservative techniques are indicated or approximating restricted range of motion if more aggressive techniques are indicated.
3. The clinician is at the patient's side, facing the humeroulnar joint with the patient's forearm, between the clinician's upper arm and trunk.
4. The stabilizing hand grips the distal humerus from the lateral side.
5. The mobilizing/manipulating hand grips the proximal ulna from the medial side.

Procedure
1. The clinician applies a grade I traction to the joint.
2. The stabilizing hand holds the humerus in position.
3. The mobilizing/manipulating hand glides the proximal ulna in a lateral direction while the clinician's trunk guides the motion (see Figure 4-3).

Particulars
- This technique is commonly performed with the elbow in slight flexion using a grade V manipulation.

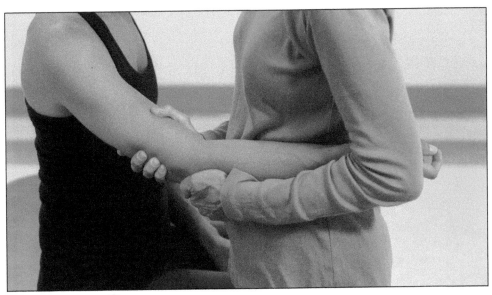

▶ **Figure 4-4** Medial glide mobilization with movement.

Medial Glide Mobilization with Movement (Figure 4-4, Video 4-4)

Purpose
- To increase pain-free range of motion into elbow flexion or extension, or wrist flexion
- To decrease pain with gripping activities
- To decrease pain from medial epicondylalgia

Positioning
1. The patient is sitting with the elbow slightly bent and the forearm supinated.
2. The clinician stands in front of and on the side of the elbow being mobilized, with the patient's forearm between the clinician's stabilizing side forearm and trunk.
3. The stabilizing hand grasps the medial distal humerus.
4. The thenar eminence of the mobilizing hand is positioned on the lateral proximal ulna.

Procedure
1. The clinician imparts a medial glide to the olecranon.
2. While maintaining the medial glide, the patient performs active or resisted elbow flexion or extension, or wrist flexion or gripping (see Figure 4-4).

Particulars
- This technique are indicated only if they can be performed without reproducing the patient's pain/symptoms.
- This technique should result in an immediate increase in range of motion and/or a decrease in pain.
- If effective (the technique results in an immediate increase in range of motion and/or decrease in pain), this technique should be repeated (~3 sets of 10).

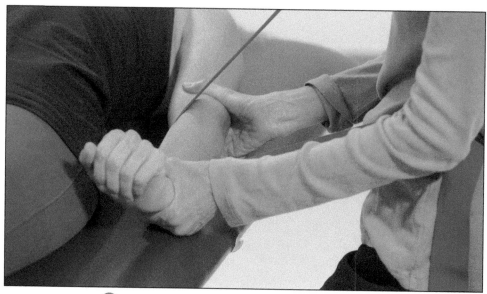

▶ **Figure 4-5** Lateral glide mobilization with movement.

Lateral Glide Mobilization with Movement (Figure 4-5, Video 4-5)
Purpose
- To increase pain-free range of motion into wrist extension and/or gripping
- To decrease pain with gripping activities
- To decrease pain from lateral epicondylalgia

Positioning
1. The patient is supine with the shoulder internally rotated, the elbow slightly flexed, and the forearm pronated.
2. The clinician stands on the side of the elbow being mobilized, facing the elbow.
3. The clinician places a mobilization belt around his or her shoulder, behind the neck and around the trunk, and around the patient's proximal forearm. The belt should be at a 90 degree angle to the forearm to ensure patient comfort with the technique.
4. The clinician places the heel of the stabilizing hand on the distal lateral humerus and the mobilizing hand on the distal posterior forearm.

Procedure
1. The clinician imparts a lateral glide to the proximal forearm with the belt. This can be accomplished by adjusting the belt such that the clinician's knees are in slight flexion before initiating the lateral glide. The clinician can then add tension to the belt by extending the knees.
2. While maintaining the lateral glide, the patient performs active or resisted wrist extension or gripping. Slight changes in the belt angle or joint glide might be needed to ensure pain free execution of the technique (see Figure 4-5).

Particulars
- This technique are indicated only if they can be performed without reproducing the patient's pain/symptoms.
- This technique should result in an immediate increase in range of motion and/or a decrease in pain.
- If effective (the technique results in an immediate increase in range of motion and/or decrease in pain), this technique should be repeated (~3 sets of 10).
- This technique has been shown to produce an increase in pain-free grip strength and pressure pain threshold compared with a placebo control group immediately after treatment in subjects with lateral epicondylalgia.[4] When added to a regimen of exercise and ultrasound, this technique reduced pain and increased grip strength for up to 12 weeks of follow-up.[5] Furthermore, when a regimen of this mobilization technique and exercise was compared with steroid injections, global improvement, grip force, and assessor's rating of severity were greater at 52 weeks follow-up.[6]

HUMERORADIAL JOINT

Osteokinematic motions:
  Flexion/extension
  Pronation/supination
Ligaments:
  Radial collateral ligament
Type of joint:
  Synovial
Joint orientation:
  Humerus: inferior
  Radius: superior
Concave joint surface:
  Radius
Resting position:
  Full extension and supination[2]
Close-packed position:
  90 degrees flexion, 5 degrees supination[2]
Capsular pattern of restriction:
  Flexion is more limited than extension[3]

Distraction (Figure 4-6, Video 4-6)

Purpose
- To examine for humeroradial joint impairment
- To increase accessory motion into humeroradial joint distraction
- To increase range of motion at the elbow joint
- To decrease pain

Positioning
1. The patient is supine.
2. The humeroradial joint is positioned in the resting position if conservative techniques are indicated or approximating restricted range of motion if more aggressive techniques are indicated.
3. The clinician is at the patient's side, facing the humeroradial joint.
4. The stabilizing hand grips the distal humerus from the anterior side.
5. The mobilizing/manipulating hand grips the distal radius, avoiding contact with the ulna.

Procedure
1. The stabilizing hand holds the humerus in position.
2. The mobilizing/manipulating hand moves the radial head distally perpendicular to the radial joint surface (see Figure 4-6).

Particulars
- This technique might be effective in correcting a humeroradial joint compression positional fault.

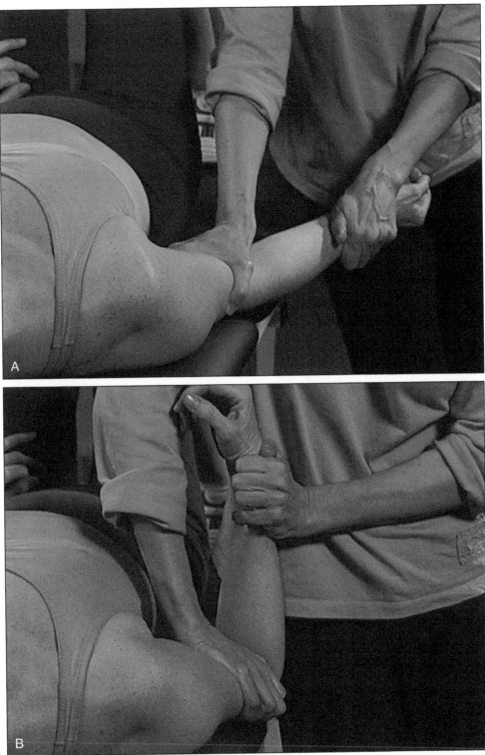

Figure 4-6 Distraction. A, Distraction performed in the resting position. B, Distraction performed approximating the restricted range of motion into flexion.

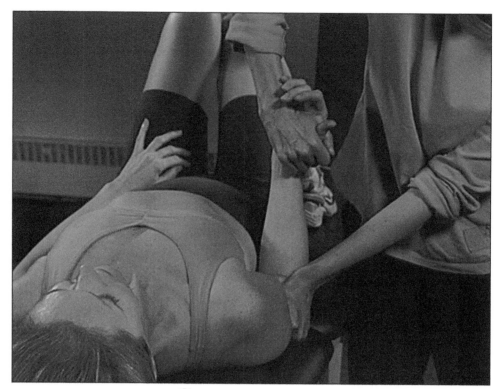

▶ **Figure 4-7** Compression.

Compression (Figure 4-7, Video 4-7)
Purpose
- To correct a humeroradial joint distraction positional fault

Positioning
1. The patient is supine.
2. The elbow joint is positioned in 90 degrees of flexion with the forearm in full supination.
3. The clinician is at the patient's side, facing the humeroradial joint.
4. The stabilizing hand supports the distal humerus.
5. The mobilizing/manipulating hand grips the patient's hand.

Procedure
1. The stabilizing hand holds the humerus in position.
2. The mobilizing/manipulating hand moves the shaft of the radius downward toward the humerus indirectly through the wrist (see Figure 4-7).

Particulars
- It is important to screen for wrist joint impairments before performing this technique.

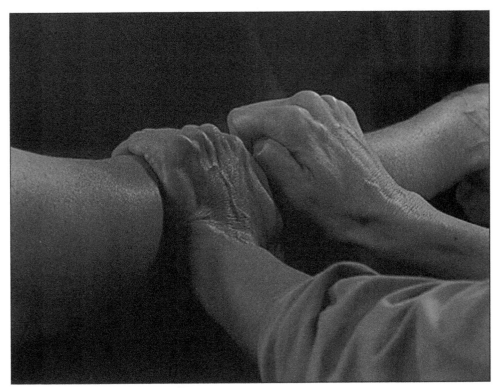

▶ **Figure 4-8** Posterior glide.

Posterior Glide (Figure 4-8, Video 4-8)

Purpose
- To examine for humeroradial joint impairment
- To increase accessory motion into humeroradial posterior glide
- To increase range of motion at the elbow joint
- To decrease pain

Positioning
1. The patient is supine with the shoulder medially rotated.
2. The humeroradial joint is positioned in the resting position if conservative techniques are indicated or approximating restricted range of motion if more aggressive techniques are indicated.
3. The clinician is at the patient's side, facing the humeroradial joint.
4. The stabilizing hand grips the distal humerus from the posterior side.
5. The mobilizing/manipulating hand grips the proximal radius from the anterior side.

Procedure
1. The clinician applies a grade I traction to the joint.
2. The stabilizing hand holds the humerus in position.
3. The mobilizing/manipulating hand glides the proximal radius in a posterior direction (see Figure 4-8).

Particulars
- The clinician should use caution in performing this technique because this motion might be hypermobile.
- This technique might be especially effective for increasing range of motion into elbow joint extension.

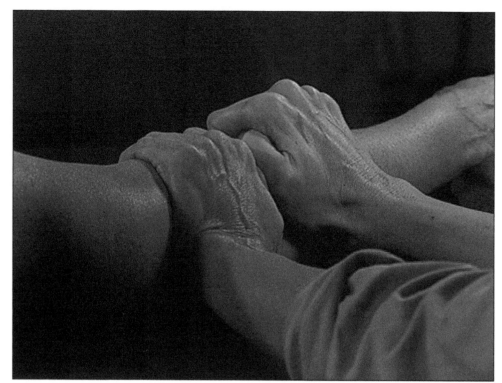

▶ **Figure 4-9** Anterior glide.

Anterior Glide (Figure 4-9, Video 4-9)

Purpose
- To examine for humeroradial joint impairment
- To increase accessory motion into humeroradial anterior glide
- To increase range of motion at the elbow joint
- To decrease pain

Positioning
1. The patient is supine with the shoulder medially rotated.
2. The humeroradial joint is positioned in the resting position if conservative techniques are indicated or approximating restricted range of motion if more aggressive techniques are indicated.
3. The clinician is at the patient's side, facing the humeroradial joint.
4. The stabilizing hand grips the distal humerus from the anterior side.
5. The mobilizing/manipulating hand grips the proximal radius from the posterior side.

Procedure
1. The clinician applies a grade I traction to the joint.
2. The stabilizing hand holds the humerus in position.
3. The mobilizing/manipulating hand glides the proximal radius in an anterior direction (see Figure 4-9).

Particulars
- The clinician should use caution in performing this technique because this motion might be hypermobile.
- This technique might be especially effective for increasing range of motion into elbow joint flexion.

PROXIMAL RADIOULNAR JOINT

Osteokinematic motion:
  Pronation/supination
Ligaments:
  Annular ligament
  Quadrate ligament
  Interosseous membrane
Joint orientation:
  Ulna: lateral, anterior
  Radius: medial, posterior
Concave joint surface:
  Ulna
Type of joint:
  Synovial
Resting position:
  70 degrees of flexion, 35 degrees of supination[2]
Close-packed position:
  Full supination or full pronation[2]
Capsular pattern of restriction:
  Pain at the end of the range of motion for pronation or supination or both[3]

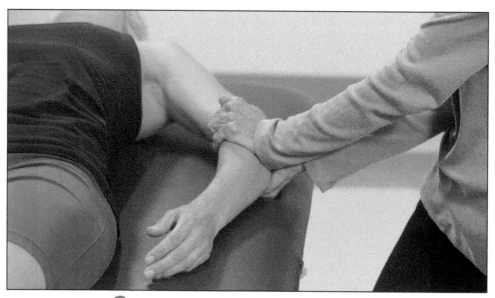

▶ **Figure 4-10** Posterior glide of the proximal radius.

Posterior Glide of the Proximal Radius (Figure 4-10, Video 4-10)

Purpose
- To examine for proximal radioulnar joint impairment
- To increase accessory motion into proximal radioulnar posterior glide
- To increase range of motion at the forearm
- To decrease pain

Positioning
1. The patient is sitting with the forearm resting on the treatment table.
2. The proximal radioulnar joint is positioned in the resting position if conservative techniques are indicated or approximating restricted range of motion if more aggressive techniques are indicated.
3. The clinician is at the patient's side, facing the proximal radioulnar joint.
4. The stabilizing hand grips the proximal ulna from the posterior surface.
5. The mobilizing/manipulating hand grips the radial head anteriorly.

Procedure
1. The stabilizing hand holds the ulna in position.
2. The mobilizing/manipulating hand glides the radial head in a posterior direction (see Figure 4-10).

Particulars
- This technique might be especially effective for increasing range of motion into forearm pronation.

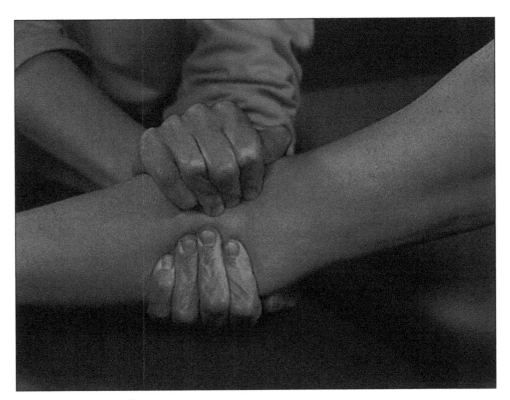

▶ **Figure 4-11** Anterior glide of the proximal radius.

Anterior Glide of the Proximal Radius (Figure 4-11, Video 4-11)

Purpose
- To examine for proximal radioulnar joint impairment
- To increase accessory motion into proximal radioulnar anterior glide
- To increase range of motion at the forearm
- To decrease pain

Positioning
1. The patient is sitting with the forearm resting on the treatment table.
2. The proximal radioulnar joint is positioned in the resting position if conservative techniques are indicated or approximating restricted range of motion if more aggressive techniques are indicated.
3. The clinician is at the patient's side, facing the proximal radioulnar joint.
4. The stabilizing hand grips the proximal ulna from the anterior surface.
5. The mobilizing/manipulating hand grips the radial head posteriorly.

Procedure
1. The stabilizing hand holds the ulna in position.
2. The mobilizing/manipulating hand glides the radial head in an anterior direction (see Figure 4-11).

Particulars
- This technique might be especially effective for increasing range of motion into forearm supination.

DISTAL RADIOULNAR JOINT

Osteokinematic motion:
  Pronation/supination
Ligaments:
  Anterior radioulnar ligament
  Posterior radioulnar ligament
  Interosseous membrane
Joint orientation:
  Ulna: lateral
  Radius: medial
Concave joint surface:
  Radius
Type of joint:
  Synovial
Resting position:
  10 degrees supination[2]
Close-packed position:
  Full supination or full pronation[2]
Capsular pattern of restriction:
  Pain at the end of the range of motion for pronation or supination or both[3]

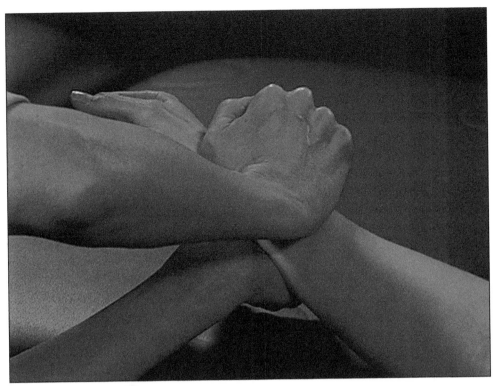

▶ **Figure 4-12** Posterior glide of the distal radius.

Posterior Glide of the Distal Radius (Figure 4-12, Video 4-12)

Purpose
- To examine for distal radioulnar joint impairment
- To increase accessory motion into distal radioulnar posterior glide
- To increase range of motion at the forearm
- To decrease pain

Positioning
1. The patient is sitting with the forearm resting on the treatment table.
2. The distal radioulnar joint is positioned in the resting position if conservative techniques are indicated or approximating restricted range of motion if more aggressive techniques are indicated.
3. The clinician is at the patient's side, facing the distal radioulnar joint.
4. The stabilizing hand grips the distal ulna from the posterior surface.
5. The mobilizing/manipulating hand grips the distal radius anteriorly.

Procedure
1. The stabilizing hand holds the ulna in position.
2. The mobilizing/manipulating hand glides the distal radius in a posterior direction (see Figure 4-12).

Particulars
- This technique might be especially effective for increasing range of motion into forearm supination.

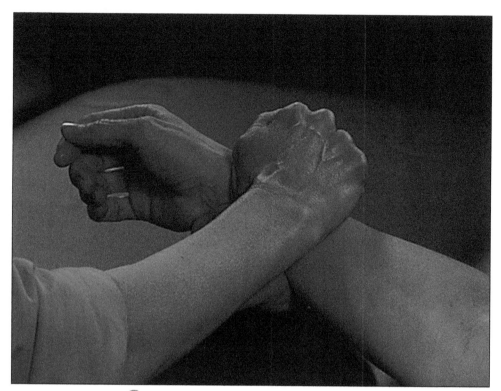

Figure 4-13 Anterior glide of the distal radius.

Anterior Glide of the Distal Radius (Figure 4-13, Video 4-13)
Purpose
- To examine for distal radioulnar joint impairment
- To increase accessory motion into distal radioulnar anterior glide
- To increase range of motion at the forearm
- To decrease pain

Positioning
1. The patient is sitting with the forearm resting on the treatment table.
2. The distal radioulnar joint is positioned in the resting position if conservative techniques are indicated or approximating restricted range of motion if more aggressive techniques are indicated.
3. The clinician is at the patient's side, facing the distal radioulnar joint.
4. The stabilizing hand grips the distal ulna from the anterior surface.
5. The mobilizing/manipulating hand grips the distal radius posteriorly.

Procedure
1. The stabilizing hand holds the ulna in position.
2. The mobilizing/manipulating hand glides the distal radius in an anterior direction (see Figure 4-13).

Particulars
- This technique might be especially effective for increasing range of motion into forearm pronation.

REFERENCES

1. Hoogvliet P, Randsdorp MS, Dingemanse R, Koes BW, Huisstede BMA. Does effectiveness of exercise therapy and mobilisation techniques offer guidance for the treatment of lateral and medial epicondylitis? A systematic review. *Br J Sports Med.* 2013;47:1112-1119.

2. Kaltenborn FM. *Manual Mobilization of the Joints: The Kaltenborn Method of Joint Examination and Treatment.* Vol 1. 6th ed. The Extremities. Oslo, Norway: Norli; 2002.

3. Cyriax J. *Textbook of Orthopaedic Medicine.* Vol 1. 8th ed. Diagnosis of Soft Tissue Lesions. London: Bailliere Tindall; 1982.

4. Vicenzino B, Paungmali A, Buratowski S, Wright A. Specific manipulative therapy treatment for chronic lateral epicondylalgia produces uniquely characteristic hypoalgesia. *Man Ther.* 2001;6:205-212.

5. Kochar M, Dogra A. Effectiveness of a specific physiotherapy regimen on patients with tennis elbow. *Physiotherapy.* 2002;88:333-341.

6. Bisset L, Beller E, Jull G, et al. Mobilisation with movement and exercise, corticosteroid injection, or wait and see for tennis elbow: randomized trial. *BMJ.* 2006; 333:939.

7. Heiser R, O'Brien VH, Schwartz DA. The use of joint mobilization to improve clinical outcomes in hand therapy: a systemic review of the literature. *J Hand Ther.* 2013;26:297-311.

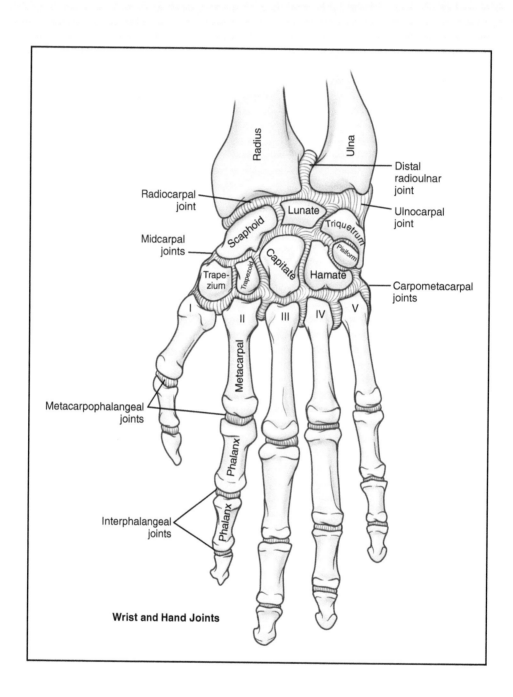

Radius

Ulna

Distal radioulnar joint

Radiocarpal joint

Ulnocarpal joint

Lunate

Triquetrum

Scaphoid

Pisiform

Midcarpal joints

Capitate

Hamate

Trapezium

Trapezoid

Carpometacarpal joints

I

II

III

IV

V

Metacarpal

Metacarpophalangeal joints

Phalanx

Phalanx

Interphalangeal joints

Wrist and Hand Joints

CHAPTER 5

The Wrist and Hand

BASICS

The wrist and hand comprise numerous small joints that are located in close proximity to one another. This proximity allows the individual to perform a wide variety of skilled activities.

Wrist Joint

The wrist comprises the radiocarpal and ulnocarpal joints, the triquetrum-pisiform articulation, and the midcarpal joints. Wrist range of motion is considered functional for most basic activities of daily living if 10 degrees of flexion and 35 degrees of extension are present because this amount of motion allows the wrist to position the hand for skilled activities.

Intermetacarpal Joints

The metacarpals are capable of gliding on one another, causing the arch of the hand to increase and decrease. The axis for this motion is the third metacarpal.

Thumb and Finger Joints

There is a relatively large amount of motion at the thumb and finger joints, allowing for a wide variety of functional hand movements. The amount of range of motion considered functional is highly task dependent.

Of all the joints in the human body, the trapeziometacarpal joint is considered the most important because it allows an individual to grasp objects. The trapezium is flexed, abducted, and medially rotated in relation to the other carpal bones; therefore, it does not lie in the same plane as the joints of the fingers. Flexion and extension therefore occur in a plane approximately parallel to the plane of the palm of the hand, and abduction and adduction in a plane approximately perpendicular to this plane. Opposition occurs at the trapeziometacarpal and metacarpophalangeal articulations, although most of this motion occurs at the trapeziometacarpal joint. Movement into opposition, a prerequisite for grasping motion, combines trapeziometacarpal flexion, abduction, and rotation. A fair amount of ligamentous laxity at the trapeziometacarpal joint must be present for functional opposition to occur.

SPECIFIC PATHOLOGY AND WRIST AND HAND JOINT MOBILIZATION/ MANIPULATION

Carpal Tunnel Syndrome

In a 2013 systematic review addressing the efficacy of wrist manipulation and multi-modal therapy for treatment of carpal tunnel syndrome, the investigators concluded that there is fair evidence to support this intervention strategy.[1]

Fracture of the Distal Radius

Three separate studies addressed the effectiveness of wrist joint mobilization in patients who were status post distal radial fracture. In all three studies, subjects demonstrated improvements in wrist range of motion compared with pretreatment measurements[2-4] and with a placebo treatment[4] for up to 6 weeks posttreatment. In two of these studies, function also improved,[2,3] as did pain,[2] compared with pretreatment measurements.

Decreased Metacarpophalangeal Joint Range of Motion

In a study of patients who had sustained a metacarpophalangeal fracture, subjects received either a home exercise program or a home exercise program with the addition of joint mobilization intervention to the metacarpophalangeal joint. The mobilization and exercise group experienced a significant increase in range of motion compared with the exercise-alone group.[5]

Lateral Epicondylalgia

In a 2013 systematic review addressing conservative interventions for patients with lateral epicondylalgia, the authors concluded that there is limited evidence to support the use of wrist manipulation to decrease pain at 6 weeks follow-up when compared with multi-modal interventions which included stretching and strengthening exercises, friction massage and ultrasound.[6]

RADIOCARPAL AND ULNOCARPAL JOINTS

Osteokinematic motions:
  Flexion/extension
  Radial/ulnar deviation
  Pronation/supination
Ligaments:
  Ulnar collateral ligament
  Radial collateral ligament
  Transverse carpal ligament
  Palmar radiocarpal ligaments
  Dorsal radiocarpal ligaments
  Intercarpal ligaments
Joint orientation:
  Radius and ulna: inferior, anterior, medial (in an ulnar direction)
  Carpals: superior, posterior, lateral (in a radial direction)
Concave joint surface:
  Radius and ulna
Type of joint:
  Synovial
Resting position:
  Slight flexion and ulnar deviation[7]
Close-packed position:
  Full extension[7]
Capsular pattern of restriction:
  Flexion and extension equally limited[8]

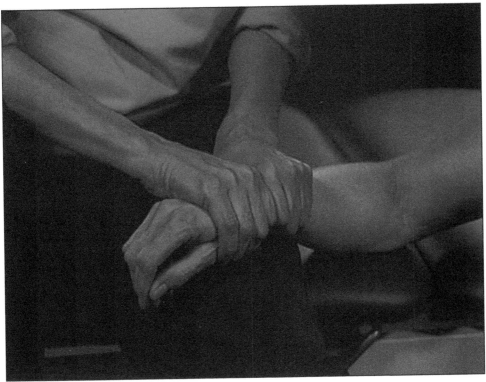

▶ **Figure 5-1** Distraction.

Distraction (Figure 5-1, Video 5-1)

Purpose

- To examine for radiocarpal and ulnocarpal joint impairment
- To increase accessory motion into radiocarpal and ulnocarpal joint distraction
- To increase range of motion at the wrist joint
- To decrease pain

Positioning

1. The patient is sitting with the anterior surface of the forearm on the treatment table and the hand off the table.
2. The radiocarpal and ulnocarpal joints are positioned in the resting position if conservative techniques are indicated or approximating restricted range of motion if more aggressive techniques are indicated.
3. The clinician is facing the radiocarpal and ulnocarpal joints.
4. The stabilizing hand grips the distal radius and ulna from the posterior side.
5. The mobilizing/manipulating hand grips the proximal row of carpals from the posterior side.

Procedure

1. The stabilizing hand holds the radius and ulna to the treatment table.
2. The mobilizing/manipulating hand moves the proximal row of carpals distally perpendicular to the radioulnar joint surface (see Figure 5-1).

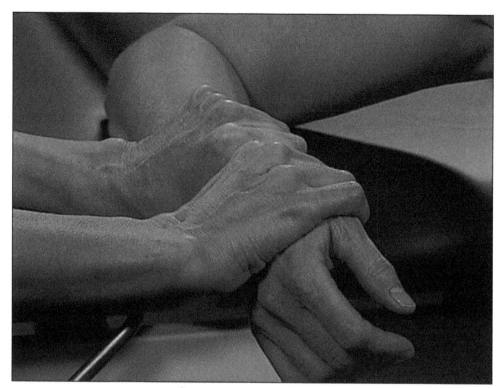

▶ **Figure 5-2** Posterior glide.

Posterior Glide (Figure 5-2, Video 5-2)

Purpose
- To examine for radiocarpal and ulnocarpal joint impairment
- To increase accessory motion into radiocarpal and ulnocarpal joint posterior glide
- To increase range of motion at the wrist joint
- To decrease pain

Positioning
1. The patient is sitting with the medial (ulnar) surface of the forearm on the treatment table and the hand off the table.
2. The radiocarpal and ulnocarpal joints are positioned in the resting position if conservative techniques are indicated or approximating restricted range of motion if more aggressive techniques are indicated.
3. The clinician is facing the radiocarpal and ulnocarpal joints.
4. The stabilizing hand grips the distal radius and ulna from the posterior side.
5. The mobilizing/manipulating hand grips the proximal row of carpals from the posterior side.

Procedure
1. The clinician applies a grade I traction to the joint.
2. The stabilizing hand holds the radius and ulna to the treatment table.
3. The mobilizing/manipulating hand glides the proximal row of carpals in a posterior direction (see Figure 5-2).

Particulars
- This technique might be especially effective for increasing range of motion into wrist joint flexion.

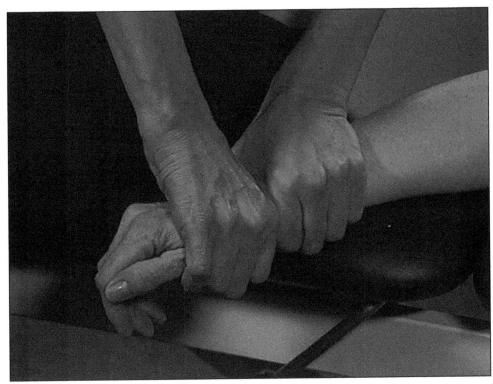

Figure 5-3 Anterior glide.

Anterior Glide (Figure 5-3, Video 5-3)

Purpose
- To examine for radiocarpal and ulnocarpal joint impairment
- To increase accessory motion into radiocarpal and ulnocarpal joint anterior glide
- To increase range of motion at the wrist joint
- To decrease pain

Positioning
1. The patient is sitting with the anterior surface of the forearm on the treatment table and the hand off the table.
2. The radiocarpal and ulnocarpal joints are positioned in the resting position if conservative techniques are indicated or approximating restricted range of motion if more aggressive techniques are indicated.
3. The clinician is facing the radiocarpal and ulnocarpal joints.
4. The stabilizing hand grips the distal radius and ulna from the posterior side.
5. The mobilizing/manipulating hand grips the proximal row of carpals from the posterior side.

Procedure
1. The clinician applies a grade I traction to the joint.
2. The stabilizing hand holds the radius and ulna to the treatment table.
3. The mobilizing/manipulating hand glides the proximal row of carpals in an anterior direction (see Figure 5-3).

Particulars
- This technique might be especially effective for increasing range of motion into wrist joint extension.

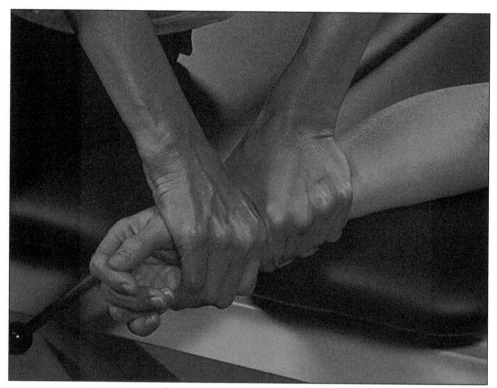

▶ **Figure 5-4** Medial (ulnar) glide.

Medial (Ulnar) Glide (Figure 5-4, Video 5-4)

Purpose
- To examine for radiocarpal and ulnocarpal joint impairment
- To increase accessory motion into radiocarpal and ulnocarpal joint medial (ulnar) glide
- To increase range of motion at the wrist joint
- To decrease pain

Positioning
1. The patient is sitting with the medial (ulnar) surface of the forearm on the treatment table and the hand off the table.
2. The radiocarpal and ulnocarpal joints are positioned in the resting position if conservative techniques are indicated or approximating restricted range of motion if more aggressive techniques are indicated.
3. The clinician is facing the radiocarpal and ulnocarpal joints.
4. The stabilizing hand grips the distal radius and ulna from the anterior side.
5. The mobilizing/manipulating hand grips the proximal row of carpals from the lateral (radial) side.

Procedure
1. The clinician applies a grade I traction to the joint.
2. The stabilizing hand holds the radius and ulna to the treatment table.
3. The mobilizing/manipulating hand glides the proximal row of carpals in a medial (ulnar) direction (see Figure 5-4).

Particulars
- This technique might be especially effective for increasing range of motion into wrist joint radial deviation.

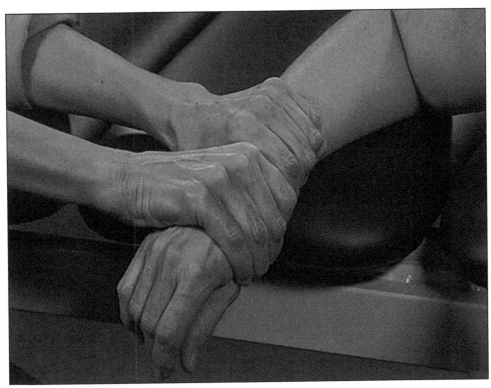

▶ **Figure 5-5** Lateral (radial) glide.

Lateral (Radial) Glide (Figure 5-5, Video 5-5)

Purpose
- To examine for radiocarpal and ulnocarpal joint impairment
- To increase accessory motion into radiocarpal and ulnocarpal joint lateral (radial) glide
- To increase range of motion at the wrist joint
- To decrease pain

Positioning
1. The patient is sitting with the anterior surface of the forearm on the treatment table and the hand off the table.
2. The radiocarpal and ulnocarpal joints are positioned in the resting position if conservative techniques are indicated or approximating restricted range of motion if more aggressive techniques are indicated.
3. The clinician is facing the radiocarpal and ulnocarpal joints.
4. The stabilizing hand grips the distal radius and ulna from the posterior side.
5. The mobilizing/manipulating hand grips the proximal row of carpals from the medial (ulnar) side.

Procedure
1. The clinician applies a grade I traction to the joint.
2. The stabilizing hand holds the radius and ulna to the treatment table.
3. The mobilizing/manipulating hand glides the proximal row of carpals in a lateral (radial) direction (see Figure 5-5).

Particulars
- This technique might be especially effective for increasing range of motion into wrist joint ulnar deviation.

Specific Radiocarpal and Ulnocarpal Joint Posterior Glides (Figure 5-6, Video 5-6)

Purpose
- To examine for radiocarpal and ulnocarpal joint impairment
- To increase accessory motion into radiocarpal and ulnocarpal joint posterior glide
- To increase range of motion at the wrist joint
- To decrease pain

Positioning
1. The patient is sitting with the anterior surface of the forearm on the treatment table and the hand off the table.
2. The radiocarpal and ulnocarpal joints are positioned in the resting position if conservative techniques are indicated or approximating restricted range of motion if more aggressive techniques are indicated.
3. The clinician is facing the radiocarpal and ulnocarpal joints.
4. The stabilizing hand grips the distal radius or ulna with the thumb on the posterior surface and the index finger on the anterior surface.
5. The mobilizing/manipulating hand grips the proximal row carpal bone with the thumb on the posterior surface and the index finger on the anterior surface.

Procedure
1. The stabilizing hand holds the radius or ulna in position.
2. The mobilizing/manipulating hand glides the scaphoid in a posterior direction on the radius, the lunate in a posterior direction on the radius, and the triquetrum in a posterior direction on the ulna (see Figure 5-6).

Particulars
- The clinician should use caution in performing these techniques because some of these motions might be hypermobile.
- These techniques might be especially effective for increasing range of motion into wrist joint flexion.

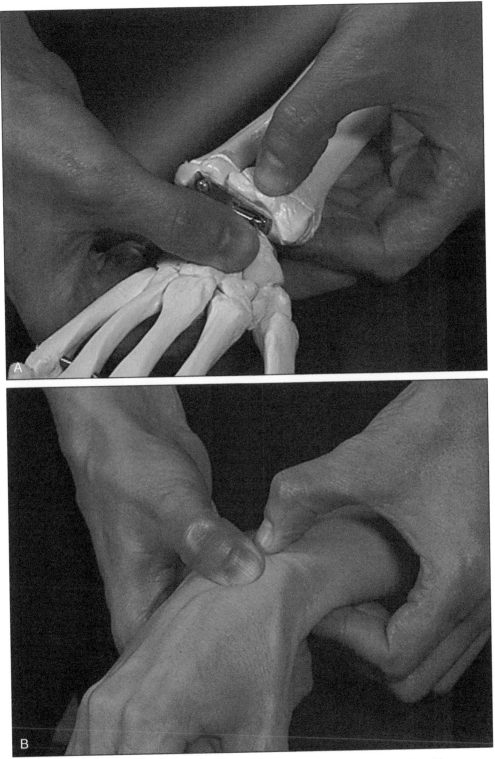

Figure 5-6 **A** and **B,** Specific radiocarpal and ulnocarpal joint posterior glides.

Specific Radiocarpal and Ulnocarpal Joint Anterior Glides (Figure 5-7, Video 5-7)

Purpose

- To examine for radiocarpal and ulnocarpal joint impairment
- To increase accessory motion into radiocarpal and ulnocarpal joint anterior glide
- To increase range of motion at the wrist joint
- To decrease pain

Positioning

1. The patient is sitting with the anterior surface of the forearm on the treatment table and the hand off the table.
2. The radiocarpal and ulnocarpal joints are positioned in the resting position if conservative techniques are indicated or approximating restricted range of motion if more aggressive techniques are indicated.
3. The clinician is facing the radiocarpal and ulnocarpal joints.
4. The stabilizing hand grips the distal radius or ulna with the thumb on the posterior surface and the index finger on the anterior surface.
5. The mobilizing/manipulating hand grips the proximal row carpal bone with the thumb on the posterior surface and the index finger on the anterior surface.

Procedure

1. The stabilizing hand holds the radius or ulna in position.
2. The mobilizing/manipulating hand glides the scaphoid in an anterior direction on the radius, the lunate in an anterior direction on the radius, and the triquetrum in an anterior direction on the ulna (see Figure 5-7).

Particulars

- The clinician should use caution in performing these techniques because some of these motions might be hypermobile.
- Gliding the lunate on the radius commonly is performed using a grade V manipulation and can be performed with both of the clinician's thumbs on the lunate.
- The radiolunate technique might be effective in correcting a radiolunate joint positional fault.
- These techniques might be especially effective for increasing range of motion into wrist joint extension.

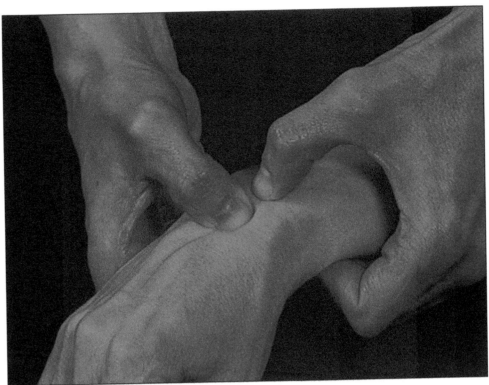

▶ **Figure 5-7** Specific radiocarpal and ulnocarpal joint anterior glides.

Specific Proximal Row Carpal Joint Posterior Glides (Figure 5-8, Video 5-8)

Purpose

- To examine for proximal row carpal joint impairment
- To increase accessory motion into proximal row carpal joint posterior glide
- To increase range of motion at the wrist joint
- To decrease pain

Positioning

1. The patient is sitting with the anterior surface of the forearm on the treatment table and the hand off the table.
2. The radiocarpal and ulnocarpal joints are positioned in the resting position if conservative techniques are indicated or approximating restricted range of motion if more aggressive techniques are indicated.
3. The clinician is facing the proximal row of carpal joints.
4. The stabilizing hand grips the one carpal bone with the thumb on the posterior surface and the index finger on the anterior surface.
5. The mobilizing/manipulating hand grips the other carpal bone with the thumb on the posterior surface and the index finger on the anterior surface.

Procedure

1. The stabilizing hand holds the one carpal bone in position.
2. The mobilizing/manipulating hand glides the scaphoid in a posterior direction on the lunate and the triquetrum in a posterior direction on the lunate (see Figure 5-8).

Particulars

- The clinician should use caution in performing these techniques because these motions might be hypermobile.

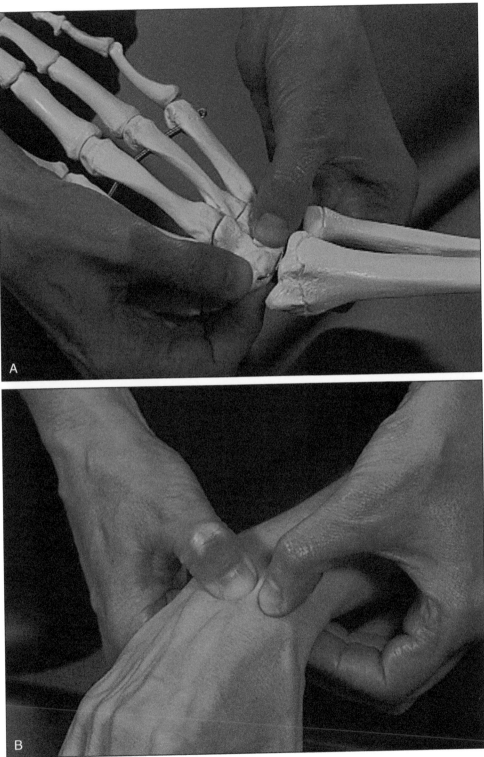

Figure 5-8 **A** and **B,** Specific proximal row carpal joint posterior glides.

Specific Proximal Row Carpal Joint Anterior Glides (Figure 5-9, Video 5-9)

Purpose

- To examine for proximal row carpal joint impairment
- To increase accessory motion into proximal row carpal joint anterior glide
- To increase range of motion at the wrist joint
- To decrease pain

Positioning

1. The patient is sitting with the anterior surface of the forearm on the treatment table and the hand off the table.
2. The radiocarpal and ulnocarpal joints are positioned in the resting position if conservative techniques are indicated or approximating restricted range of motion if more aggressive techniques are indicated.
3. The clinician is facing the proximal row of carpal joints.
4. The stabilizing hand grips the one carpal bone with the thumb on the posterior surface and the index finger on the anterior surface.
5. The mobilizing/manipulating hand grips the other carpal bone with the thumb on the posterior surface and the index finger on the anterior surface.

Procedure

1. The stabilizing hand holds the one carpal bone in position.
2. The mobilizing/manipulating hand glides the scaphoid in an anterior direction on the lunate and the triquetrum in an anterior direction on the lunate (see Figure 5-9).

Particulars

- The clinician should use caution in performing these techniques because these motions might be hypermobile.

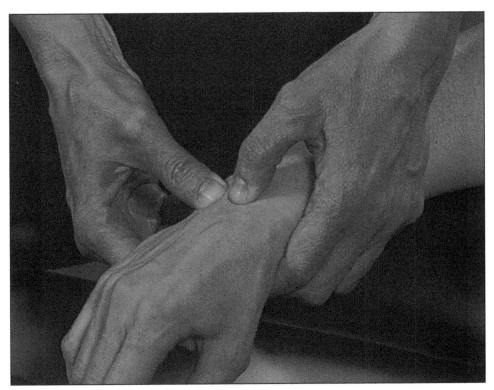

▶ **Figure 5-9** Specific proximal row carpal joint anterior glides.

Specific Triquetrum-Pisiform Joint Lateral (Radial) and Medial (Ulnar) Glides (Figure 5-10, Video 5-10)

Purpose

- To examine for triquetrum-pisiform joint impairment
- To increase accessory motion into triquetrum-pisiform lateral (radial) and medial (ulnar) glide
- To decrease pain

Positioning

1. The patient is sitting with the posterior surface of the forearm, wrist, and hand on the treatment table.
2. The radiocarpal and ulnocarpal joints are positioned in the resting position if conservative techniques are indicated or approximating restricted range of motion if more aggressive techniques are indicated.
3. The clinician is facing the pisiform.
4. The stabilizing hand grips the lateral (radial) and medial (ulnar) surfaces of the wrist with the thumb and index finger.
5. The mobilizing/manipulating hand grips the lateral (radial) and medial (ulnar) surfaces of the pisiform with the thumb and index finger.

Procedure

1. The stabilizing hand holds the scaphoid, lunate, and triquetrum in position.
2. The mobilizing/manipulating hand glides the pisiform in a lateral (radial) direction on the triquetrum and the pisiform in a medial (ulnar) direction on the triquetrum (see Figure 5-10).

Particulars

- The clinician should use caution in performing this technique because this motion might be hypermobile (especially if the patient is a clinician who frequently performs spinal mobilization/manipulation techniques with the pisiform).

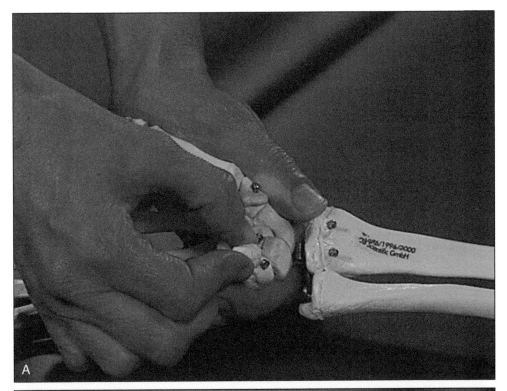

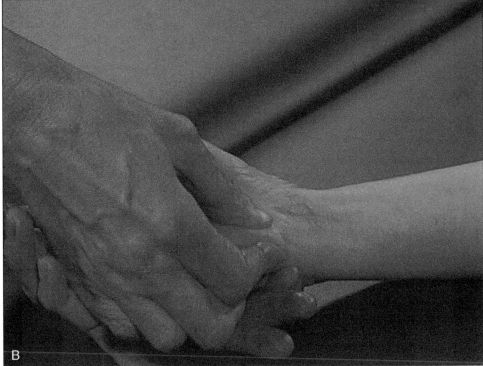

Figure 5-10 **A** and **B,** Specific triquetrum-pisiform joint lateral (radial) and medial (ulnar) glides.

MIDCARPAL JOINTS

Osteokinematic motions:
    Flexion/extension
    Radial/ulnar deviation
Ligaments:
    Radial collateral ligament
    Dorsal radiocarpal ligament
    Volar radiocarpal ligament
    Intercarpal ligament
Joint orientation:
    Proximal row: inferior
    Distal row: superior
Concave joint surface:
    Varies, depending on the specific joint
Type of joint:
    Synovial
Resting position:
    Slight flexion and ulnar deviation[7]
Close-packed position:
    Full extension[7]
Capsular pattern of restriction:
    Flexion and extension are equally limited[8]

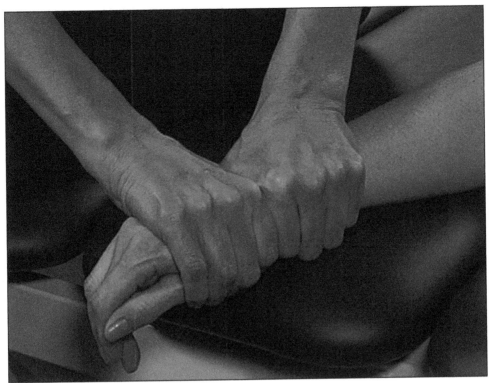

▶ **Figure 5-11** Distraction.

Distraction (Figure 5-11, Video 5-11)

Purpose

- To examine for midcarpal joint impairment
- To increase accessory motion into midcarpal joint distraction
- To increase range of motion at the wrist joint
- To decrease pain

Positioning

1. The patient is sitting with the anterior surface of the forearm on the treatment table and the hand off the table.
2. The midcarpal joints are positioned in the resting position if conservative techniques are indicated or approximating restricted range of motion if more aggressive techniques are indicated.
3. The clinician is facing the midcarpal joints.
4. The stabilizing hand grips the proximal row of carpals from the posterior side.
5. The mobilizing/manipulating hand grips the distal row of carpals from the posterior side.

Procedure

1. The stabilizing hand holds the proximal row of carpals to the treatment table.
2. The mobilizing/manipulating hand moves the distal row of carpals distally perpendicular to the proximal carpal row joint surface (see Figure 5-11).

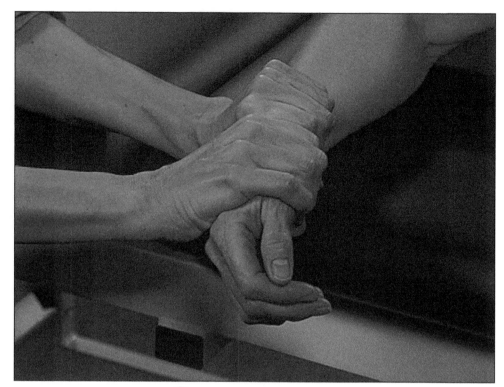

▶ **Figure 5-12** Posterior glide.

Posterior Glide (Figure 5-12, Video 5-12)

Purpose
- To examine for midcarpal joint impairment
- To increase accessory motion into midcarpal joint posterior glide
- To increase range of motion at the wrist joint
- To decrease pain

Positioning
1. The patient is sitting with the medial (ulnar) surface of the forearm on the treatment table and the hand off the table.
2. The midcarpal joints are positioned in the resting position if conservative techniques are indicated or approximating the restricted range of motion if more aggressive techniques are indicated.
3. The clinician is facing the midcarpal joints.
4. The stabilizing hand grips the proximal row of carpals from the posterior side.
5. The mobilizing/manipulating hand grips the distal row of carpals from the posterior side.

Procedure
1. The clinician applies a grade I traction to the joint.
2. The stabilizing hand holds the proximal row of carpals to the treatment table.
3. The mobilizing/manipulating hand glides the distal row of carpals in a posterior direction (see Figure 5-12).

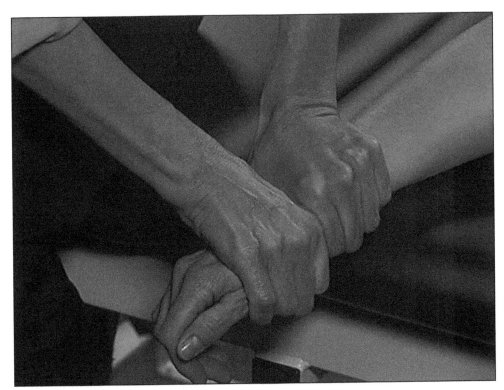

▶ **Figure 5-13** Anterior glide.

Anterior Glide (Figure 5-13, Video 5-13)

Purpose
- To examine for midcarpal joint impairment
- To increase accessory motion into midcarpal joint anterior glide
- To increase range of motion at the wrist joint
- To decrease pain

Positioning
1. The patient is sitting with the anterior surface of the forearm on the treatment table and the hand off the table.
2. The midcarpal joints are positioned in the resting position if conservative techniques are indicated or approximating restricted range of motion if more aggressive techniques are indicated.
3. The clinician is facing the midcarpal joints.
4. The stabilizing hand grips the proximal row of carpals from the posterior side.
5. The mobilizing/manipulating hand grips the distal row of carpals from the posterior side.

Procedure
1. The clinician applies a grade I traction to the joint.
2. The stabilizing hand holds the proximal row of carpals to the treatment table.
3. The mobilizing/manipulating hand glides the distal row of carpals in an anterior direction (see Figure 5-13).

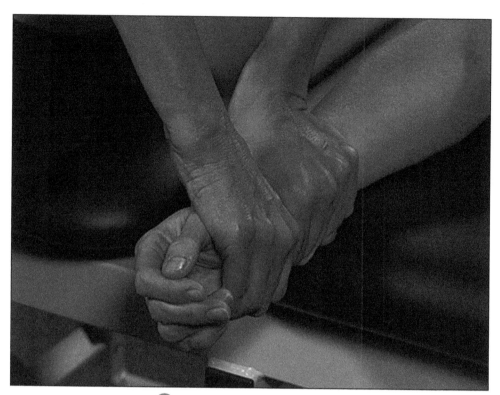

▶ **Figure 5-14** Medial (ulnar) glide.

Medial (Ulnar) Glide (Figure 5-14, Video 5-14)
Purpose
- To examine for midcarpal joint impairment
- To increase accessory motion into midcarpal joint medial (ulnar) glide
- To increase range of motion at the wrist joint
- To decrease pain

Positioning
1. The patient is sitting with the medial (ulnar) surface of the forearm on the treatment table and the hand off the table.
2. The midcarpal joints are positioned in the resting position if conservative techniques are indicated or approximating restricted range of motion if more aggressive techniques are indicated.
3. The clinician is facing the midcarpal joints.
4. The stabilizing hand grips the proximal row of carpals from the anterior side.
5. The mobilizing/manipulating hand grips the distal row of carpals from the lateral (radial) side.

Procedure
1. The clinician applies a grade I traction to the joint.
2. The stabilizing hand holds the proximal row of carpals to the treatment table.
3. The mobilizing/manipulating hand glides the distal row of carpals in a medial (ulnar) direction (see Figure 5-14).

Particulars
- This technique might be especially effective for increasing range of motion into wrist joint radial deviation.

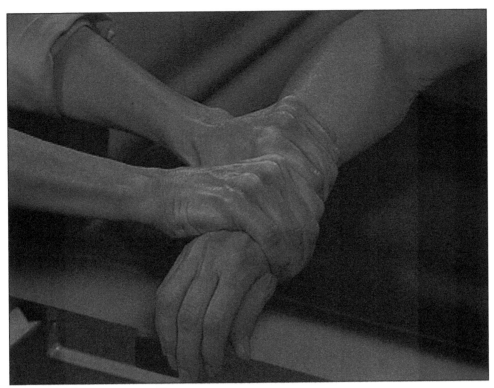

Figure 5-15 Lateral (radial) glide.

Lateral (Radial) Glide (Figure 5-15, Video 5-15)

Purpose
- To examine for midcarpal joint impairment
- To increase accessory motion into midcarpal joint lateral (radial) glide
- To increase range of motion at the wrist joint
- To decrease pain

Positioning
1. The patient is sitting with the anterior surface of the forearm on the treatment table and the hand off the table.
2. The midcarpal joints are positioned in the resting position if conservative techniques are indicated or approximating restricted range of motion if more aggressive techniques are indicated.
3. The clinician is facing the midcarpal joints.
4. The stabilizing hand grips the proximal row of carpals from the posterior side.
5. The mobilizing/manipulating hand grips the distal row of carpals from the medial (ulnar) side.

Procedure
1. The clinician applies a grade I traction to the joint.
2. The stabilizing hand holds the proximal row of carpals to the treatment table.
3. The mobilizing/manipulating hand glides the distal row of carpals in a lateral (radial) direction (see Figure 5-15).

Particulars
- This technique might be especially effective for increasing range of motion into wrist joint ulnar deviation.

Specific Midcarpal Joint Posterior Glide Mobilizations/Manipulations (Figure 5-16, Video 5-16)

Purpose

- To examine for midcarpal joint impairment
- To increase accessory motion into midcarpal joint posterior glide
- To increase range of motion at the wrist joint
- To decrease pain

Positioning

1. The patient is sitting with the anterior surface of the forearm on the treatment table and the hand off the table.
2. The midcarpal joints are positioned in the resting position if conservative techniques are indicated or approximating restricted range of motion if more aggressive techniques are indicated.
3. The clinician is facing the midcarpal joints.
4. The stabilizing hand grips the proximal row carpal bone with the thumb on the posterior surface and the index finger on the anterior surface.
5. The mobilizing/manipulating hand grips the distal row carpal bone with the thumb on the posterior surface and the index finger on the anterior surface.

Procedure

1. The stabilizing hand holds the proximal row carpal bone in position.
2. The mobilizing/manipulating hand glides the trapezium and trapezoid in a posterior direction on the scaphoid, the capitate in a posterior direction on the lunate, and the hamate in a posterior direction on the triquetrum (see Figure 5-16).

Particulars

- The clinician should use caution in performing these techniques because these motions might be hypermobile.

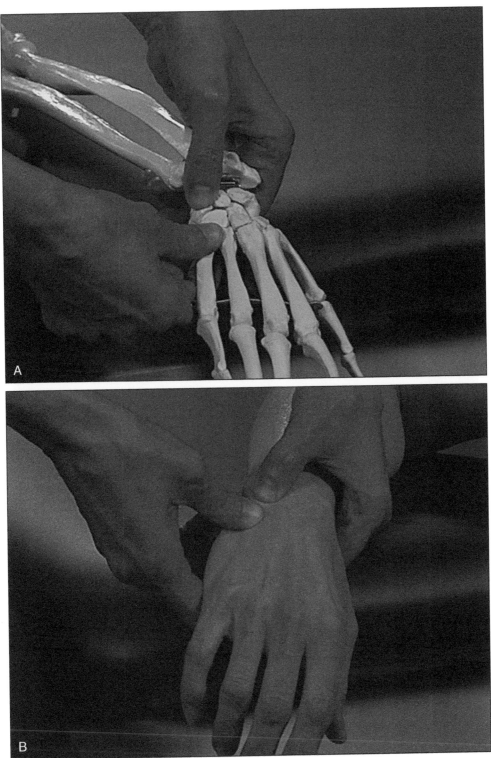

Figure 5-16 **A** and **B,** Specific midcarpal joint posterior glide mobilizations/manipulations.

Specific Midcarpal Joint Anterior Glide Mobilizations/Manipulations (Figure 5-17, Video 5-17)

Purpose

- To examine for midcarpal joint impairment
- To increase accessory motion into midcarpal joint anterior glide
- To increase range of motion at the wrist joint
- To decrease pain

Positioning

1. The patient is sitting with the anterior surface of the forearm on the treatment table and the hand off the table.
2. The midcarpal joints are positioned in the resting position if conservative techniques are indicated or approximating restricted range of motion if more aggressive techniques are indicated.
3. The clinician is facing the midcarpal joints.
4. The stabilizing hand grips the proximal row carpal bone with the thumb on the posterior surface and the index finger on the anterior surface.
5. The mobilizing/manipulating hand grips the distal row carpal bone with the thumb on the posterior surface and the index finger on the anterior surface.

Procedure

1. The stabilizing hand holds the proximal row carpal bone in position.
2. The mobilizing/manipulating hand glides the trapezium and trapezoid in an anterior direction on the scaphoid, the capitate in an anterior direction on the lunate, and the hamate in an anterior direction on the triquetrum (see Figure 5-17).

Particulars

- The clinician should use caution in performing these techniques because these motions might be hypermobile.
- Gliding the capitate on the lunate commonly is performed using a grade V manipulation.
- The lunate-capitate technique might be effective in correcting a lunate-capitate joint positional fault.

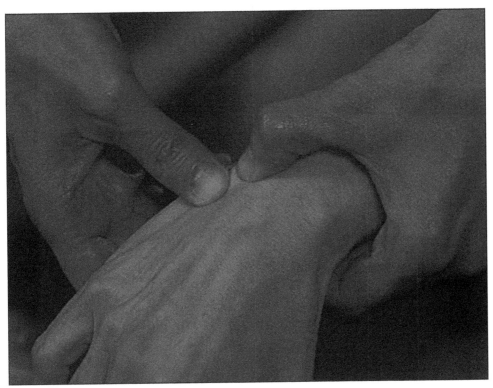

Figure 5-17 Specific midcarpal joint anterior glide mobilizations/manipulations.

Specific Distal Row Carpal Joint Posterior Glide Mobilizations/Manipulations
(Figure 5-18, Video 5-18)

Purpose
- To examine for distal row carpal joint impairment
- To increase accessory motion into distal row carpal joint posterior glide
- To increase range of motion at the wrist joint
- To decrease pain

Positioning
1. The patient is sitting with the anterior surface of the forearm on the treatment table and the hand off the table.
2. The midcarpal joints are positioned in the resting position if conservative techniques are indicated or approximating restricted range of motion if more aggressive techniques are indicated.
3. The clinician is facing the distal row of carpal joints.
4. The stabilizing hand grips the one carpal bone with the thumb on the posterior surface and the index finger on the anterior surface.
5. The mobilizing/manipulating hand grips the other carpal bone with the thumb on the posterior surface and the index finger on the anterior surface.

Procedure
1. The stabilizing hand holds the one carpal bone in position.
2. The mobilizing/manipulating hand glides the trapezoid in a posterior direction on the capitate and the hamate in a posterior direction on the capitate (see Figure 5-18).

Particulars
- The clinician should use caution in performing these techniques because these motions might be hypermobile.

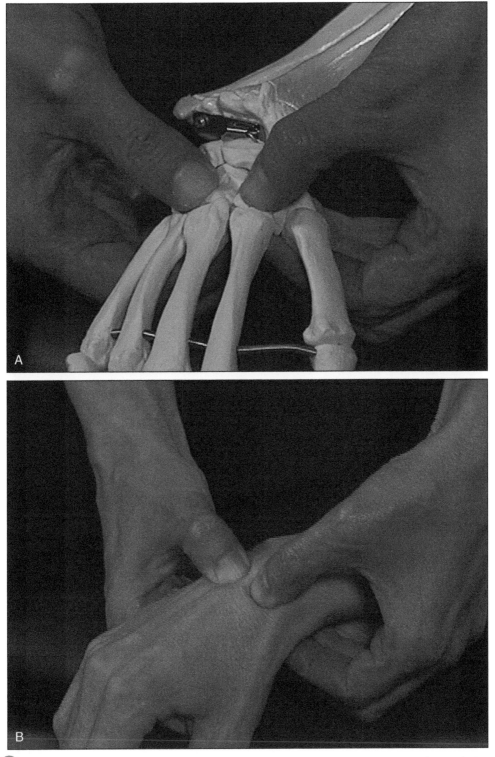

Figure 5-18 **A** and **B,** Specific distal row carpal joint posterior glide mobilizations/manipulations.

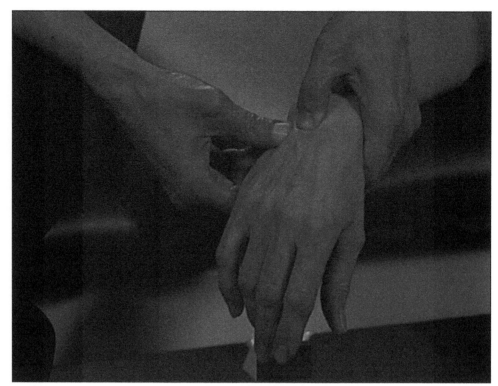

▶ **Figure 5-19** Specific distal row carpal joint anterior glide mobilizations/manipulations.

Specific Distal Row Carpal Joint Anterior Glide Mobilizations/Manipulations (Figure 5-19, Video 5-19)
Purpose
- To examine for distal row carpal joint impairment
- To increase accessory motion into distal row carpal joint anterior glide
- To increase range of motion at the wrist joint
- To decrease pain

Positioning
1. The patient is sitting with the anterior surface of the forearm on the treatment table and the hand off the table.
2. The midcarpal joints are positioned in the resting position if conservative techniques are indicated or approximating restricted range of motion if more aggressive techniques are indicated.
3. The clinician is facing the distal row of carpal joints.
4. The stabilizing hand grips the one carpal bone with the thumb on the posterior surface and the index finger on the anterior surface.
5. The mobilizing/manipulating hand grips the other carpal bone with the thumb on the posterior surface and the index finger on the anterior surface.

Procedure
1. The stabilizing hand holds the one carpal bone in position.
2. The mobilizing/manipulating hand glides the trapezoid in an anterior direction on the capitate and the hamate in an anterior direction on the capitate (see Figure 5-19).

Particulars
- The clinician should use caution in performing these techniques because these motions might be hypermobile.

TRAPEZIOMETACARPAL JOINT

Osteokinematic motions:
   Flexion/extension
   Abduction/adduction
   Medial/lateral rotation
Ligament:
   Capsular ligament
Joint orientation:
   Trapezium: inferior, anterior, lateral
   Metacarpal: superior, posterior, medial
   *Note that the trapezium and first metacarpal are rotated approximately 90 degrees in relation to the palm of the
      hand.
Concave joint surface:
   Trapezium concave posterior to anterior
   First metacarpal concave lateral (radial) to medial (ulnar)
Type of joint:
   Synovial
Resting position:
   Midway between flexion and extension and abduction and adduction[7]
Close-packed position:
   Full opposition[7]
Capsular pattern of restriction:
   Limitation in abduction and extension and no limitation in flexion[8]

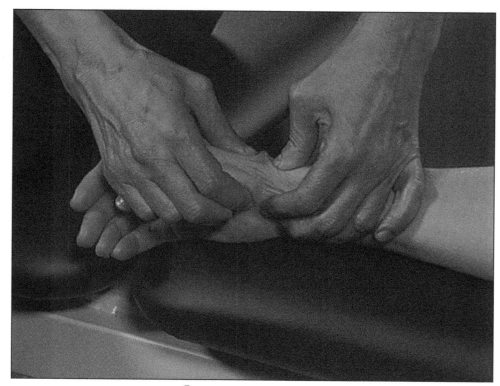

Figure 5-20 Distraction.

Distraction (Figure 5-20, Video 5-20)

Purpose

- To examine for trapeziometacarpal joint impairment
- To increase accessory motion into trapeziometacarpal joint distraction
- To increase range of motion at the trapeziometacarpal joint
- To decrease pain

Positioning

1. The patient is sitting with the medial (ulnar) surface of the forearm on the treatment table.
2. The trapeziometacarpal joint is positioned in the resting position if conservative techniques are indicated or approximating restricted range of motion if more aggressive techniques are indicated.
3. The clinician is facing the trapeziometacarpal joint.
4. The stabilizing hand grips the trapezium with the thumb on the lateral (radial) surface and the index finger on the medial (ulnar) surface.
5. The mobilizing/manipulating hand grips the proximal metacarpal with the thumb on the lateral (radial) surface (the back of the thumb) and the index finger on the medial (ulnar) surface (the front of the thumb).

Procedure

1. The stabilizing hand holds the trapezium in position.
2. The mobilizing/manipulating hand moves the metacarpal distally perpendicular to the trapezium and metacarpal joint surfaces (see Figure 5-20).

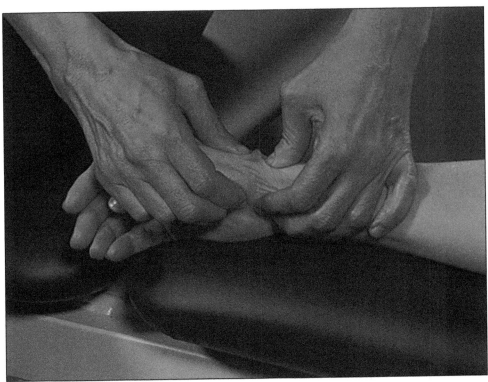

▶ **Figure 5-21** Posterior glide.

Posterior Glide (Figure 5-21, Video 5-21)

Purpose
- To examine for trapeziometacarpal joint impairment
- To increase accessory motion into trapeziometacarpal joint posterior glide
- To increase range of motion at the trapeziometacarpal joint
- To decrease pain

Positioning
1. The patient is sitting with the medial (ulnar) surface of the forearm on the treatment table.
2. The trapeziometacarpal joint is positioned in the resting position if conservative techniques are indicated or approximating restricted range of motion if more aggressive techniques are indicated.
3. The clinician is facing the trapeziometacarpal joint.
4. The stabilizing hand grips the trapezium, with the thumb as close to the posterior surface (the back of the hand) and the index finger as close to the anterior surface (the palm of the hand) as possible.
5. The mobilizing/manipulating hand grips the proximal metacarpal with the thumb and index fingers on the posterior and anterior surfaces (sides) of the metacarpal.

Procedure
1. The clinician applies a grade I traction to the joint.
2. The stabilizing hand holds the trapezium in position.
3. The mobilizing/manipulating hand glides the metacarpal in a posterior direction (toward the back of the hand) (see Figure 5-21).

Particulars
- This technique might be especially effective for increasing range of motion into trapeziometacarpal joint abduction.
- This technique, when combined with an anterior glide mobilization technique, exercise, and neural mobilization, was shown to decrease pain in patients with carpometacarpal joint osteoarthritis at 1- and 2-month follow-up compared with a sham-treatment group.[9]

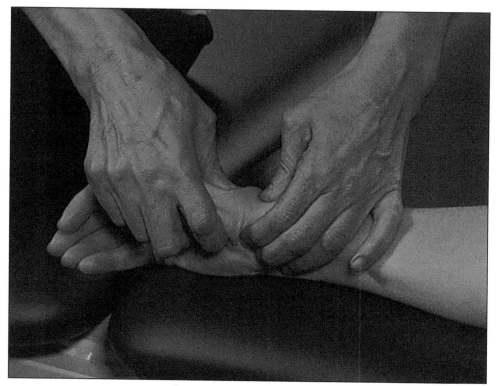

▶ Figure 5-22 Anterior glide.

Anterior Glide (Figure 5-22, Video 5-22)
Purpose
- To examine for trapeziometacarpal joint impairment
- To increase accessory motion into trapeziometacarpal joint anterior glide
- To increase range of motion at the trapeziometacarpal joint
- To decrease pain

Positioning
1. The patient is sitting with the medial (ulnar) surface of the forearm on the treatment table.
2. The trapeziometacarpal joint is positioned in the resting position if conservative techniques are indicated or approximating restricted range of motion if more aggressive techniques are indicated.
3. The clinician is facing the trapeziometacarpal joint.
4. The stabilizing hand grips the trapezium with the thumb as close to the posterior surface (the back of the hand) and the index finger as close to the anterior surface (the palm of the hand) as possible.
5. The mobilizing/manipulating hand grips the proximal metacarpal with the thumb and index fingers on the posterior and anterior surfaces (sides) of the metacarpal.

Procedure
1. The clinician applies a grade I traction to the joint.
2. The stabilizing hand holds the trapezium in position.
3. The mobilizing/manipulating hand glides the metacarpal in an anterior direction (toward the palm of the hand) (see Figure 5-22).

Particulars
- This technique might be especially effective for increasing range of motion into trapeziometacarpal joint adduction.
- This technique, when combined with a posterior glide mobilization technique, exercise, and neural mobilization, was shown to decrease pain in patients with carpometacarpal joint osteoarthritis at 1- and 2-month follow-up compared with a sham-treatment group.[9]

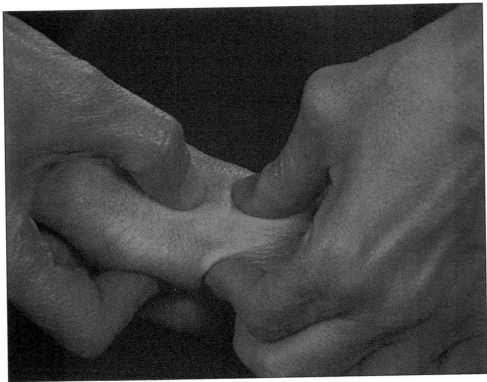

Figure 5-23 Medial (ulnar) glide.

Medial (Ulnar) Glide (Figure 5-23, Video 5-23)

Purpose
- To examine for trapeziometacarpal joint impairment
- To increase accessory motion into trapeziometacarpal joint medial (ulnar) glide
- To increase range of motion at the trapeziometacarpal joint
- To decrease pain

Positioning
1. The patient is sitting with the medial (ulnar) surface of the forearm on the treatment table.
2. The trapeziometacarpal joint is positioned in the resting position if conservative techniques are indicated or approximating restricted range of motion if more aggressive techniques are indicated.
3. The clinician is facing the trapeziometacarpal joint.
4. The stabilizing hand grips the trapezium with the thumb on the lateral (radial) surface and the index finger on the medial (ulnar) surface.
5. The mobilizing/manipulating hand grips the proximal metacarpal with the thumb on the lateral (radial) surface (the back of the thumb) and the index finger on the medial (ulnar) surface (the front of the thumb).

Procedure
1. The clinician applies a grade I traction to the joint.
2. The stabilizing hand holds the trapezium in position.
3. The mobilizing/manipulating hand glides the metacarpal in a medial (ulnar) direction (toward the front of the metacarpal) (see Figure 5-23).

Particulars
- This technique might be especially effective for increasing range of motion into trapeziometacarpal joint flexion.

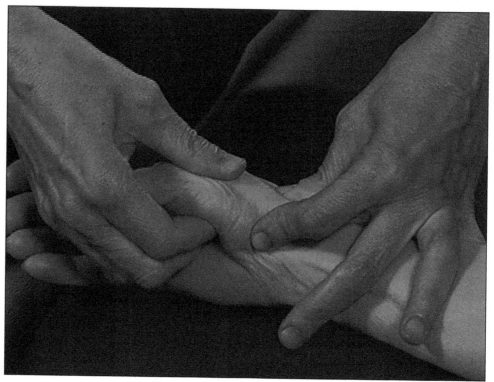

▶ **Figure 5-24** Lateral (radial) glide.

Lateral (Radial) Glide (Figure 5-24, Video 5-24)

Purpose
- To examine for trapeziometacarpal joint impairment
- To increase accessory motion into trapeziometacarpal joint lateral (radial) glide
- To increase range of motion at the trapeziometacarpal joint
- To decrease pain

Positioning
1. The patient is sitting with the medial (ulnar) surface of the forearm on the treatment table.
2. The trapeziometacarpal joint is positioned in the resting position if conservative techniques are indicated or approximating restricted range of motion if more aggressive techniques are indicated.
3. The clinician is facing the trapeziometacarpal joint.
4. The stabilizing hand grips the trapezium with the thumb on the lateral (radial) surface and the index finger on the medial (ulnar) surface.
5. The mobilizing/manipulating hand grips the proximal metacarpal with the thumb on the lateral (radial) surface (the back of the thumb) and the index finger on the medial (ulnar) surface (the front of the thumb).

Procedure
1. The clinician applies a grade I traction to the joint.
2. The stabilizing hand holds the trapezium in position.
3. The mobilizing/manipulating hand glides the metacarpal in a lateral (radial) direction (toward the back of the metacarpal) (see Figure 5-24).

Particulars
- This technique might be especially effective for increasing range of motion into trapeziometacarpal joint extension.

INTERMETACARPAL JOINTS TWO THROUGH FIVE

Osteokinematic motion:
>   Increasing/decreasing the arch of the hand

Ligaments:
>   Palmar interosseous ligament
>   Dorsal interosseous ligament

Joint orientation:
>   Medial metacarpal: lateral
>   Lateral metacarpal: medial

Concave joint surface:
>   None; these are plane joints

Type of joint:
>   Synarthrosis

Resting position:
>   Unknown[7]

Close-packed position:
>   Unknown[7]

Capsular pattern of restriction:
>   None, not a synovial joint

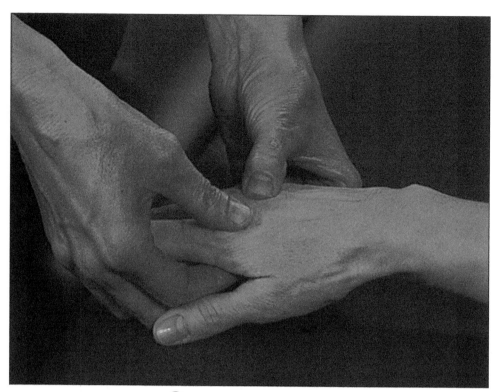

▶ **Figure 5-25** Posterior glide.

Posterior Glide (Figure 5-25, Video 5-25)
Purpose
- To examine for intermetacarpal joint impairment
- To increase accessory motion into intermetacarpal posterior glide, using the third metacarpal as a reference point
- To increase range of motion at the palm of the hand
- To decrease pain

Positioning
1. The patient is sitting with the palm down.
2. The hand is in a relaxed position.
3. The clinician is facing the intermetacarpal joints.
4. The stabilizing hand grips the midshaft of one metacarpal with the thumb on the posterior surface and the index finger on the anterior surface.
5. The mobilizing/manipulating hand grips the midshaft of the other metacarpal with the thumb on the posterior surface and the index finger on the anterior surface.

Procedure
1. The clinician applies a grade I traction to the joint.
2. The stabilizing hand holds one metacarpal in position.
3. The mobilizing/manipulating hand glides the second metacarpal in a posterior direction on the third metacarpal, the fourth metacarpal in a posterior direction on the third metacarpal, and the fifth metacarpal in a posterior direction on the fourth metacarpal (see Figure 5-25).

Particulars
- This technique might be especially effective for increasing range of motion into decreasing the arch of the hand.

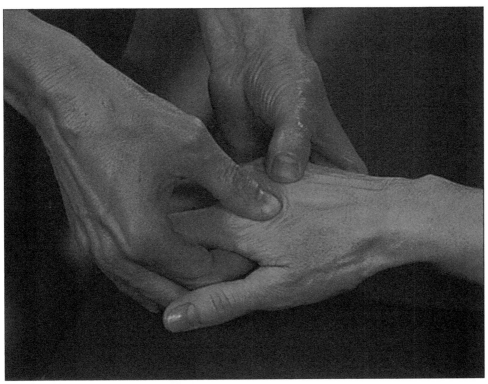

▶ **Figure 5-26** Anterior glide.

Anterior Glide (Figure 5-26, Video 5-26)

Purpose
- To examine for intermetacarpal joint impairment
- To increase accessory motion into intermetacarpal anterior glide, using the third metacarpal as a reference point
- To increase range of motion at the palm of the hand
- To decrease pain

Positioning
1. The patient is sitting with the palm down.
2. The hand is in a relaxed position.
3. The clinician is facing the intermetacarpal joints.
4. The stabilizing hand grips the midshaft of the one metacarpal with the thumb on the posterior surface and the index finger on the anterior surface.
5. The mobilizing/manipulating hand grips the midshaft of the other metacarpal with the thumb on the posterior surface and the index finger on the anterior surface.

Procedure
1. The clinician applies a grade I traction to the joint.
2. The stabilizing hand holds one metacarpal in position.
3. The mobilizing/manipulating hand glides the second metacarpal in an anterior direction on the third metacarpal, the fourth metacarpal in an anterior direction on the third metacarpal, and the fifth metacarpal in an anterior direction on the fourth metacarpal (see Figure 5-26).

Particulars
- This technique might be especially effective for increasing range of motion into increasing the arch of the hand.

FIRST METACARPOPHALANGEAL JOINT

Osteokinematic motion:
  Flexion/extension
Ligaments:
  Collateral ligament
  Palmar ligament
  Deep transverse ligament
Joint orientation:
  Metacarpals: inferior, anterior, lateral
  Phalanges: superior, posterior, medial
Concave joint surface:
  Phalanx
Type of joint:
  Synovial
Resting position:
  Slight flexion[7]
Close-packed position:
  Full extension[7]
Capsular pattern of restriction:
  Flexion is more limited than extension[8]

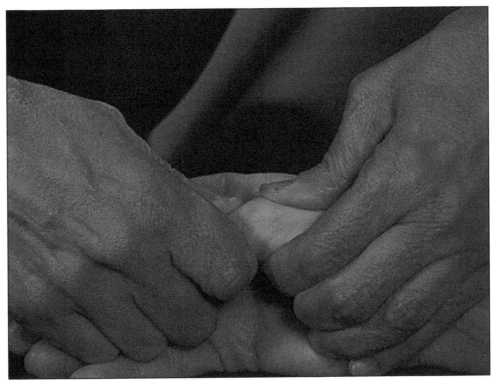

Figure 5-27 Distraction.

Distraction (Figure 5-27, Video 5-27)

Purpose
- To examine for thumb metacarpophalangeal joint impairment
- To increase accessory motion into thumb metacarpophalangeal joint distraction
- To increase range of motion at the metacarpophalangeal joint of the thumb
- To decrease pain

Positioning
1. The patient is sitting with the medial (ulnar) surface of the forearm on the treatment table.
2. The metacarpophalangeal joint of the thumb is positioned in the resting position if conservative techniques are indicated or approximating restricted range of motion if more aggressive techniques are indicated.
3. The clinician is facing the metacarpophalangeal joint of the thumb.
4. The stabilizing hand grips the head of the first metacarpal with the thumb on the lateral (radial) surface and the index finger on the medial (ulnar) surface.
5. The mobilizing/manipulating hand grips the proximal end of the first proximal phalanx with the thumb on the lateral (radial) surface and the index finger on the medial (ulnar) surface.

Procedure
1. The stabilizing hand holds the metacarpal in position.
2. The mobilizing/manipulating hand moves the proximal phalanx distally perpendicular to the proximal phalanx joint surface (see Figure 5-27).

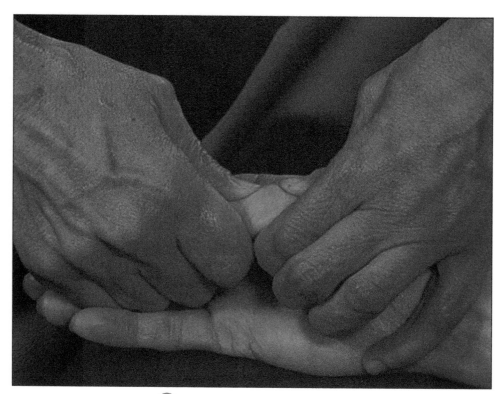

▶ **Figure 5-28** Medial (ulnar) glide.

Medial (Ulnar) Glide (Figure 5-28, Video 5-28)

Purpose
- To examine for thumb metacarpophalangeal joint impairment
- To increase accessory motion into thumb metacarpophalangeal joint medial (ulnar) glide
- To increase range of motion at the metacarpophalangeal joint of the thumb
- To decrease pain

Positioning
1. The patient is sitting with the medial (ulnar) surface of the forearm on the treatment table.
2. The metacarpophalangeal joint of the thumb is positioned in the resting position if conservative techniques are indicated or approximating restricted range of motion if more aggressive techniques are indicated.
3. The clinician is facing the metacarpophalangeal joint of the thumb.
4. The stabilizing hand grips the head of the first metacarpal with the thumb on the lateral (radial) surface and the index finger on the medial (ulnar) surface.
5. The mobilizing/manipulating hand grips the proximal end of the first proximal phalanx with the thumb on the lateral (radial) surface and the index finger on the medial (ulnar) surface.

Procedure
1. The clinician applies a grade I traction to the joint.
2. The stabilizing hand holds the metacarpal in position.
3. The mobilizing/manipulating hand glides the proximal phalanx in a medial (ulnar) direction (see Figure 5-28).

Particulars
- This technique might be especially effective for increasing range of motion into first metacarpophalangeal joint flexion.

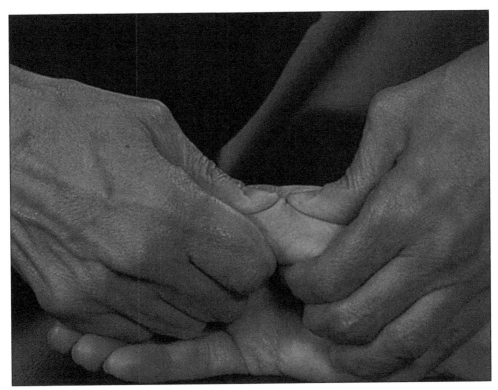

▶ **Figure 5-29** Lateral (radial) glide.

Lateral (Radial) Glide (Figure 5-29, Video 5-29)

Purpose
- To examine for thumb metacarpophalangeal joint impairment
- To increase accessory motion into thumb metacarpophalangeal joint lateral (radial) glide
- To increase range of motion at the metacarpophalangeal joint of the thumb
- To decrease pain

Positioning
1. The patient is sitting with the medial (ulnar) surface of the forearm on the treatment table.
2. The metacarpophalangeal joint of the thumb is positioned in the resting position if conservative techniques are indicated or approximating restricted range of motion if more aggressive techniques are indicated.
3. The clinician is facing the metacarpophalangeal joint of the thumb.
4. The stabilizing hand grips the head of the first metacarpal with the thumb on the lateral (radial) surface and the index finger on the medial (ulnar) surface.
5. The mobilizing/manipulating hand grips the proximal end of the first proximal phalanx with the thumb on the lateral (radial) surface and the index finger on the medial (ulnar) surface.

Procedure
1. The clinician applies a grade I traction to the joint.
2. The stabilizing hand holds the metacarpal in position.
3. The mobilizing/manipulating hand glides the proximal phalanx in a lateral (radial) direction (see Figure 5-29).

Particulars
- This technique might be especially effective for increasing range of motion into first metacarpophalangeal joint extension.

METACARPOPHALANGEAL JOINTS TWO THROUGH FIVE

Osteokinematic motions:
  Flexion/extension
  Radial/ulnar deviation
Ligaments:
  Collateral ligament
  Palmar ligament
  Deep transverse ligament
Joint orientation:
  Metacarpals: inferior
  Phalanges: superior
Concave joint surface:
  Phalanx
Type of joint:
  Synovial
Resting position:
  Slight flexion and slight ulnar deviation[7]
Close-packed position:
  Full flexion[7]
Capsular pattern of restriction:
  Flexion is more limited than extension[8]

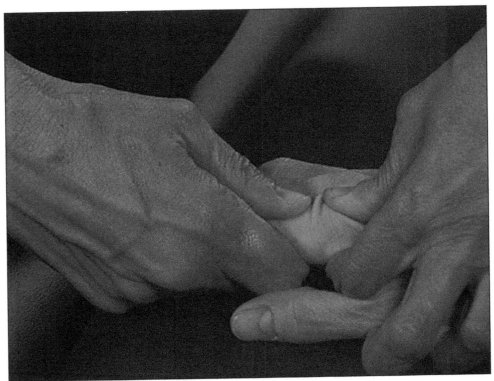

▶ **Figure 5-30** Distraction.

Distraction (Figure 5-30, Video 5-30)

Purpose
- To examine for digits two through five metacarpophalangeal joint impairment
- To increase accessory motion into metacarpophalangeal joint distraction of digits two through five
- To increase range of motion at the metacarpophalangeal joints of digits two through five
- To decrease pain

Positioning
1. The patient is sitting with the palm down.
2. The metacarpophalangeal joints of digits two through five are positioned in the resting position if conservative techniques are indicated or approximating restricted range of motion if more aggressive techniques are indicated.
3. The clinician is facing the metacarpophalangeal joints of digits two through five.
4. The stabilizing hand grips the head of the metacarpal with the thumb on the posterior surface and the index finger on the anterior surface.
5. The mobilizing/manipulating hand grips the proximal end of the proximal phalanx with the thumb on the posterior surface and the index finger on the anterior surface.

Procedure
1. The stabilizing hand holds the metacarpal in position.
2. The mobilizing/manipulating hand moves the proximal phalanx distally perpendicular to the proximal phalanx joint surface (see Figure 5-30).

Particulars
- This technique, in combination with home exercises and anterior and posterior metacarpophalangeal joint mobilizations, has been shown to increase metacarpophalangeal range of motion in patients with metacarpal fractures when measured after 1 week of treatment.[5]

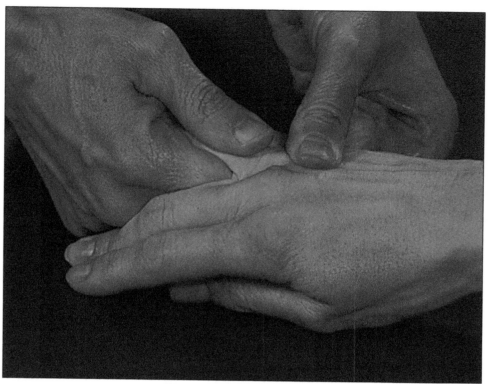

Figure 5-31 Posterior glide.

Posterior Glide (Figure 5-31, Video 5-31)
Purpose
- To examine for digits two through five metacarpophalangeal joint impairment
- To increase accessory motion into digits two through five metacarpophalangeal joint posterior glide
- To increase range of motion at the metacarpophalangeal joints of digits two through five
- To decrease pain

Positioning
1. The patient is sitting with the palm down.
2. The metacarpophalangeal joints of digits two through five are positioned in the resting position if conservative techniques are indicated or approximating restricted range of motion if more aggressive techniques are indicated.
3. The clinician is facing the metacarpophalangeal joints of digits two through five.
4. The stabilizing hand grips the head of the metacarpal with the thumb on the posterior surface and the index finger on the anterior surface.
5. The mobilizing/manipulating hand grips the proximal end of the proximal phalanx with the thumb on the posterior surface and the index finger on the anterior surface.

Procedure
1. The clinician applies a grade I traction to the joint.
2. The stabilizing hand holds the metacarpal in position.
3. The mobilizing/manipulating hand glides the proximal phalanx in a posterior direction (see Figure 5-31).

Particulars
- This technique might be especially effective for increasing range of motion into digits two through five metacarpophalangeal joint extension.
- This technique, in combination with home exercises and distraction and anterior glide metacarpophalangeal joint mobilizations, has been shown to increase metacarpophalangeal range of motion in patients with metacarpal fractures when measured after 1 week of treatment.[5]

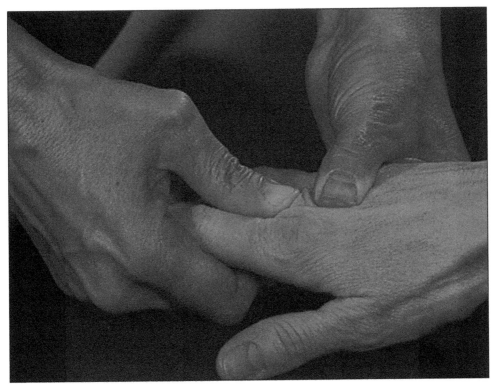

Figure 5-32 Anterior glide.

Anterior Glide (Figure 5-32, Video 5-32)

Purpose
- To examine for digits two through five metacarpophalangeal joint impairment
- To increase accessory motion into digits two through five metacarpophalangeal joint anterior glide
- To increase range of motion at the metacarpophalangeal joints of digits two through five
- To decrease pain

Positioning
1. The patient is sitting with the palm down.
2. The metacarpophalangeal joints of digits two through five are positioned in the resting position if conservative techniques are indicated or approximating restricted range of motion if more aggressive techniques are indicated.
3. The clinician is facing the metacarpophalangeal joints of digits two through five.
4. The stabilizing hand grips the head of the metacarpal with the thumb on the posterior surface and the index finger on the anterior surface.
5. The mobilizing/manipulating hand grips the proximal end of the proximal phalanx with the thumb on the posterior surface and the index finger on the anterior surface.

Procedure
1. The clinician applies a grade I traction to the joint.
2. The stabilizing hand holds the metacarpal in position.
3. The mobilizing/manipulating hand glides the proximal phalanx in an anterior direction (see Figure 5-32).

Particulars
- This technique might be especially effective for increasing range of motion into digits two through five metacarpophalangeal joint flexion.
- This technique, in combination with home exercises and distraction and posterior glide metacarpophalangeal joint mobilizations, has been shown to increase metacarpophalangeal range of motion in patients with metacarpal fractures when measured after 1 week of treatment.[5]

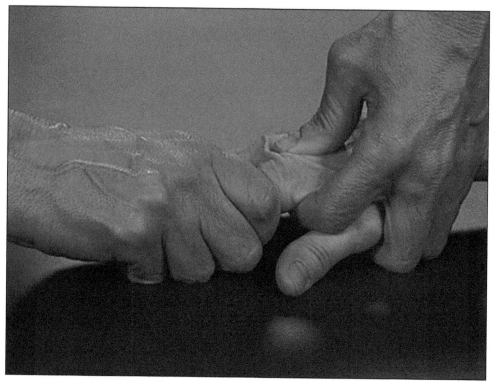

Figure 5-33 Medial (ulnar) glide.

Medial (Ulnar) Glide (Figure 5-33, Video 5-33)

Purpose
- To examine for digits two through five metacarpophalangeal joint impairment
- To increase accessory motion into digits two through five metacarpophalangeal joint medial (ulnar) glide
- To increase range of motion at the metacarpophalangeal joints of digits two through five
- To decrease pain

Positioning
1. The patient is sitting with the palm down.
2. The metacarpophalangeal joints of digits two through five are positioned in the resting position if conservative techniques are indicated or approximating restricted range of motion if more aggressive techniques are indicated.
3. The clinician is facing the metacarpophalangeal joints of digits two through five.
4. The stabilizing hand grips the head of the metacarpal with the thumb on the posteromedial surface and the index finger on the anteromedial surface.
5. The mobilizing/manipulating hand grips the proximal end of the proximal phalanx on the lateral (radial) and medial (ulnar) surfaces.

Procedure
1. The clinician applies a grade I traction to the joint.
2. The stabilizing hand holds the metacarpal in position.
3. The mobilizing/manipulating hand glides the proximal phalanx in a medial (ulnar) direction (see Figure 5-33).

Particulars
- This technique might be especially effective for increasing range of motion into digits two through five metacarpophalangeal joint ulnar deviation.

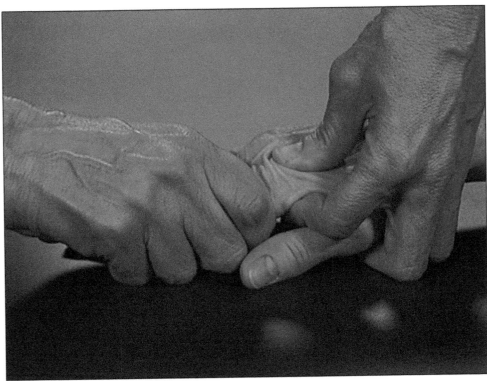

▶ **Figure 5-34** Lateral (radial) glide.

Lateral (Radial) Glide (Figure 5-34, Video 5-34)

Purpose
- To examine for digits two through five metacarpophalangeal joint impairment
- To increase accessory motion into digits two through five metacarpophalangeal joint lateral (radial) glide
- To increase range of motion at the metacarpophalangeal joints of digits two through five
- To decrease pain

Positioning
1. The patient is sitting with the palm down.
2. The metacarpophalangeal joints of digits two through five are positioned in the resting position if conservative techniques are indicated or approximating restricted range of motion if more aggressive techniques are indicated.
3. The clinician is facing the metacarpophalangeal joints of digits two through five.
4. The stabilizing hand grips the head of the metacarpal with the thumb on the posterolateral surface and the index finger on the anterolateral surface.
5. The mobilizing/manipulating hand grips the proximal end of the proximal phalanx on the lateral (radial) and medial (ulnar) surfaces.

Procedure
1. The clinician applies a grade I traction to the joint.
2. The stabilizing hand holds the metacarpal in position.
3. The mobilizing/manipulating hand glides the proximal phalanx in a lateral (radial) direction (see Figure 5-34).

Particulars
- This technique might be especially effective for increasing range of motion into digits two through five metacarpophalangeal joint radial deviation.

INTERPHALANGEAL JOINTS OF FINGERS ONE THROUGH FIVE

Osteokinematic motion:
    Flexion/extension
Ligaments:
    Palmar ligament
    Medial collateral ligament
    Lateral collateral ligament
Joint orientation:
    Proximal phalanx: inferior
    Distal phalanx: superior
Concave joint surface:
    Distal phalanx
Type of joint:
    Synovial
Resting position:
    Slight flexion[7]
Close-packed position:
    Full extension[7]
Capsular pattern of restriction:
    Flexion is more limited than extension[8]

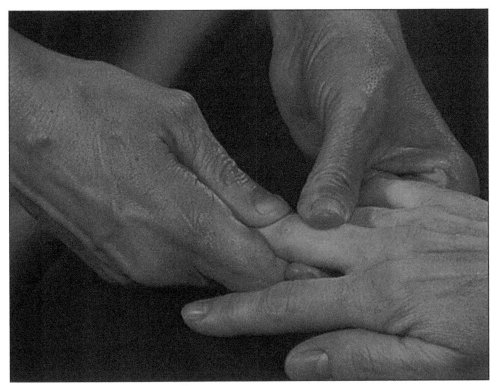

▶ **Figure 5-35** Distraction.

Distraction (Figure 5-35, Video 5-35)

Purpose
- To examine for finger interphalangeal joint impairment
- To increase accessory motion into finger interphalangeal joint distraction
- To increase range of motion at the interphalangeal joints of the fingers
- To decrease pain

Positioning
1. The patient is sitting with the palm down.
2. The interphalangeal joints are positioned in the resting position if conservative techniques are indicated or approximating restricted range of motion if more aggressive techniques are indicated.
3. The clinician is facing the interphalangeal joints.
4. The stabilizing hand grips the distal end of the more proximal phalanx with the thumb on the posterior surface and the index finger on the anterior surface. If the thumb interphalangeal joint is being mobilized/manipulated, the clinician's thumb grips the lateral (radial) surface, and the index finger grips the medial (ulnar) surface.
5. The mobilizing/manipulating hand grips the proximal end of the more distal phalanx with the thumb on the posterior surface and the index finger on the anterior surface. If the thumb interphalangeal joint is being mobilized/manipulated, the clinician's thumb grips the lateral (radial) surface, and the index finger grips the medial (ulnar) surface.

Procedure
1. The stabilizing hand holds the proximal phalanx in position.
2. The mobilizing/manipulating hand moves the distal phalanx distally perpendicular to the distal phalanx joint surface (see Figure 5-35).
3. The clinician could wear surgical gloves to reduce slippage against the patient's skin.

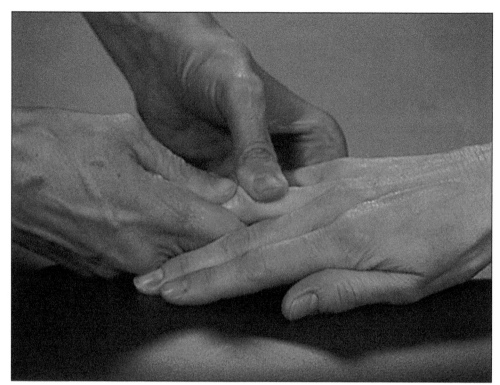

▶ **Figure 5-36** Posterior glide.

Posterior Glide (Figure 5-36, Video 5-36)

Purpose
- To examine for finger interphalangeal joint impairment
- To increase accessory motion into finger interphalangeal posterior glide
- To increase range of motion at the interphalangeal joints of the fingers
- To decrease pain

Positioning
1. The patient is sitting with the palm down.
2. The interphalangeal joints are positioned in the resting position if conservative techniques are indicated or approximating restricted range of motion if more aggressive techniques are indicated.
3. The clinician is facing the interphalangeal joints.
4. The stabilizing hand grips the distal end of the more proximal phalanx with the thumb on the posterior surface and the index finger on the anterior surface. If the thumb interphalangeal joint is being mobilized/manipulated, the clinician's thumb grips the lateral (radial) surface and the index finger grips the medial (ulnar) surface.
5. The mobilizing/manipulating hand grips the proximal end of the more distal phalanx with the thumb on the posterior surface and the index finger on the anterior surface. If the thumb interphalangeal joint is being mobilized/manipulated, the clinician's thumb grips the lateral (radial) surface and the index finger grips the medial (ulnar) surface.

Procedure
1. The clinician applies a grade I traction to the joint.
2. The stabilizing hand holds the proximal phalanx in position.
3. The mobilizing/manipulating hand glides the distal phalanx in a posterior direction. If the thumb interphalangeal joint is being mobilized/manipulated, the distal phalanx is glided in a lateral (radial) direction (see Figure 5-36).
4. The clinician could wear surgical gloves to reduce slippage against the patient's skin.

Particulars
- This technique might be especially effective for increasing range of motion into interphalangeal joint extension.

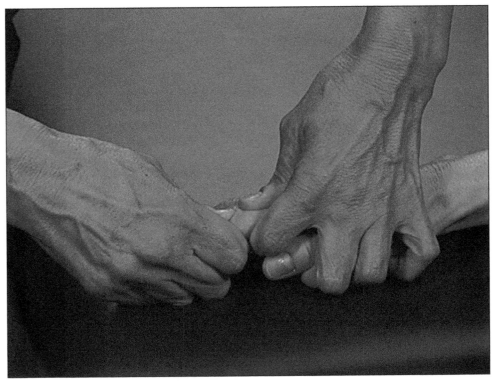

Figure 5-37 Anterior glide.

Anterior Glide (Figure 5-37, Video 5-37)

Purpose
- To examine for finger interphalangeal joint impairment
- To increase accessory motion into finger interphalangeal anterior glide
- To increase range of motion at the interphalangeal joints of the fingers
- To decrease pain

Positioning
1. The patient is sitting with the palm down.
2. The interphalangeal joints are positioned in the resting position if conservative techniques are indicated or approximating restricted range of motion if more aggressive techniques are indicated.
3. The clinician is facing the interphalangeal joints.
4. The stabilizing hand grips the distal end of the more proximal phalanx with the thumb on the posterior surface and the index finger on the anterior surface. If the thumb interphalangeal joint is being mobilized/manipulated, the clinician's thumb grips the lateral (radial) surface and the index finger grips the medial (ulnar) surface.
5. The mobilizing/manipulating hand grips the proximal end of the more distal phalanx with the thumb on the posterior surface and the index finger on the anterior surface. If the thumb interphalangeal joint is being mobilized/manipulated, the clinician's thumb grips the lateral (radial) surface and the index finger grips the medial (ulnar) surface.

Procedure
1. The clinician applies a grade I traction to the joint.
2. The stabilizing hand holds the proximal phalanx in position.
3. The mobilizing/manipulating hand glides the distal phalanx in an anterior direction. If the thumb interphalangeal joint is being mobilized/manipulated, the distal phalanx is glided in a medial (ulnar) direction (see Figure 5-37).
4. The clinician could wear surgical gloves to reduce slippage against the patient's skin.

Particulars
- This technique might be especially effective for increasing range of motion into interphalangeal joint flexion.

REFERENCES

1. Brantingham JW, Cassa TK, Bonnefin D, et al. Manipulative and multimodal therapy for upper extremity and temporomandibular disorders: a systematic review. *J Manipulative Physiol Ther*. 2013;36: 143-201.

2. Kay S, Haensel N, Stiller K. The effect of passive mobilisation following fractures involving the distal radius: a randomised study. *Aust J Phys Ther*. 2000;46: 93-101.

3. Naik VC, Chitra J, Khatri S. Effectiveness of Maitland versus Mulligan mobilization technique following post-surgical management of Colles fracture; randomized clinical trial. *Indian J Physiother Occup Ther*. 2007;1:14-19.

4. Taylor NF, Bennell KL. The effectiveness of passive joint mobilization on the return of active wrist extension following Colles fracture: a clinical trial. *N Z J Physiother*. 1994;April:24-28.

5. Randall T, Portney L, Harris BA. Effects of joint mobilization on joint stiffness and active motion of the metacarpophalangeal joint. *J Orthop Sports Phys Ther*. 1992;16:30-36.

6. Hoogvliet P, Randsdorp MS, Dingemanse R, Koes BW, Huisstede BMA. Does effectiveness of exercise therapy and mobilisation techniques offer guidance for the treatment of lateral and medial epicondylitis? a systemic review. *Br J Sports Med*. 2013;47: 1112-1119.

7. Kaltenborn FM. *Manual Mobilization of the Joints: The Kaltenborn Method of Joint Examination and Treatment*, Vol. I. 6th ed. The Extremities. Oslo, Norway: Norli; 2002.

8. Cyriax J. *Textbook of Orthopaedic Medicine*, Vol. 1. 8th ed. Diagnosis of Soft Tissue Lesions. London: Bailliere Tindall; 1982.

9. Villafane JH, Cleland JA, Fernandez-De-Las-Penas C. The effectiveness of a manual therapy and exercise protocol in patients with thumb carpometacarpal osterarthritis: a randomized controlled trial. *J Orthop Sports Phys Ther*. 2013;43:204-213.

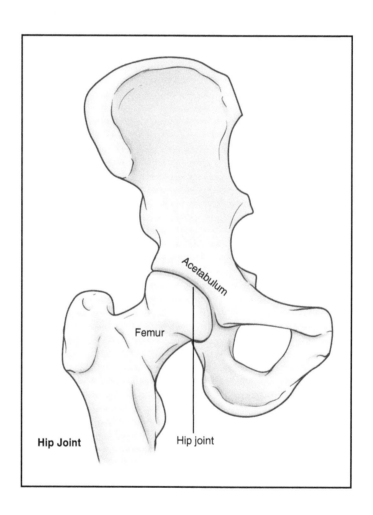

Acetabulum

Femur

Hip Joint

Hip joint

CHAPTER 6

The Hip Joint

BASICS

Hip

The hip is a ball-and-socket joint with a compressed anterior-to-posterior diameter. Its construction is similar to that of the glenohumeral joint, but the hip is far more stable. This increased stability is due to negative intracapsular atmospheric pressure, a stronger joint capsule, a more spherical femoral head, and a deeper socket made even deeper by the labrum, which provides greater joint surface contact area than at the glenohumeral joint. Most basic activities of daily living occur between 0 and 120 degrees of hip flexion and between 0 and 20 degrees of lateral rotation and abduction.

SPECIFIC PATHOLOGY AND HIP JOINT MOBILIZATION/MANIPULATION

Hip Osteoarthritis

In one clinical practice guideline and 2 systematic reviews, investigators reported on the efficacy of joint mobilization/ manipulation for the treatment of patients with hip osteoarthritis. The clinical practice guideline, published in 2009, comprised recommendations for treatment with manual therapy, which included joint mobilization/ manipulation interventions for patients with mild hip osteoarthritis. Expected outcomes included only short-term improvements in function, pain, and range of motion but were based on moderate evidence.[1] In the 2013 systematic review, the authors corroborated these findings, concluding that manual therapy is an effective intervention for reducing pain and disability short term.[2] In the other systematic review, published earlier in 2012, the authors reported exclusively on joint manipulation. They concluded that there is fair evidence to support manipulation with multi-modal interventions for treatment of hip osteoarthritis for short term outcomes, and limited evidence for long term outcomes.[6]

Nonarthritic Hip Joint Pain

In a 2014 clinical practice guideline, the authors evaluated the clinical literature addressing physical therapy evaluation and intervention procedures for patients with nonarthritic hip joint pain, which included femoroacetabular impingement, osseous abnormalities, structural instability, labral tears, osteochondral lesions, loose bodies, ligamentum teres ligament injuries, and septic conditions. In relation to joint mobilization/manipulation interventions, the investigators recommended that, assuming there are no contraindications to these techniques and there is evidence suggesting that capsular restrictions are causing hip mobility impairments, joint mobilization/ manipulation might be indicated. The investigators recommended using caution when considering joint mobilization/manipulation if osseous abnormalities are present. These recommendations were based on expert opinion.[3]

HIP JOINT

Osteokinematic motions:
   Flexion/extension
   Abduction/adduction
   Medial/lateral rotation
Ligaments:
   Iliofemoral (Y) ligament
   Ischiofemoral ligament
   Pubofemoral ligament
   Ligamentum teres
   Zona orbicularis
   Transverse ligament
Joint orientation:
   Acetabulum: inferior, lateral, anterior
   Femur: superior, medial, anterior
Concave joint surface:
   Acetabulum
Type of joint:
   Synovial
Resting position:
   30 degrees flexion, 30 degrees abduction, and slight lateral rotation[4]
Close-packed position:
   Full extension, abduction, and medial rotation[4]
Capsular pattern of restriction:
   Flexion, abduction, and medial rotation are grossly limited; extension is slightly limited[5]

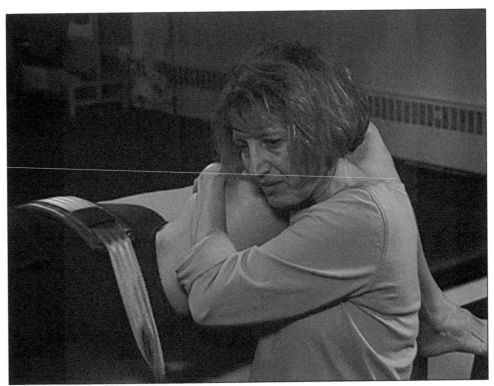

▶ **Figure 6-1** Distraction.

Distraction (Figure 6-1, Video 6-1)

Purpose
- To examine for hip joint impairment
- To increase accessory motion into hip joint distraction
- To increase range of motion at the hip joint
- To decrease pain

Positioning
1. The patient is supine with the leg positioned over the clinician's shoulder.
2. The clinician can wrap a belt around the patient's pelvis and the treatment table to help stabilize the pelvis.
3. The hip joint is positioned as close to the resting position as possible if conservative techniques are indicated or approximating restricted range of motion if more aggressive techniques are indicated.
4. The clinician is at the patient's side, facing the patient's hip.
5. Both hands are positioned on the medial surface of the proximal thigh.

Procedure
1. Both hands move the femoral head inferior, lateral, and anterior, while the clinician elevates the shoulder, moving the femur perpendicular to the joint surface of the acetabulum (see Figure 6-1).

Particulars
- This technique is commonly performed using a grade V manipulation.

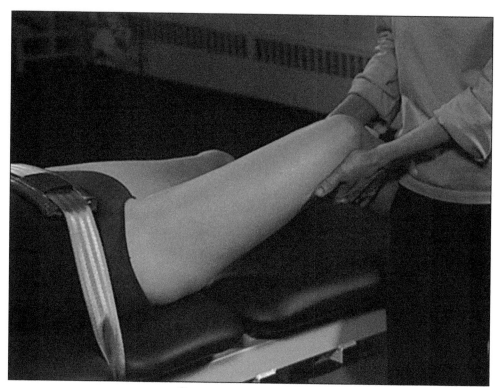

▶ **Figure 6-2** Inferior glide.

Inferior Glide (Figure 6-2, Video 6-2)
Purpose
- To examine for hip joint impairment
- To increase accessory motion into hip joint inferior glide
- To increase range of motion at the hip joint
- To decrease pain

Positioning
1. The patient is supine.
2. The clinician can wrap a belt around the patient's pelvis and the treatment table to help stabilize the pelvis.
3. The hip joint is positioned in the resting position if conservative techniques are indicated or approximating restricted range of motion if more aggressive techniques are indicated.
4. The clinician is at the patient's foot, facing the patient's hip.
5. Both hands grip the distal thigh.

Procedure
1. The clinician applies a grade I traction to the joint.
2. Both hands glide the femoral head in an inferior direction as the clinician leans away from the joint (see Figure 6-2).

Particulars
- It is important to screen for sacroiliac joint impairments before performing this technique.
- This technique is commonly performed using a grade V manipulation.
- This technique is also called a long-axis distraction.
- This technique might be especially effective for increasing range of motion into hip joint abduction.

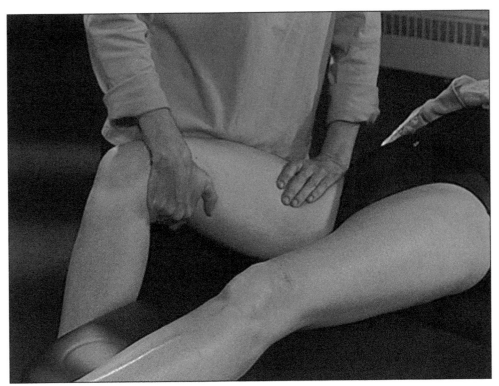

▶ **Figure 6-3** Posterior glide.

Posterior Glide (Figure 6-3, Video 6-3)

Purpose
- To examine for hip joint impairment
- To increase accessory motion into hip joint posterior glide
- To increase range of motion at the hip joint
- To decrease pain

Positioning
1. The patient is supine.
2. The hip joint is positioned in the resting position if conservative techniques are indicated or approximating restricted range of motion if more aggressive techniques are indicated.
3. The clinician is at the patient's knee, facing the patient's hip.
4. The mobilizing/manipulating hand is positioned on the anterior surface of the proximal thigh.
5. The guiding hand is positioned on the posterior surface of the distal thigh.

Procedure
1. The clinician applies a grade I traction to the joint.
2. The mobilizing/manipulating hand glides the femur in a posterior direction.
3. The guiding hand controls the position of the femur (see Figure 6-3).

Particulars
- It is important to screen for sacroiliac joint impairments before performing this technique.
- This technique might be especially effective for increasing range of motion into hip joint flexion and medial rotation.

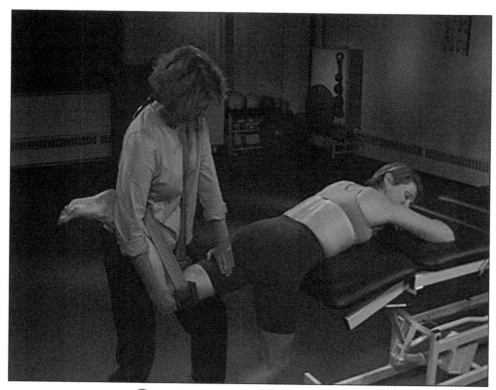

▶ **Figure 6-4** Anterior glide: first technique.

Anterior Glide: First Technique (Figure 6-4, Video 6-4)

Purpose
- To examine for hip joint impairment
- To increase accessory motion into hip joint anterior glide
- To increase range of motion at the hip joint
- To decrease pain

Positioning
1. The patient is prone with the pelvis on the treatment table and the legs off the end of the table.
2. The clinician can wrap a belt around the patient's thigh and the clinician's shoulder to help control the motion.
3. The hip joint is positioned in the resting position if conservative techniques are indicated or approximating restricted range of motion if more aggressive techniques are indicated.
4. The clinician is at the foot of the treatment table, facing the patient's hip.
5. The patient's leg is supported between the clinician's arm and trunk.
6. The mobilizing/manipulating hand is positioned on the posterior surface of the proximal thigh.
7. The guiding hand is positioned on the anterior surface of the distal thigh.

Procedure
1. The clinician applies a grade I traction to the joint.
2. The mobilizing/manipulating hand glides the femur in an anterior direction as the clinician leans on the patient's thigh.
3. The guiding hand controls the position of the thigh (see Figure 6-4).

Particulars
- It is important to screen for sacroiliac joint impairments before performing this technique.
- This technique might be especially effective for increasing range of motion into hip joint extension and lateral rotation.

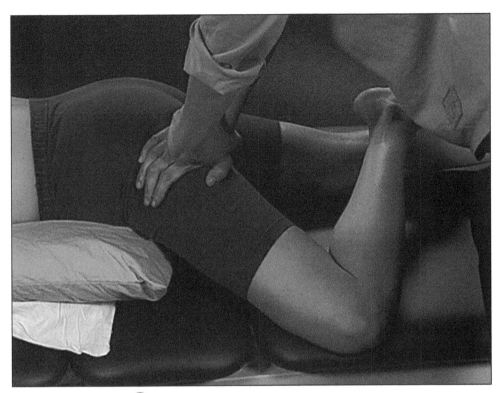

▶ **Figure 6-5** Anterior glide: second technique.

Anterior Glide: Second Technique (Figure 6-5, Video 6-5)

Purpose
- To examine for hip joint impairment
- To increase accessory motion into hip joint anterior glide
- To increase range of motion at the hip joint
- To decrease pain

Positioning
1. The patient is prone with one or more pillows under the trunk and the hip positioned in abduction and lateral rotation.
2. The clinician is at the side of the treatment table, facing the patient's hip.
3. The mobilizing/manipulating hand is positioned over the guiding hand.
4. The guiding hand is positioned on the posterolateral surface of the proximal thigh.

Procedure
1. The clinician applies a grade I traction to the joint.
2. The mobilizing/manipulating hand glides the femur in an anterior direction as the clinician leans on the patient's thigh.
3. The guiding hand controls the position of the mobilizing hand (see Figure 6-5).

Particulars
- This technique might be especially effective for increasing range of motion into hip joint extension and lateral rotation.
- If the patient has pain or insufficient range of motion preventing the patient from being positioned with the hip in abduction and lateral rotation, the clinician can position the patient with the knee off the treatment table.

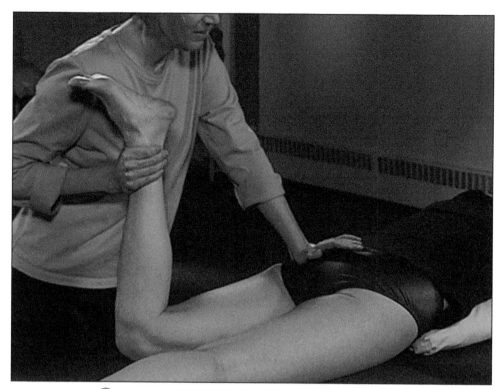

▶ Figure 6-6 Posterolateral glide of the femur on the pelvis.

Posterolateral Glide of the Femur on the Pelvis (Figure 6-6, Video 6-6)

Purpose
- To examine for hip joint impairment
- To increase accessory motion into hip joint posterolateral glide
- To increase range of motion at the hip joint
- To decrease pain

Positioning
1. The patient is prone with the knee on the side being treated flexed to 90 degrees.
2. The hip joint is positioned in as close to resting position as possible if conservative techniques are indicated or approximating restricted range of motion if more aggressive techniques are indicated.
3. The clinician is at the patient's side, facing the patient's hip.
4. The stabilizing hand grips the ankle and controls the amount of hip rotation.
5. The mobilizing/manipulating hand is positioned over the midpoint of the posterior surface of the ilium.

Procedure
1. The stabilizing hand holds the leg in position.
2. The mobilizing/manipulating hand glides the pelvis in an anteromedial direction, thereby imparting a posterolateral force to the femur on the pelvis (see Figure 6-6).

Particulars
- It is important to screen for sacroiliac joint impairments before performing this technique.
- This technique might be especially effective for increasing range of motion into hip joint medial rotation, in part because approximating the restricted range of motion for medial rotation is performed easily by moving the lower leg toward the clinician.

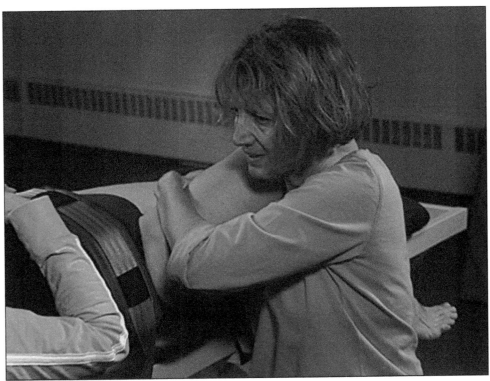

Figure 6-7 Lateral glide.

Lateral Glide (Figure 6-7, Video 6-7)

Purpose
- To examine for hip joint impairment
- To increase accessory motion into hip joint lateral glide
- To increase range of motion at the hip joint
- To decrease pain

Positioning
1. The patient is supine with the leg positioned over the clinician's shoulder.
2. The clinician can wrap a belt around the patient's pelvis and treatment table to help stabilize the pelvis.
3. The hip joint is positioned as close to the resting position as possible if conservative techniques are indicated or approximating restricted range of motion if more aggressive techniques are indicated.
4. The clinician is at the patient's side, facing the patient's hip.
5. Both hands are positioned on the medial surface of the proximal thigh.

Procedure
1. The clinician applies a grade I traction to the joint.
2. Both hands glide the femur in a lateral direction (see Figure 6-7).

Particulars
- This technique might be especially effective for increasing range of motion into hip joint adduction and medial rotation.

REFERENCES

1. Cibulka MT, White DM, Woehrle J, et al. Hip pain and mobility deficits—hip osteoarthritis: clinical practice guidelines linked to the International Classification of Functioning, Disability, and Health from the Orthopaedic Section of the American Physical Therapy Association. *J Orthop Sports Phys Ther.* 2009;39:A1-A25.

2. Romeo A, Parazza S, Boschi N, Nava T, Vanti C. Manual therapy and therapeutic exercise in the treatment of osteoarthritis of the hip: a systematic review. *Reumatismo.* 2013;65:63-74.

3. Enseki K, Harris-Hayes M, White DM, et al. Nonarthritic hip joint pain clinical practice guidelines linked to the International Classification of Functioning, Disability and Health from the Orthopaedic Section of the American Physical Therapy Association. *J Orthop Sports Phys Ther.* 2014;44:A1-A32.

4. Kaltenborn FM. *Manual Mobilization of the Joints: The Kaltenborn Method of Joint Examination and Treatment*, Vol. I. 6th ed. The Extremities. Oslo, Norway: Norli; 2002.

5. Cyriax J. *Textbook of Orthopaedic Medicine*, Vol. 1. 8th ed. Diagnosis of Soft Tissue Lesions. London: Bailliere Tindall; 1982.

6. Brantingham JW, Bonnefin D, Perle SM, et al. Manipulative therapy for lower extremity conditions: update of a literature review. *J Manipulative Physiol Ther.* 2012;35:127-166.

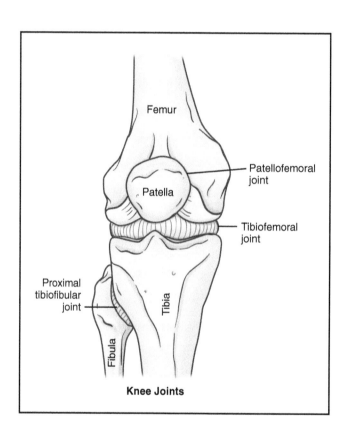

Knee Joints

CHAPTER 7

The Knee

BASICS

The knee joint consists of two sets of articulating surfaces, the tibiofemoral joint and the patellofemoral joint. To perform most basic activities of daily living, these two joints must allow at least 120 degrees of knee flexion to occur.

Tibiofemoral Joint

Flexion at the knee is accompanied by medial rotation of the tibia, and extension is accompanied by lateral rotation. Lateral rotation occurs during the last 30 degrees of extension. This rotational motion is caused by tightening of ligamentous structures and the configuration of the two articular surfaces.

Patellofemoral Joint

The patellofemoral joint moves 5 to 7 cm superiorly in the femoral groove as the knee extends. It also is believed to move from a lateral position to a more medial position and back to a more lateral position as the knee moves from full flexion to full extension.

SPECIFIC PATHOLOGY AND KNEE JOINT MOBILIZATION/MANIPULATION

Knee Osteoarthritis

In a 2011 systematic review of the efficacy of manual therapy for treatment of knee osteoarthritis, only one study was included that addressed joint mobilization/manipulation. The investigators of this study concluded that subjects did not attain greater improvements in pain or function compared with treatment with nonsteroidal antiinflammatory medications.[1] In a 2012 systematic review, the authors specifically evaluated the efficacy of thrust manipulation. The authors concluded that there was fair evidence supporting manipulation and multimodal interventions for short term outcomes, but limited evidence for long term outcomes.[4]

TIBIOFEMORAL JOINT

Osteokinematic motions:
    Flexion/extension
    Medial/lateral rotation
Ligaments:
    Tibial collateral ligament
    Fibular collateral ligament
    Anterior cruciate ligament
    Posterior cruciate ligament
    Oblique ligament
    Arcuate popliteal ligament
Joint orientation:
    Femur: inferior
    Tibia: superior
Concave joint surface:
    Tibia
Type of joint:
    Synovial
Resting position:
    25 to 40 degrees of flexion[2]
Close-packed position:
    Full extension[2]
Capsular pattern of restriction:
    Gross limitations in flexion accompanied by slight limitations in extension[3]

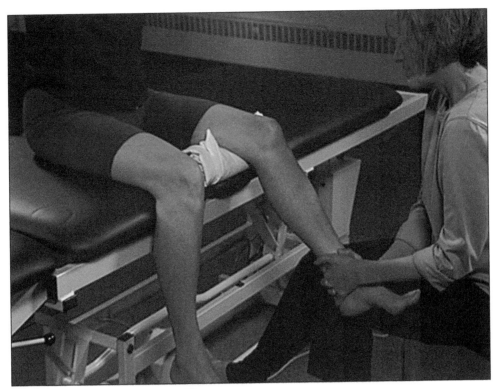

Figure 7-1 Distraction.

Distraction (Figure 7-1, Video 7-1)
Purpose
- To examine for tibiofemoral joint impairment
- To increase accessory motion into tibiofemoral joint distraction
- To increase range of motion at the knee joint
- To decrease pain

Positioning
1. The patient is sitting with the knee off the edge of the treatment table.
2. The tibiofemoral joint is positioned in the resting position if conservative techniques are indicated or approximating restricted range of motion if more aggressive techniques are indicated.
3. The clinician is at the patient's foot, facing the patient's knee.
4. Both hands grip the distal tibia from the medial and lateral sides.

Procedure
1. Both hands move the tibia distally perpendicular to the tibial joint surface (see Figure 7-1).

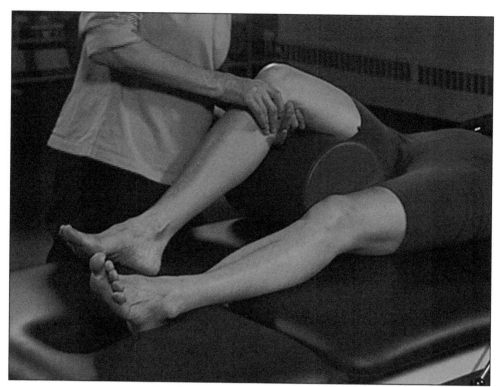

▶ Figure 7-2 Posterior glide.

Posterior Glide (Figure 7-2, Video 7-2)

Purpose

- To examine for tibiofemoral joint impairment
- To increase accessory motion into tibiofemoral joint posterior glide
- To increase range of motion at the tibiofemoral joint
- To decrease pain

Positioning

1. The patient is supine.
2. The tibiofemoral joint is positioned in the resting position if conservative techniques are indicated or approximating restricted range of motion if more aggressive techniques are indicated.
3. The clinician is at the side of the patient's leg, facing the patient's knee.
4. The stabilizing hand supports the femur from the posterior side.
5. The mobilizing/manipulating hand grips the proximal tibia from the anterior side.

Procedure

1. The clinician applies a grade I traction to the joint.
2. The stabilizing hand holds the femur in position.
3. The mobilizing/manipulating hand glides the tibia in a posterior direction (see Figure 7-2).

Particulars

- This technique might be especially effective for increasing range of motion into knee joint flexion.

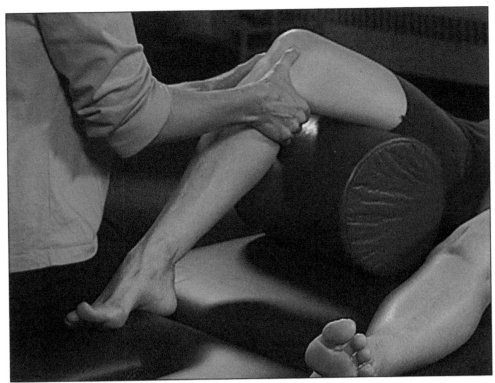

Figure 7-3 Anterior glide of the tibia on the femur: first technique.

Anterior Glide of the Tibia on the Femur: First Technique (Figure 7-3, Video 7-3)

Purpose
- To examine for tibiofemoral joint impairment
- To increase accessory motion into tibiofemoral joint anterior glide
- To increase range of motion at the tibiofemoral joint
- To decrease pain

Positioning
1. The patient is supine.
2. The tibiofemoral joint is positioned in the resting position if conservative techniques are indicated or approximating restricted range of motion if more aggressive techniques are indicated.
3. The clinician is at the patient's foot, facing the patient's knee.
4. Both hands grip the proximal tibia from the posterior side with the fingers while simultaneously positioning the thumbs over the anterior surface of the distal femur.

Procedure
1. Both hands glide the tibia in an anterior direction while stabilizing the femur with the thumbs (see Figure 7-3).

Particulars
- This technique might be especially effective for increasing range of motion into knee joint extension.

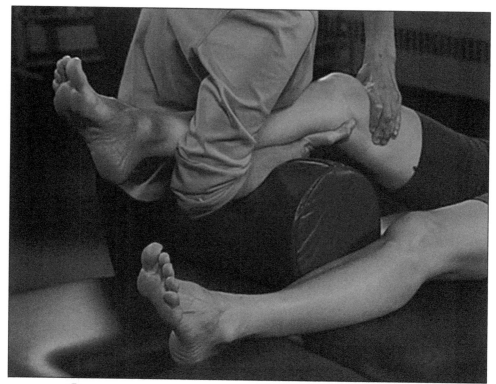

Figure 7-4 Anterior glide of the tibia on the femur: second technique.

Anterior Glide of the Tibia on the Femur: Second Technique (Figure 7-4, Video 7-4)
Purpose
- To examine for tibiofemoral joint impairment
- To increase accessory motion into tibiofemoral joint anterior glide
- To increase range of motion at the tibiofemoral joint
- To decrease pain

Positioning
1. The patient is supine.
2. The tibiofemoral joint is positioned in the resting position if conservative techniques are indicated or approximating restricted range of motion if more aggressive techniques are indicated.
3. The clinician is at the side of the patient's leg, facing the patient's knee.
4. The stabilizing hand grips the proximal tibia posteriorly.
5. The mobilizing/manipulating hand is positioned over the anterior surface of the distal femur.

Procedure
1. The clinician applies a grade I traction to the joint.
2. The stabilizing hand holds the tibia in position.
3. The mobilizing/manipulating hand glides the femur in a posterior direction, thereby imparting an anterior force to the tibia on the femur (see Figure 7-4).

Particulars
- This technique might be especially effective for increasing range of motion into knee joint extension.

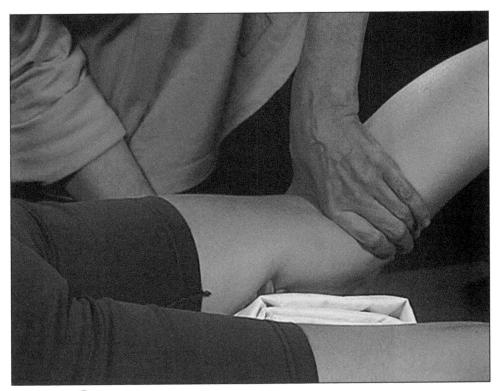

Figure 7-5 Anterior glide of the tibia on the femur: third technique.

Anterior Glide of the Tibia on the Femur: Third Technique (Figure 7-5, Video 7-5)

Purpose
- To examine for tibiofemoral joint impairment
- To increase accessory motion into tibiofemoral joint anterior glide
- To increase range of motion at the tibiofemoral joint
- To decrease pain

Positioning
1. The patient is prone with a small pillow positioned under the distal femur to protect the patellofemoral joint.
2. The tibiofemoral joint is positioned in the resting position if conservative techniques are indicated or approximating restricted range of motion if more aggressive techniques are indicated.
3. The clinician is at the side of the patient's leg, facing the patient's knee.
4. The stabilizing hand grips the distal femur from the anterior side.
5. The mobilizing/manipulating hand is positioned over the posterior surface of the proximal tibia.

Procedure
1. The clinician applies a grade I traction to the joint.
2. The stabilizing hand holds the femur in position.
3. The mobilizing/manipulating hand glides the tibia in an anterior direction (see Figure 7-5).

Particulars
- This technique might be especially effective for increasing range of motion into knee joint extension.

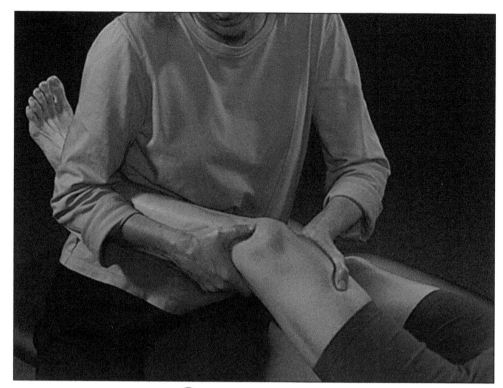

▶ **Figure 7-6** Medial glide.

Medial Glide (Figure 7-6, Video 7-6)

Purpose
- To examine for tibiofemoral joint impairment
- To increase accessory motion into tibiofemoral joint medial glide
- To increase range of motion at the tibiofemoral joint
- To decrease pain

Positioning
1. The patient is supine.
2. The tibiofemoral joint is positioned in the resting position if conservative techniques are indicated or approximating restricted range of motion if more aggressive techniques are indicated.
3. The clinician is between the patient's knees with the patient's lower leg between the clinician's arm and trunk.
4. The stabilizing hand grips the distal femur from the medial side.
5. The mobilizing/manipulating hand grips the proximal tibia and fibula from the lateral side and supports the lateral lower leg with the forearm.

Procedure
1. The clinician applies a grade I traction to the joint.
2. The stabilizing hand holds the femur in position.
3. The mobilizing/manipulating hand glides the proximal tibia in a medial direction indirectly through the fibula, while the trunk guides the motion (see Figure 7-6).

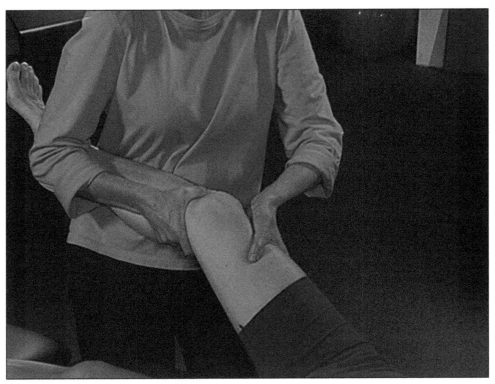

Figure 7-7 Lateral glide.

Lateral Glide (Figure 7-7, Video 7-7)

Purpose
- To examine for tibiofemoral joint impairment
- To increase accessory motion into tibiofemoral joint lateral glide
- To increase range of motion at the tibiofemoral joint
- To decrease pain

Positioning
1. The patient is supine.
2. The tibiofemoral joint is positioned in the resting position if conservative techniques are indicated or approximating restricted range of motion if more aggressive techniques are indicated.
3. The clinician is at the side of the treatment table, facing the patient's knee with the patient's lower leg between the clinician's arm and trunk.
4. The stabilizing hand grips the distal femur from the lateral side.
5. The mobilizing/manipulating hand grips the proximal tibia from the medial side and supports the medial lower leg with the forearm.

Procedure
1. The clinician applies a grade I traction to the joint.
2. The stabilizing hand holds the femur in position.
3. The mobilizing/manipulating hand glides the proximal tibia in a lateral direction while the trunk guides the motion (see Figure 7-7).

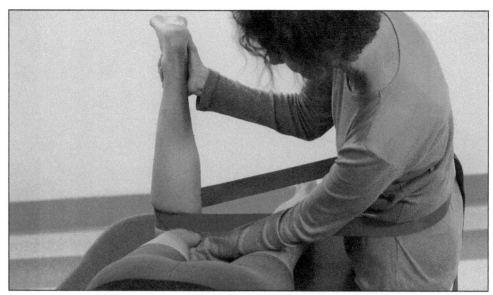

▶ **Figure 7-8** Medial glide mobilization with movement.

Medial Glide Mobilization with Movement (Figure 7-8, Video 7-8)

Purpose
- To increase pain-free range of motion into knee flexion
- To decrease medial knee joint pain

Positioning
1. The patient is prone with the knee flexed to around midrange.
2. The clinician stands on the side opposite the knee being mobilized, facing the knee.
3. The clinician places a mobilization belt around his or her hips and the patient's proximal tibia/fibula.
4. The clinician places the heel of the stabilizing hand on the medial distal femur and the heel of the mobilizing hand on the medial malleolus of the leg being mobilized.

Procedure
1. The clinician imparts a medial glide to the proximal tibia by leaning back onto the belt.
2. While maintaining the medial glide, the patient slowly moves the knee into flexion.
3. The clinician applies overpressure into flexion.
4. The clinician maintains the medial glide while the patient moves the knee to the starting position.
5. The clinician continually adjusts his or her own position in relation to the patient's position, to maintain the joint mobilization force during joint movement (see Figure 7-8).

Particulars
- This technique is indicated only if it can be performed without reproducing the patient's pain/symptoms.
- This technique should result in an immediate increase in range of motion and/or decrease in pain.
- If effective (the technique results in an immediate increase in range of motion and/or decrease in pain), this technique should be repeated (~3 sets of 10).

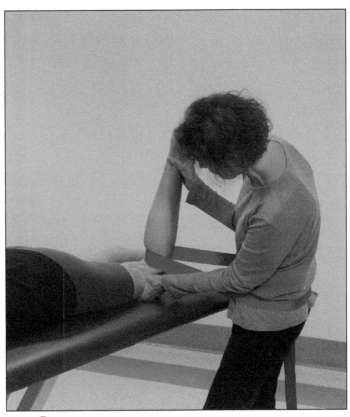

▶ **Figure 7-9** Lateral glide mobilization with movement.

Lateral Glide Mobilization with Movement (Figure 7-9, Video 7-9)

Purpose
- To increase pain-free range of motion into knee flexion
- To decrease lateral knee joint pain

Positioning
1. The patient is prone with the knee flexed to around midrange.
2. The clinician stands on the side of the knee being mobilized, facing the knee.
3. The clinician places a mobilization belt around his or her hips and the patient's proximal tibia.
4. The clinician places the heel of the stabilizing hand on the lateral distal femur and the heel of the mobilizing hand on the lateral malleolus of the leg being mobilized.

Procedure
1. The clinician imparts a lateral glide to the proximal tibia by leaning back onto the belt.
2. While maintaining the lateral glide, the patient slowly moves the knee into flexion.
3. The clinician applies overpressure into flexion.
4. The clinician maintains the lateral glide while the patient moves the knee to the starting position.
5. The clinician continually adjusts his or her own position in relation to the patient's position, to maintain the joint mobilization force during joint movement (see Figure 7-9).

Particulars
- This technique is indicated only if it can be performed without reproducing the patient's pain/symptoms.
- This technique should result in an immediate increase in range of motion and/or decrease in pain.
- If effective (the technique results in an immediate increase in range of motion and/or decrease in pain), this technique should be repeated (~3 sets of 10).

PATELLOFEMORAL JOINT

Osteokinematic motion:
    Flexion/extension
Ligament:
    Patellofemoral ligament
Joint orientation:
    Patella: posterior
    Femur: anterior
Concave joint surface:
    Femur
Type of joint:
    Synovial
Resting position:
    25 to 40 degrees of flexion[2], although most clinicians consider full extension or slight flexion to be the resting position
Close-packed position:
    Full extension[2]
Capsular pattern of restriction:
    Not described by Cyriax[3]

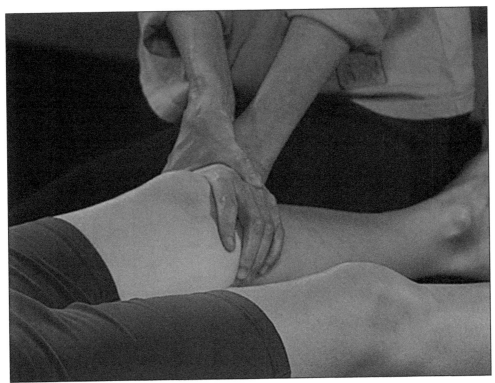

▶ **Figure 7-10** Superior glide.

Superior Glide (Figure 7-10, Video 7-10)

Purpose
- To examine for patellofemoral joint impairment
- To increase accessory motion into patellofemoral joint superior glide
- To increase range of motion at the patellofemoral joint
- To decrease pain

Positioning
1. The patient is supine.
2. The knee is positioned in full extension or slight flexion if conservative techniques are indicated or approximating restricted range of motion if more aggressive techniques are indicated and the patient does not experience an increase in symptoms from the increased compressive forces on the patellofemoral joint when it is positioned in flexion.
3. The clinician is at the patient's lower leg, facing the patellofemoral joint.
4. The mobilizing/manipulating hand is positioned with either the web space or the heel of the hand on the inferior surface of the patella.
5. The guiding hand is positioned over the mobilizing/manipulating hand.

Procedure
1. The mobilizing/manipulating hand glides the patella in a superior direction, taking care to avoid compressing the patella into the femur.
2. The guiding hand controls the position of the mobilizing/manipulating hand (see Figure 7-10).

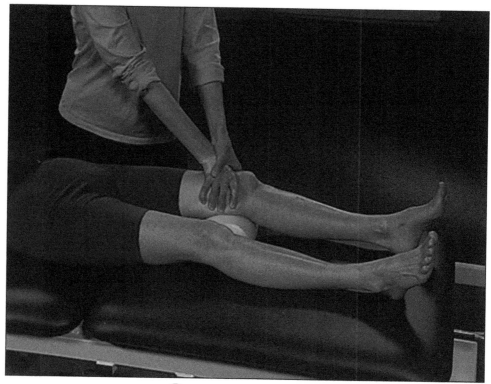

▶ **Figure 7-11** Inferior glide.

Inferior Glide (Figure 7-11, Video 7-11)

Purpose
- To examine for patellofemoral joint impairment
- To increase accessory motion into patellofemoral joint inferior glide
- To increase range of motion at the patellofemoral joint
- To decrease pain

Positioning
1. The patient is supine.
2. The knee is positioned in full extension or slight flexion if conservative techniques are indicated or approximating restricted range of motion if more aggressive techniques are indicated and the patient does not experience an increase in symptoms from the increased compressive forces on the patellofemoral joint when it is positioned in flexion.
3. The clinician is at the patient's hip, facing the patellofemoral joint.
4. The mobilizing/manipulating hand is positioned with either the web space or the heel of the hand on the superior surface of the patella.
5. The guiding hand is positioned over the mobilizing/manipulating hand.

Procedure
1. The mobilizing/manipulating hand glides the patella in an inferior direction, taking care to avoid compressing the patella into the femur as much as possible by attempting to position the web space or the heel of the hand under the patella before initiating the technique.
2. The guiding hand controls the position of the mobilizing/manipulating hand (see Figure 7-11).

Particulars
- This technique might be especially effective for increasing range of motion into knee joint flexion.

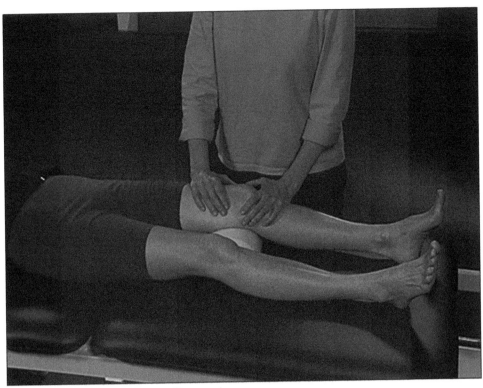

▶ Figure 7-12 Medial glide.

Medial Glide (Figure 7-12, Video 7-12)

Purpose
- To examine for patellofemoral joint impairment
- To increase accessory motion into patellofemoral joint medial glide
- To increase range of motion at the patellofemoral joint
- To decrease pain

Positioning
1. The patient is supine.
2. The knee is positioned in full extension or slight flexion if conservative techniques are indicated or approximating restricted range of motion if more aggressive techniques are indicated and the patient does not experience an increase in symptoms from the increased compressive forces on the patellofemoral joint when it is positioned in flexion.
3. The clinician is at the side of the patient's leg, facing the patellofemoral joint.
4. The stabilizing hand is positioned with the fingers on the medial surface of the distal femur.
5. The mobilizing hand or hands are positioned with both thumbs or the heel of one hand on the lateral surface of the patella.

Procedure
1. The stabilizing hand holds the femur in position.
2. The mobilizing/manipulating hand or hands glide the patella in a medial direction, taking care to avoid compressing the patella into the femur (see Figure 7-12).

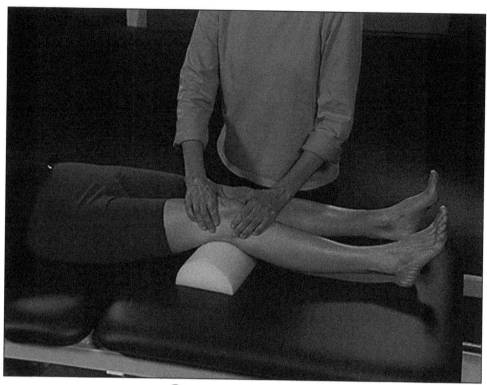

Figure 7-13 Lateral glide.

Lateral Glide (Figure 7-13, Video 7-13)

Purpose
- To examine for patellofemoral joint impairment
- To increase accessory motion into patellofemoral joint lateral glide
- To increase range of motion at the patellofemoral joint
- To decrease pain

Positioning
1. The patient is supine.
2. The knee is positioned in full extension or slight flexion if conservative techniques are indicated or approximating restricted range of motion if more aggressive techniques are indicated and the patient does not experience an increase in symptoms from the increased compressive forces on the patellofemoral joint when it is positioned in flexion.
3. The clinician is at the side of the patient's unaffected leg, facing the patellofemoral joint.
4. The stabilizing hand is positioned with the fingers on the lateral surface of the distal femur.
5. The mobilizing/manipulating hand or hands are positioned with both thumbs or the heel of one hand on the medial surface of the patella.

Procedure
1. The stabilizing hand holds the femur in position.
2. The mobilizing/manipulating hand or hands glide the patella in a lateral direction, taking care to avoid compressing the patella into the femur (see Figure 7-13).

Particulars
- The clinician should use caution in performing this technique because this motion might be hypermobile. If it is, performing a lateral glide mobilization/manipulation technique might cause the patella to dislocate.

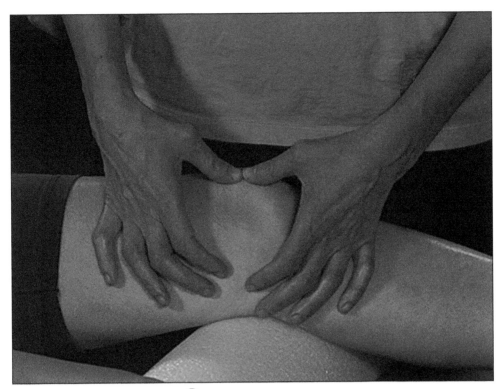

▶ **Figure 7-14** Medial tilt.

Medial Tilt (Figure 7-14, Video 7-14)

Purpose

- To examine for patellofemoral joint impairment
- To increase accessory motion into patellofemoral joint medial tilt
- To increase range of motion at the patellofemoral joint
- To decrease pain

Positioning

1. The patient is supine.
2. The knee is positioned in full extension or slight flexion.
3. The clinician is at the side of the patient's leg, facing the patellofemoral joint.
4. The stabilizing hands are positioned with the palm of the hands and fingers on the distal femur and proximal tibia.
5. The mobilizing/manipulating hand or hands are positioned with both thumbs on the medial surface of the patella.

Procedure

1. The stabilizing hand holds the femur in position.
2. The mobilizing/manipulating hand or hands glide the medial surface of the patella in a posterior direction, tilting the anterior surface of the patella toward the midline of the body (see Figure 7-14).

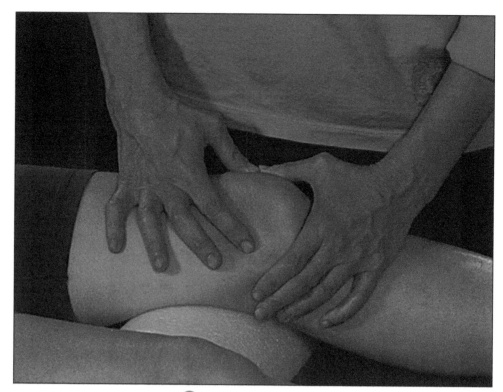

▶ **Figure 7-15** Lateral tilt.

Lateral Tilt (Figure 7-15, Video 7-15)

Purpose

- To examine for patellofemoral joint impairment
- To increase accessory motion into patellofemoral joint lateral tilt
- To increase range of motion at the patellofemoral joint
- To decrease pain

Positioning

1. The patient is supine.
2. The knee is positioned in full extension or slight flexion.
3. The clinician is at the side of the patient's leg, facing the patellofemoral joint.
4. The stabilizing hands are positioned with the palm of the hands and fingers on the distal femur and proximal tibia.
5. The mobilizing/manipulating hand or hands are positioned with both thumbs on the lateral surface of the patella.

Procedure

1. The stabilizing hand holds the femur in position.
2. The mobilizing/manipulating hand or hands glide the lateral surface of the patella in a posterior direction, tilting the anterior surface of the patella away from the midline of the body (see Figure 7-15).

REFERENCES

1. French HP, Brennan A, White B, Cusack T. Manual therapy for osteoarthritis of the hip or knee—a systemic review. *Man Ther.* 2011;16:109-117.

2. Kaltenborn FM. *Manual Mobilization of the Joints: The Kaltenborn Method of Joint Examination and Treatment,* Vol I: The Extremities. 6th ed. Oslo, Norway: Norli; 2002.

3. Cyriax J. *Textbook of Orthopaedic Medicine,* Vol I: Diagnosis of Soft Tissue Lesions. 8th ed. London: Bailliere Tindall; 1982.

4. Brantingham JW, Bonnefin D, Perle SM, et al. Manipulative therapy for lower extremity conditions: update of a literature review. *J Manipulative Physiol Ther.* 2012;35:127-166.

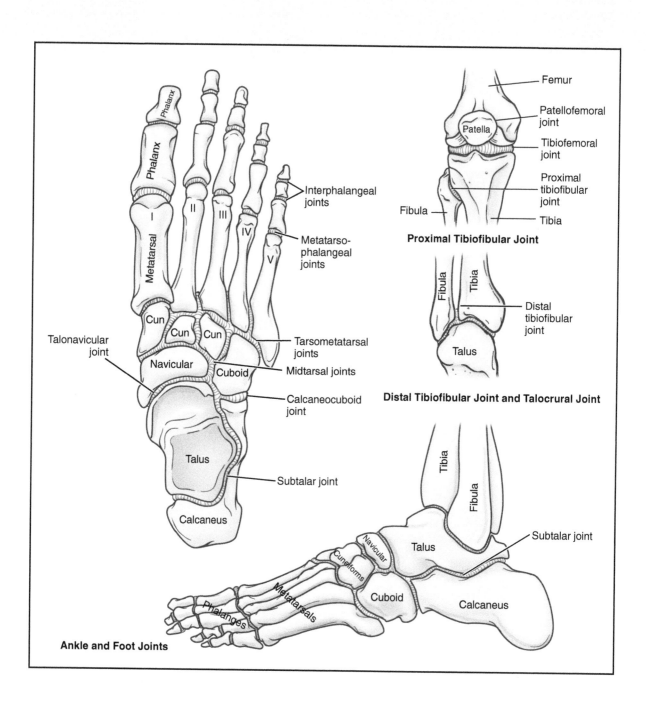

Interphalangeal joints

Metatarso-phalangeal joints

Talonavicular joint

Tarsometatarsal joints

Midtarsal joints

Calcaneocuboid joint

Subtalar joint

Phalanx

Phalanx

Phalanx

I

II

III

IV

V

Metatarsal

Cun

Cun

Cun

Navicular

Cuboid

Talus

Calcaneus

Proximal Tibiofibular Joint

Femur

Patellofemoral joint

Patella

Tibiofemoral joint

Proximal tibiofibular joint

Fibula

Tibia

Distal Tibiofibular Joint and Talocrural Joint

Fibula

Tibia

Distal tibiofibular joint

Talus

Tibia

Fibula

Navicular

Cuneiforms

Talus

Subtalar joint

Phalanges

Metatarsals

Cuboid

Calcaneus

Ankle and Foot Joints

CHAPTER 8

The Lower Leg, Ankle, and Foot

BASICS

Joints of the lower leg consist of the proximal and distal tibiofibular articulations. Motion at these articulations is minimal.

Ankle and foot motion are described as triplanar. The combined motions of dorsiflexion/abduction/eversion and plantar flexion/adduction/inversion occur together but to a different extent at each of the following joints in the ankle and foot: talocrural joint, subtalar joint, midtarsal joints, and metatarsophalangeal joints. These composite motions are called pronation and supination. These movements at the ankle and foot allow for a flexible base of support that accommodates to changes in tibial rotation and produces a smooth transition from supination to pronation and back to supination during the stance phase of gait.

Range of motion is considered functional in the talocrural and subtalar joints for most basic activities of daily living if 10 to 20 degrees of dorsiflexion is present, 20 to 30 degrees of plantar flexion is present, and 6 to 10 degrees of motion is present and equally divided between inversion/adduction and eversion/abduction. Approximately 65 to 70 degrees of extension at the first metatarsophalangeal joint is necessary for push-off during the end of the stance phase of gait. Slightly less than 65 degrees of extension is necessary for normal gait at the other metatarsophalangeal joints.

Anatomic terminology in the ankle and the foot is often inconsistent. Thus far, in this text, superior and inferior have referred to movement or positioning toward the head and foot, respectively. The exception to this rule is at the foot, where dorsal indicates movement or positioning toward the top of the foot (or toward the head) and plantar indicates movement or positioning toward the bottom of the foot. In this text, medial and lateral always indicate movement or positioning toward or away from the midline of the body, not the midline of the limb.

Proximal and Distal Tibiofibular Joints

The interosseous membrane connects the tibia and the fibula. Movement at the two joints is interrelated in a manner similar to that of the proximal and distal radioulnar joints of the forearm and likely affects movement at both the knee and ankle.

Talocrural Joint

The talocrural joint comprises the tibia and fibula and their articulation with the talus. Although triplanar motion occurs at this articulation, dorsiflexion and plantar flexion are the primary motions.

Subtalar Joint

Inversion and eversion are the primary motions occurring at the subtalar joint, which consists of the articulation between the talus and the calcaneus.

Midtarsal Joints

The midtarsal joints consist of the talonavicular and calcaneocuboid joints and the cuneiform articulations. Plantar flexion and dorsiflexion and inversion and eversion predominate at these joints.

Intermetatarsal Joints

The metatarsals move on one another, causing the transverse arch of the foot to increase and flatten. The axis for this motion is the second metatarsal.

Toe Joints

Toe flexion and extension occur at the metatarsophalangeal and interphalangeal joints. The metatarsophalangeal joints also are capable of moving into abduction and adduction, although these movements are not considered important for functional activities.

SPECIFIC PATHOLOGY AND LOWER LEG, ANKLE, AND FOOT JOINT MOBILIZATION/MANIPULATION

Lateral Ankle Sprains

A 2014 systematic review of eight articles[1] addressed the efficacy of joint mobilization/manipulation in patients with lateral ankle sprains. In relation to acute ankle sprains, the authors concluded that joint mobilization/manipulation decreased pain and increased range of motion short term. For subjects with subacute or chronic lateral ankle sprains, the investigators similarly concluded that mobilization/manipulation resulted in a reduction in pain and an improvement in range of motion, especially into dorsiflexion. Only one study included in the systematic review followed subjects long term. In this study, subjects who received talocrural joint distraction manipulations experienced greater improvements in pain, dorsiflexion range of motion, and function compared with a sham intervention.

In a second, 2012 systematic review, the authors reported specifically on the efficacy of thrust manipulation. They concluded that there was fair evidence to support manipulation and multi-modal interventions for the short term management of lateral ankle sprains, but only fair evidence for long term outcomes.[10]

These findings are similar to those outlined in a clinical practice guideline for ankle ligament sprains,[2] in which the authors recommended joint mobilization, specifically posterior glide talocrural mobilizations within the pain-free range of motion, to reduce swelling, improve pain-free ankle and foot mobility, and normalize gait for patients with acute ankle sprains. These recommendations were based on moderate evidence. In the subacute and chronic stages of injury, mobilization and manipulation, including mobilization with movement, were recommended based on strong evidence to improve dorsiflexion range of motion, proprioception, and weight-bearing tolerance.

The role of the tibiofibular joint in ankle sprains has been a subject of debate. Results of one early study suggested that a tibiofibular positional fault was present in approximately one third of subjects with symptoms of a lateral ankle sprain.[3] Investigators theorized that a tibiofibular positional fault in which the fibula was positioned anterior on the tibia thereby placing slack on the anterior talofibular ligament, might be mimicking lateral ankle sprains in some patients. This hypotheses was not supported in a recent study in which there were no differences in range of motion, balance, or function in subjects who received a proximal or distal tibiofibular joint thrust manipulation to correct the positional fault compared with a control group.[4]

PROXIMAL TIBIOFIBULAR JOINT

Osteokinematic motion:
  None
Ligaments:
  Posterior tibiofibular ligament
  Anterior tibiofibular ligament
Joint orientation:
  Tibia: lateral, posterior, inferior
  Fibula: medial, anterior, superior
Concave joint surface:
  Fibula
Type of joint:
  Synovial
Resting position:
  0 degrees of plantar flexion[5]
Close-packed position:
  Full dorsiflexion[5]
Capsular pattern:
  Pain with contracting the "biceps" (presumably, the rectus femoris) muscle[6]

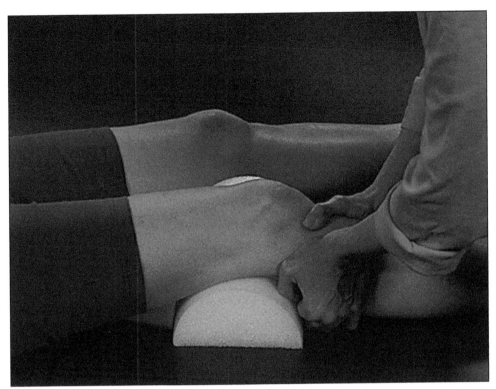

Figure 8-1 Posterior glide of the proximal fibula.

Posterior Glide of the Proximal Fibula (Figure 8-1, Video 8-1)

Purpose
- To examine for proximal tibiofibular joint impairment
- To increase accessory motion into proximal tibiofibular joint posterior glide
- To decrease pain

Positioning
1. The patient is supine with the knee supported by a small pillow.
2. The proximal tibiofibular joint is positioned in the resting position.
3. The clinician is at the side of the patient's leg, facing the patient's knee.
4. The stabilizing hand grips the proximal tibia from the medial and posterior side.
5. The mobilizing/manipulating hand is positioned with the heel of the hand on the anterior surface of the fibular head, taking care to avoid contact with the common fibular nerve.

Procedure
1. The stabilizing hand holds the tibia in position.
2. The mobilizing/manipulating hand glides the proximal fibula in a posterior direction (see Figure 8-1).

Particulars
- This technique might be effective in correcting a proximal tibiofibular joint positional fault.

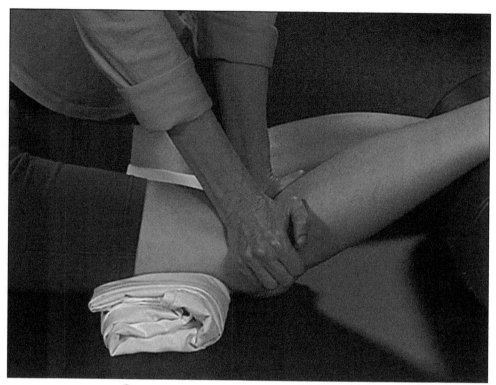

▶ **Figure 8-2** Anterior glide of the proximal fibula.

Anterior Glide of the Proximal Fibula (Figure 8-2, Video 8-2)
Purpose
- To examine for proximal tibiofibular joint impairment
- To increase accessory motion into proximal tibiofibular joint anterior glide
- To decrease pain

Positioning
1. The patient is prone with the foot supported by a pillow and a towel roll under the distal thigh to protect the patel-lofemoral joint.
2. The proximal tibiofibular joint is positioned in the resting position.
3. The clinician is at the side of the patient's unaffected leg, facing the patient's knees.
4. The stabilizing hand grips the proximal tibia from the anterior and medial side.
5. The mobilizing/manipulating hand is positioned with the heel of the hand on the posterior surface of the fibular head, taking care to avoid contact with the common fibular nerve.

Procedure
1. The stabilizing hand holds the tibia in position.
2. The mobilizing/manipulating hand glides the proximal fibula in an anterior direction (see Figure 8-2).

Particulars
- This technique might be effective in correcting a proximal tibiofibular joint positional fault.

DISTAL TIBIOFIBULAR JOINT

Osteokinematic motion:
   None
Ligaments:
   Anterior tibiofibular ligament
   Posterior tibiofibular ligament
   Inferior transverse ligament
   Interosseous membrane
Joint orientation:
   Tibia: lateral, posterior
   Fibula: medial, anterior
Concave joint surface:
   Tibia
Type of joint:
   Syndesmosis
Resting position:
   Not described by Kaltenborn
Close-packed position:
   Not described by Kaltenborn[5]
Capsular pattern of restriction:
   Pain with performing a "springing" manipulation on the ankle[6]

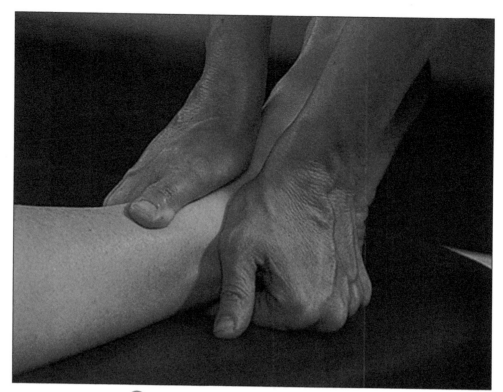

▶ **Figure 8-3** Posterior glide of the distal fibula.

Posterior Glide of the Distal Fibula (Figure 8-3, Video 8-3)
Purpose
- To examine for distal tibiofibular joint impairment
- To increase accessory motion into distal tibiofibular joint posterior glide
- To decrease pain

Positioning
1. The patient is supine.
2. The distal tibiofibular joint is positioned in a neutral position.
3. The clinician is at the foot of the treatment table, facing the patient's lower leg.
4. The stabilizing hand grips the distal tibia.
5. The mobilizing/manipulating hand is positioned with the heel of the hand over the anterior surface of the lateral malleolus (distal fibula).

Procedure
1. The stabilizing hand holds the tibia in position.
2. The mobilizing/manipulating hand glides the lateral malleolus (distal fibula) in a posterior direction (see Figure 8-3).

Particulars
- This technique might be effective in correcting a distal tibiofibular joint positional fault.

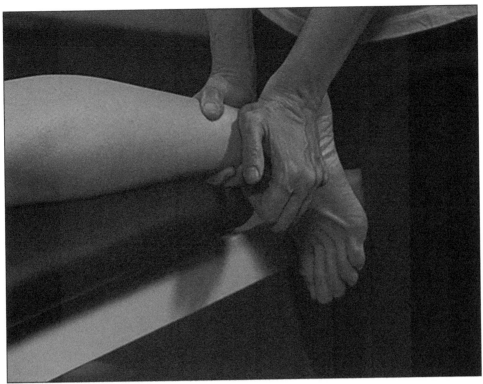

▶ **Figure 8-4** Anterior glide of the distal fibula.

Anterior Glide of the Distal Fibula (Figure 8-4, Video 8-4)

Purpose
- To examine for distal tibiofibular joint impairment
- To increase accessory motion into distal tibiofibular joint anterior glide
- To decrease pain

Positioning
1. The patient is prone.
2. The distal tibiofibular joint is positioned in a neutral position.
3. The clinician is at the foot of the treatment table, facing the patient's lower leg.
4. The stabilizing hand grips the distal tibia.
5. The mobilizing/manipulating hand is positioned with the heel of the hand over the posterior surface of the lateral malleolus (distal fibula).

Procedure
1. The stabilizing hand holds the tibia in position.
2. The mobilizing/manipulating hand glides the lateral malleolus (distal fibula) in an anterior direction (see Figure 8-4).

Particulars
- This technique might be effective in correcting a distal tibiofibular joint positional fault.

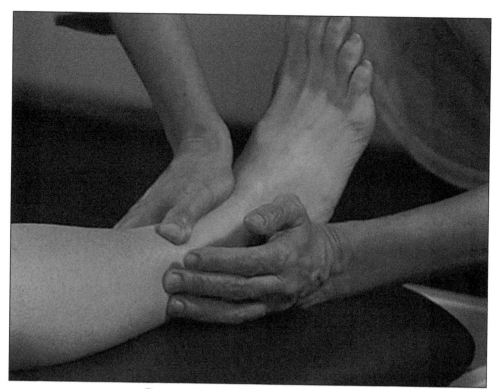

▶ **Figure 8-5** Superior glide of the fibula.

Superior Glide of the Fibula (Figure 8-5, Video 8-5)

Purpose
- To examine for impairment at the tibiofibular joints
- To increase accessory motion into tibiofibular joint superior glide
- To decrease pain

Positioning
1. The patient is supine.
2. The tibiofibular joints are positioned in a neutral position.
3. The clinician is at the foot of the treatment table, facing the patient's lower leg.
4. The stabilizing hand grips the distal tibia.
5. The mobilizing/manipulating hand is positioned with the heel of the hand on the inferior surface of the lateral malleolus (distal fibula).

Procedure
1. The stabilizing hand holds the tibia in position.
2. The mobilizing/manipulating hand glides the fibula in a superior direction (see Figure 8-5).

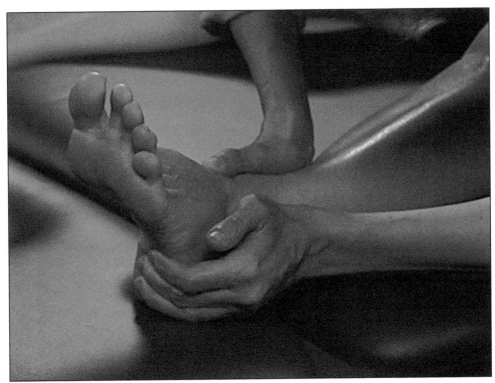

Figure 8-6 Inferior glide of the fibula.

Inferior Glide of the Fibula (Figure 8-6, Video 8-6)

Purpose
- To examine for impairment at the tibiofibular joints
- To increase accessory motion into tibiofibular joint inferior glide
- To decrease pain

Positioning
1. The patient is supine.
2. The tibiofibular joints are positioned in a neutral position.
3. The clinician is at the side of the patient's leg, facing the patient's foot.
4. The stabilizing hand grips the distal tibia.
5. The mobilizing/manipulating hand is positioned with the heel of the hand on the superior surface of the lateral malleolus (distal fibula).

Procedure
1. The stabilizing hand holds the tibia in position.
2. The mobilizing/manipulating hand glides the fibula in an inferior direction (see Figure 8-6).

TALOCRURAL JOINT

Osteokinematic motions:

    Dorsiflexion/plantar flexion

    Inversion/eversion

    Abduction/adduction

Ligaments:

    Medial collateral ligament/deltoid ligament (anterior tibiotalar, posterior tibiotalar, tibiocalcaneal, tibionavicular)

    Lateral collateral ligament (anterior talofibular, posterior talofibular, calcaneofibular)

Joint orientation:

    Tibia: inferior, lateral

    Fibula: medial

    Talus: superior, medial, lateral

Concave joint surface:

    Tibia and fibula

Type of joint:

    Synovial

Resting position:

    10 degrees plantar flexion and midway between inversion and eversion[5]

Close-packed position:

    Full dorsiflexion[5]

Capsular pattern of restriction:

    If the calf muscles are not tight, plantar flexion is more limited than dorsiflexion, whereas if the calf muscles are tight, the capsular pattern is simply limitation into plantar flexion[6]

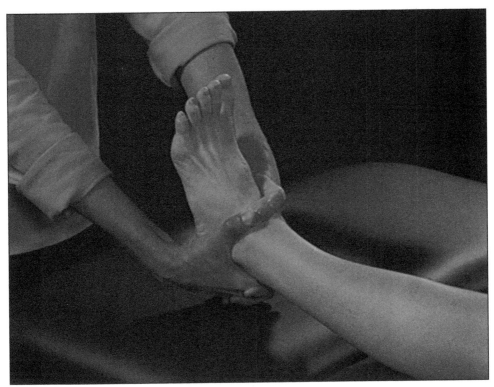

Figure 8-7 Distraction.

Distraction (Figure 8-7, Video 8-7)

Purpose
- To examine for talocrural joint impairment
- To increase accessory motion into talocrural joint distraction
- To increase range of motion at the talocrural joint
- To decrease pain

Positioning
1. The patient is supine with the knee in extension.
2. The talocrural joint is positioned in the resting position if conservative techniques are indicated or approximating restricted range of motion if more aggressive techniques are indicated.
3. The clinician is at the foot of the treatment table, facing the patient's foot.
4. Both hands grip the proximal talus with fingers intertwined.
5. The clinician's arms are lined up parallel to the patient's leg.

Procedure
1. Both hands move the talus in a direction perpendicular to the tibia and fibula joint surfaces as the clinician leans away from the joint (see Figure 8-7).

Particulars
- It is important to screen for tibiofemoral joint impairments before performing this technique.
- This technique is commonly performed using a grade V manipulation.

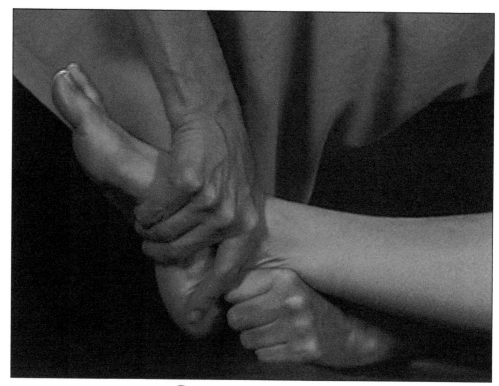

▶ **Figure 8-8** Posterior glide.

Posterior Glide (Figure 8-8, Video 8-8)

Purpose
- To examine for talocrural joint impairment
- To increase accessory motion into talocrural joint posterior glide
- To increase range of motion at the talocrural joint
- To decrease pain

Positioning
1. The patient is supine with the foot positioned over the edge of the treatment table.
2. The talocrural joint is positioned in the resting position if more conservative techniques are indicated or approximating restricted range of motion if more aggressive techniques are indicated.
3. The clinician is at the foot of the treatment table, facing the patient's foot.
4. The stabilizing hand grips the posterior surface of the distal lower leg at the malleoli.
5. The mobilizing/manipulating hand grips the talus at the anterior surface.

Procedure
1. The clinician applies a grade I traction to the joint.
2. The stabilizing hand holds the distal lower leg in position.
3. The mobilizing/manipulating hand glides the talus in a posterior direction (see Figure 8-8).

Particulars
- This technique might be especially effective for increasing range of motion into ankle joint dorsiflexion.

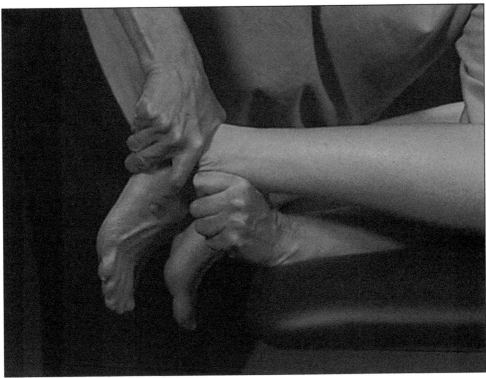

Figure 8-9 Anterior glide of the talus on the tibia and fibula: first technique.

Anterior Glide of the Talus on the Tibia and Fibula: First Technique (Figure 8-9, Video 8-9)

Purpose
- To examine for talocrural joint impairment
- To increase accessory motion into talocrural joint anterior glide
- To increase range of motion at the talocrural joint
- To decrease pain

Positioning
1. The patient is prone with the foot positioned off the edge of the treatment table.
2. The talocrural joint is positioned in the resting position if conservative techniques are indicated or approximating restricted range of motion if more aggressive techniques are indicated.
3. The clinician is at the foot of the treatment table, facing the patient's foot.
4. The stabilizing hand grips the anterior surface of the distal lower leg at the malleoli.
5. The mobilizing/manipulating hand grips the talus at the posterior surface if the ankle is in the resting position or the calcaneus at the posterior surface if the foot is in too much plantar flexion to allow contact with the talus.

Procedure
1. The clinician applies a grade I traction to the joint.
2. The stabilizing hand holds the distal lower leg in position.
3. The mobilizing/manipulating hand glides the talus in an anterior direction, either directly or through the calcaneus (see Figure 8-9).

Particulars
- This technique might be especially effective for increasing range of motion into ankle joint plantar flexion.

Anterior Glide of the Talus on the Tibia and Fibula: Second Technique (Figure 8-10, Video 8-10)

Purpose

- To examine for talocrural joint impairment
- To increase accessory motion into talocrural joint anterior glide
- To increase range of motion at the talocrural joint
- To decrease pain

Positioning

1. The patient is supine.
2. The talocrural joint is positioned in the resting position if more conservative techniques are indicated or approximating restricted range of motion if more aggressive techniques are indicated.
3. The clinician is at the foot of the treatment table, facing the patient's foot.
4. The stabilizing hand grips the talus at the posterior surface.
5. The mobilizing/manipulating hand grips the anterior surface of the distal lower leg at the malleoli.

Procedure

1. The clinician applies a grade I traction to the joint.
2. The stabilizing hand holds the talus in position.
3. The mobilizing/manipulating hand glides the tibia and fibula in a posterior direction, thereby imparting an anterior force to the talus on the tibia and fibula (see Figure 8-10).

Particulars

- This technique might be especially effective for increasing range of motion into ankle joint plantar flexion.
- When approximating the restricted range of motion into plantar flexion, the clinician stabilizes the calcaneus, thereby indirectly imparting a stabilizing force to the talus.

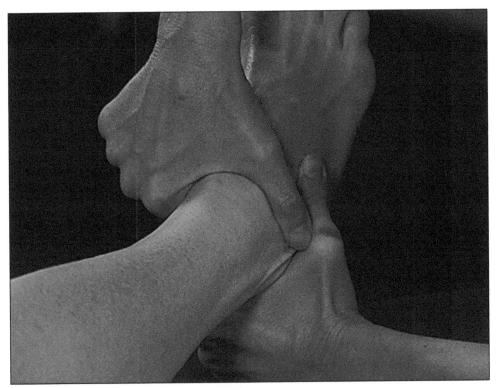

Figure 8-10 Anterior glide of the talus on the tibia and fibula: second technique.

Anterior Glide of the Talus Mobilization with Movement (Figure 8-11, Video 8-11)

Purpose
- To increase pain-free range of motion into ankle plantar flexion
- To decrease pain with ankle plantar flexion

Positioning
1. The patient is supine with the knee flexed to 90 degrees, the calcaneus on the treatment table, and the ankle joint in neutral.
2. The clinician stands at the foot of the treatment table, facing the foot being mobilized.
3. The clinician places the palm or web space of one hand on the anterior surface of the distal tibia and fibula and the web space of the other hand on the anterior surface of the talus.

Procedure
1. The clinician glides the tibia and fibula in a posterior direction.
2. While holding this position, the clinician then rolls/glides the talus in an anterior and inferior direction. This mobilization force is similar to performing an anterior draw test (see Figure 8-11).

Particulars
- This mobilization with movement technique is unique in that it is a passive range-of-motion technique—the patient will have difficult actively plantarflexing the ankle if the technique is being performed correctly.
- Adjustment of the glide out of the sagittal plane may be necessary at times to increase range of motion.
- This technique are indicated only if they can be performed without reproducing the patient's pain/symptoms.
- This technique should result in an immediate increase in pain-free range of motion into plantar flexion.
- If effective (the technique results in an immediate increase in range of motion and/or decrease in pain), this technique should be repeated (~3 sets of 10).

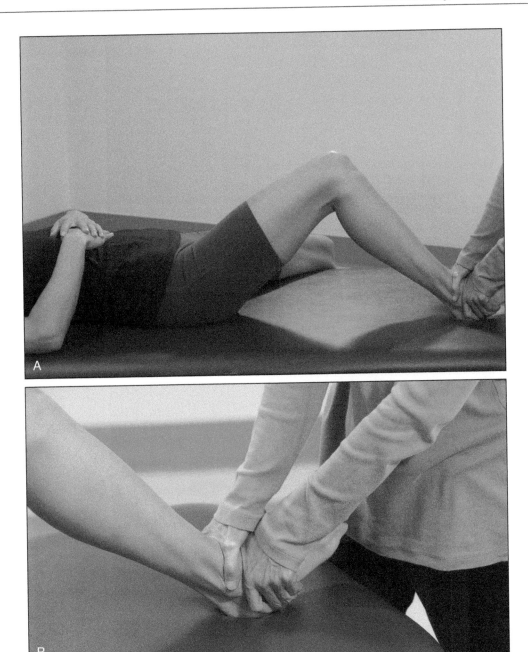

Figure 8-11 **A** and **B,** Anterior glide of the talus mobilization with movement.

Anterior Glide of the Tibia and Fibula on the Talus Mobilization with Movement (Figure 8-12, Video 8-12)

Purpose
- To increase pain-free range of motion into ankle dorsiflexion
- To decrease pain with ankle dorsiflexion

Positioning
1. The patient is standing with the knee bent and the plantar surface of the foot on a chair.
2. The clinician is positioned kneeling in front of the patient. The clinician wraps a mobilization strap around the patient's distal tibia and fibula approximately 2-3″ above the insertion of the Achilles tendon and the clinician's hips such that the belt forms a 90 degree angle with the lower leg.
3. The clinician's mobilizing hand is positioned with the web space around the anterior talus.

Procedure
1. The clinician holds the talus in position.
2. While the clinician holds the talus in position, the patient slowly flexes the knee, thereby dorsiflexing the ankle.
3. While the patient flexes the knee, the clinician guides the movement of the tibia and fibula in an anterior direction by leaning back on the mobilization strap, imparting an anterior glide to the tibia and fibula on the talus.
4. The clinician maintains the talus in position while the patient moves the leg to the starting position.
5. The clinician continually adjusts his or her own position in relation to the patient's position to maintain the joint mobilization force during joint movement (see Figure 8-12).

Particulars
- This technique are indicated only if they can be performed without reproducing the patient's pain/symptoms.
- The patient may need to move out of the sagittal slightly, e.g., ask the patient to angle toward the clinician's left or right shoulder to ensure pain-free execution of the technique.
- This technique should result in an immediate increase in pain-free range of motion into dorsiflexion.
- If effective (the technique results in an immediate increase in range of motion and/or decrease in pain), this technique should be repeated (~3 sets of 10).
- In three different studies in which subjects served as their own controls this technique has been shown to increase weight-bearing range of motion into dorsiflexion immediately after treatment in subjects with lateral ankle sprains,[7] subacute ankle sprains,[8] and recurrent ankle sprains,[9] respectively. In one of these studies,[8] the investigators reported no change in pressure or thermal pain threshold following treatment.

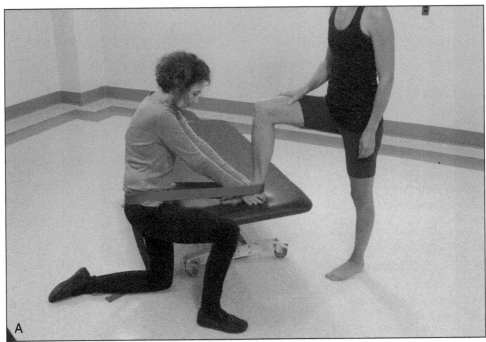

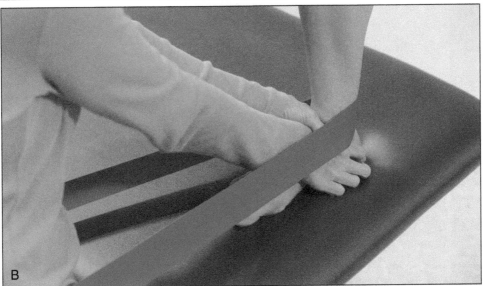

Figure 8-12 Anterior glide of the tibia on the talus mobilization with movement.

SUBTALAR JOINT

Osteokinematic motion:
   Inversion/eversion
Ligaments:
   Interosseous talocalcaneal ligament
   Cervical ligament
   Lateral talocalcaneal ligament
   Medial talocalcaneal ligament
Joint orientation:
   Talus: inferior, posterior, lateral
   Calcaneus: superior, anterior, medial
Concave joint surface:
   None, this is a plane joint
Type of joint:
   Synovial
Resting position:
   10 degrees of plantar flexion and midway between inversion and eversion[5]
Close-packed position:
   Full inversion[5]
Capsular pattern of restriction:
   Limitation in inversion[6]

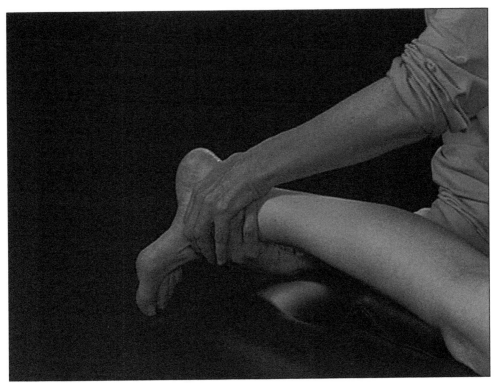

Figure 8-13 Distraction.

Distraction (Figure 8-13, Video 8-13)

Purpose
- To examine for subtalar joint impairment
- To increase accessory motion into subtalar joint distraction
- To increase range of motion at the subtalar joint
- To decrease pain

Positioning
1. The patient is prone with the foot off the treatment table.
2. The subtalar joint is positioned in the resting position if conservative techniques are indicated or approximating restricted range of motion if more aggressive techniques are indicated.
3. The clinician is at the side of the treatment table, facing the patient's foot.
4. The stabilizing hand grips the talus at the anterior surface with the web space.
5. The mobilizing/manipulating hand is positioned with the web space on the posterior and superior surface of the calcaneus and the thumb and index finger on the medial and lateral surface of the calcaneus.

Procedure
1. The stabilizing hand holds the talus in position.
2. The mobilizing/manipulating hand moves the calcaneus inferiorly in a direction perpendicular to the talocalcaneal joint surface (see Figure 8-13).

Particulars
- This technique is commonly performed using a grade V manipulation.

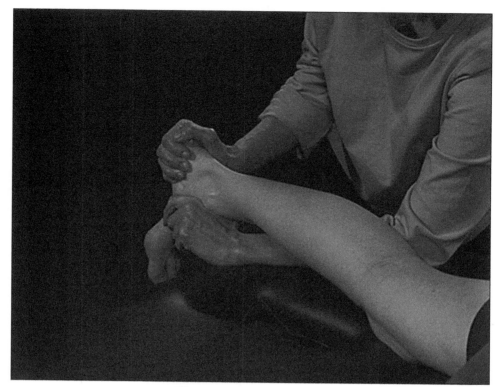

▶ **Figure 8-14** Medial glide.

Medial Glide (Figure 8-14, Video 8-14)

Purpose

- To examine for subtalar joint impairment
- To increase accessory motion into subtalar joint medial glide
- To increase range of motion at the subtalar joint
- To decrease pain

Positioning

1. The patient is prone with the foot off the treatment table.
2. The subtalar joint is positioned in the resting position if conservative techniques are indicated or approximating restricted range of motion if more aggressive techniques are indicated.
3. The clinician is at the side of the treatment table, facing the patient's foot.
4. The stabilizing hand grips the talus at the anterior and medial surface with the web space.
5. The mobilizing/manipulating hand grips the calcaneus with the heel of the hand on the lateral surface.

Procedure

1. The clinician applies a grade I traction to the joint.
2. The stabilizing hand holds the talus in position.
3. The mobilizing/manipulating hand glides the calcaneus in a medial direction (see Figure 8-14).

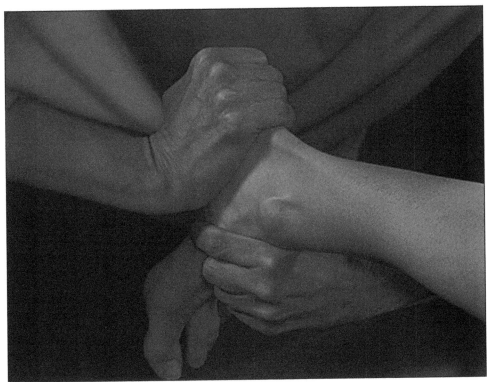

▶ **Figure 8-15** Lateral glide.

Lateral Glide (Figure 8-15, Video 8-15)

Purpose
- To examine for subtalar joint impairment
- To increase accessory motion into subtalar joint lateral glide
- To increase range of motion at the subtalar joint
- To decrease pain

Positioning
1. The patient is prone with the foot off the treatment table.
2. The subtalar joint is positioned in the resting position if conservative techniques are indicated or approximating restricted range of motion if more aggressive techniques are indicated.
3. The clinician is at the side of the treatment table, facing the patient's foot.
4. The stabilizing hand grips the talus at the anterior and lateral surface with the web space.
5. The mobilizing/manipulating hand grips the calcaneus with the heel of the hand on the medial surface.

Procedure
1. The clinician applies a grade I traction to the joint.
2. The stabilizing hand holds the talus in position.
3. The mobilizing/manipulating hand glides the calcaneus in a lateral direction (see Figure 8-15).

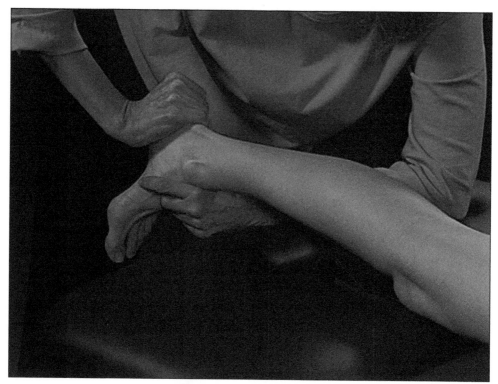

▶ **Figure 8-16** Medial tilt.

Medial Tilt (Figure 8-16, Video 8-16)

Purpose
- To examine for subtalar joint impairment
- To increase accessory motion into subtalar joint medial tilt
- To increase range of motion at the subtalar joint
- To decrease pain

Positioning
1. The patient is prone with the foot off the treatment table.
2. The subtalar joint is positioned in the resting position.
3. The clinician is at the side of the treatment table, facing the patient's foot.
4. The stabilizing hand grips the talus at the anterior and lateral surface with the web space.
5. The mobilizing/manipulating hand grips the calcaneus with the heel of the hand on the medial surface.

Procedure
1. The stabilizing hand holds the talus in position.
2. The mobilizing/manipulating hand tilts the calcaneus in a valgus direction (see Figure 8-16).

Particulars
- This technique might be especially effective for increasing range of motion into subtalar joint eversion.

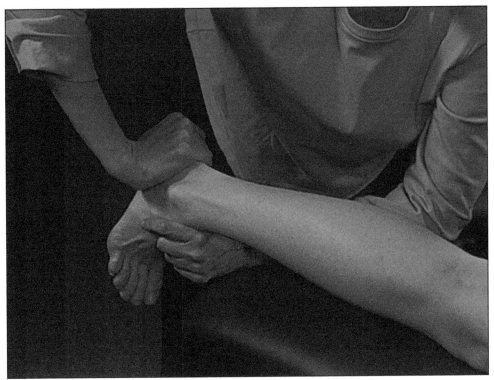

Figure 8-17 Lateral tilt.

Lateral Tilt (Figure 8-17, Video 8-17)

Purpose
- To examine for subtalar joint impairment
- To increase accessory motion into subtalar joint lateral tilt
- To increase range of motion at the subtalar joint
- To decrease pain

Positioning
1. The patient is prone with the foot off the treatment table.
2. The subtalar joint is positioned in the resting position.
3. The clinician is at the side of the treatment table, facing the patient's foot.
4. The stabilizing hand grips the talus at the anterior and medial surface with the web space.
5. The mobilizing/manipulating hand grips the calcaneus with the heel of the hand on the lateral surface.

Procedure
1. The stabilizing hand holds the talus in position.
2. The mobilizing/manipulating hand tilts the calcaneus in a varus direction (see Figure 8-17).

Particulars
- This technique might be especially effective for increasing range of motion into subtalar joint inversion.

MIDTARSAL JOINTS

This section discusses the talonavicular and calcaneocuboid joints.

Osteokinematic motions:
  Dorsiflexion/plantar flexion
  Inversion/eversion
Ligaments:
  Long plantar ligament
  Plantar calcaneonavicular ligament
  Bifurcate ligament
Joint orientation: talonavicular joint
  Talus: anterior, lateral
  Navicular: posterior, medial
Joint orientation: calcaneocuboid joint
  Calcaneus: anterior, medial
  Cuboid: posterior, lateral
Concave joint surface:
  None, these are plane joints
Type of joint:
  Synovial
Resting position:
  10 degrees plantar flexion and midway between inversion and eversion[5]
Close-packed position:
  Full inversion[5]
Capsular pattern of restriction:
  Limitations in dorsiflexion, plantar flexion, adduction, and inversion[6]

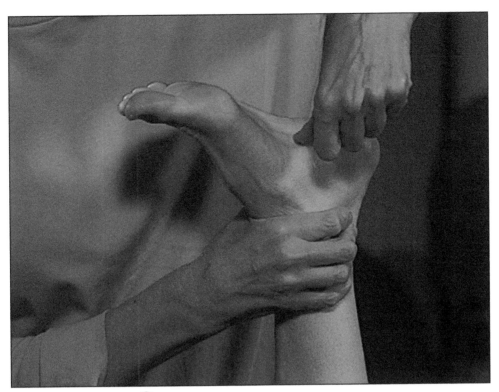

Figure 8-18 Dorsal glide of the navicular.

Dorsal Glide of the Navicular (Figure 8-18, Video 8-18)

Purpose
- To examine for talonavicular joint impairment
- To increase accessory motion into talonavicular dorsal glide
- To increase range of motion at the midtarsal joint
- To decrease pain

Positioning
1. The patient is prone with the knee flexed to 90 degrees.
2. The talonavicular joint is positioned in the resting position.
3. The clinician is facing the plantar surface of the patient's foot.
4. The stabilizing hand grips the talus at the dorsal surface with the web space.
5. The mobilizing/manipulating hand grips the navicular with the thumb on the plantar surface and the index finger on the dorsal surface.

Procedure
1. The clinician applies a grade I traction to the joint.
2. The stabilizing hand holds the talus in position.
3. The mobilizing/manipulating hand glides the navicular in a dorsal direction (see Figure 8-18).

Particulars
- The clinician should use caution in performing this technique because this motion might be hypermobile.

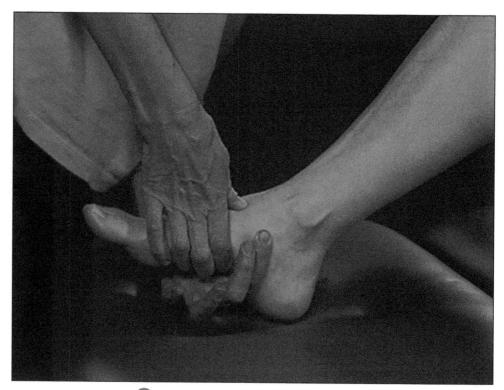

Figure 8-19 Plantar glide of the navicular.

Plantar Glide of the Navicular (Figure 8-19, Video 8-19)
Purpose
- To examine for talonavicular joint impairment
- To increase accessory motion into talonavicular plantar glide
- To increase range of motion at the midtarsal joint
- To decrease pain

Positioning
1. The patient is supine.
2. The talonavicular joint is positioned in the resting position.
3. The clinician is facing the dorsal surface of the patient's foot.
4. The stabilizing hand grips the talus at the plantar surface with the web space.
5. The mobilizing/manipulating hand grips the navicular with the thumb on the dorsal surface and the index finger on the plantar surface.

Procedure
1. The clinician applies a grade I traction to the joint.
2. The stabilizing hand holds the talus in position.
3. The mobilizing/manipulating hand glides the navicular in a plantar direction (see Figure 8-19).

Particulars
- The clinician should use caution in performing this technique because this motion might be hypermobile.

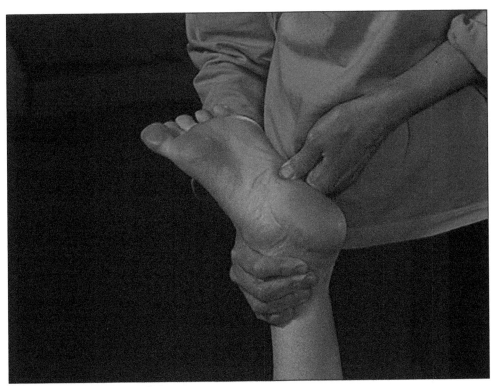

▶ **Figure 8-20** Dorsal glide of the cuboid.

Dorsal Glide of the Cuboid (Figure 8-20, Video 8-20)

Purpose
- To examine for calcaneocuboid joint impairment
- To increase accessory motion into calcaneocuboid dorsal glide
- To increase range of motion at the midtarsal joint
- To decrease pain

Positioning
1. The patient is prone with the knee flexed to 90 degrees.
2. The calcaneocuboid joint is positioned in the resting position.
3. The clinician is facing the plantar surface of the patient's foot.
4. The stabilizing hand grips the talus at the dorsal surface with the web space, indirectly stabilizing the calcaneus.
5. The mobilizing/manipulating hand grips the cuboid with the thumb on the plantar surface and the index finger on the dorsal surface.

Procedure
1. The clinician applies a grade I traction to the joint.
2. The stabilizing hand holds the calcaneus in position.
3. The mobilizing/manipulating hand glides the cuboid in a dorsal direction (see Figure 8-20).

Particulars
- The clinician should use caution in performing this technique because this motion might be hypermobile.
- This technique might be effective in correcting a calcaneocuboid joint positional fault.

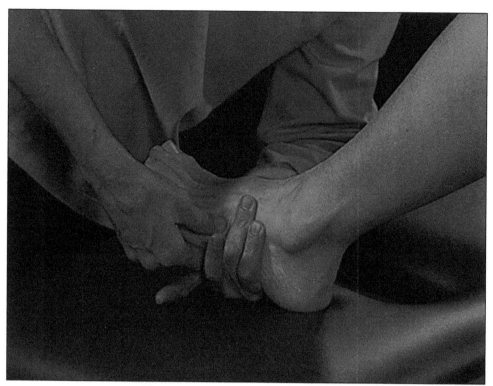

▶ **Figure 8-21** Plantar glide of the cuboid.

Plantar Glide of the Cuboid (Figure 8-21, Video 8-21)

Purpose
- To examine for calcaneocuboid joint impairment
- To increase accessory motion into calcaneocuboid plantar glide
- To increase range of motion at the midtarsal joint
- To decrease pain

Positioning
1. The patient is supine.
2. The calcaneocuboid joint is positioned in the resting position.
3. The clinician is facing the dorsal surface of the patient's foot.
4. The stabilizing hand grips the calcaneus at the plantar surface with the web space.
5. The mobilizing/manipulating hand grips the cuboid with the thumb on the dorsal surface and the index finger on the plantar surface.

Procedure
1. The clinician applies a grade I traction to the joint.
2. The stabilizing hand holds the calcaneus in position.
3. The mobilizing/manipulating hand glides the cuboid in a plantar direction (see Figure 8-21).

Particulars
- The clinician should use caution in performing this technique because this motion might be hypermobile.

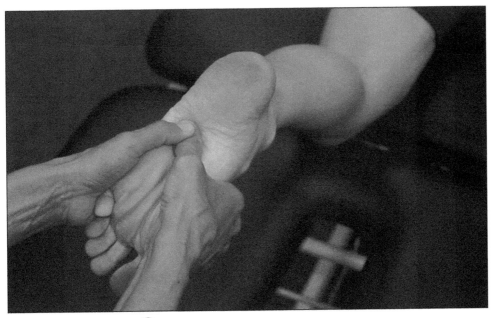

Figure 8-22 Cuboid whip/manipulation.

Cuboid Whip/Manipulation (Figure 8-22, Video 8-22)

Purpose
- To increase accessory motion into calcaneocuboid dorsal glide
- To increase range of motion at the midtarsal joint
- To decrease pain

Positioning
1. The patient is prone with the knee flexed to about 75 degrees and the ankle in slight plantar flexion.
2. The clinician is facing the plantar surface of the patient's foot.
3. The manipulating hand is positioned with the thumb over the thumb of the guiding hand and the fingers on the dorsal surface of the foot distal to the cuboid.
4. The guiding hand is positioned with the thumb over the plantar surface of the cuboid and the fingers interlacing the fingers of the manipulating hand on the dorsal surface of the foot.

Procedure
1. The manipulating hand glides the cuboid in a dorsal direction while moving the ankle slightly into plantar flexion and the knee slightly into extension.
2. The guiding hand supports the manipulating hand (see Figure 8-22).

Particulars
- The clinician should use caution in performing this technique because this motion might be hypermobile.
- This technique should be performed using grade V manipulations.
- This technique might be effective in correcting a calcaneocuboid joint positional fault,[11] also known as 'cuboid syndrome'.

INTERMETATARSAL JOINTS ONE THROUGH FIVE

Osteokinematic motion:
    Increasing/flattening the transverse arch of the foot
Ligaments:
    Transverse metatarsal ligaments
Joint orientation:
    Medial metatarsal: lateral
    Lateral metatarsal: medial
Concave joint surface:
    None, this is a plane joint
Type of joint:
    Synarthrosis
Resting position:
    Unknown[5]
Close-packed position:
    Unknown[5]
Capsular pattern of restriction:
    None, not a synovial joint

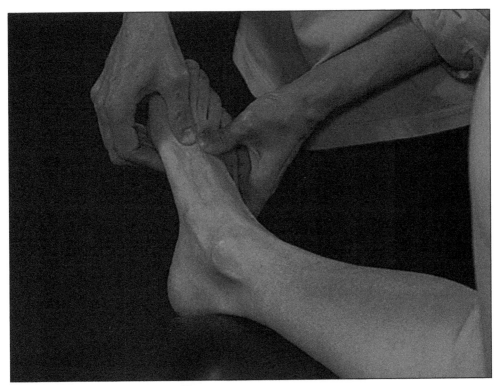

Figure 8-23 Dorsal glide.

Dorsal Glide (Figure 8-23, Video 8-23)

Purpose

- To examine for intermetatarsal joint impairment
- To increase accessory motion into intermetatarsal joint dorsal glide, using the second metatarsal as a reference point
- To increase range of motion at the intermetatarsal joints
- To decrease pain

Positioning

1. The patient is supine.
2. The foot is positioned in a neutral position.
3. The clinician is facing the dorsal surface of the patient's foot.
4. The stabilizing hand grips the midshaft of one metatarsal with the thumb on the dorsal surface and the index finger on the plantar surface.
5. The mobilizing/manipulating hand grips the midshaft of the other metatarsal with the thumb on the dorsal surface and the index finger on the plantar surface.

Procedure

1. The clinician applies a grade I traction to the joint.
2. The stabilizing hand holds one metatarsal in position.
3. The mobilizing/manipulating hand glides the first metatarsal in a dorsal direction on the second metatarsal, the third metatarsal in a dorsal direction on the second metatarsal, the fourth metatarsal in a dorsal direction on the third metatarsal, and the fifth metatarsal in a dorsal direction on the fourth metatarsal (see Figure 8-23).

Particulars

- This technique might be especially effective for increasing range of motion into flattening the transverse arch of the foot.

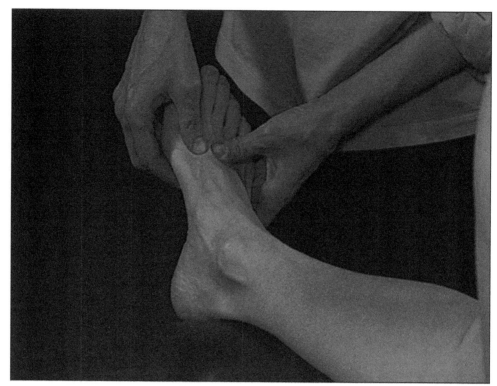

▶ **Figure 8-24** Plantar glide.

Plantar Glide (Figure 8-24, Video 8-24)
Purpose
- To examine for intermetatarsal joint impairment
- To increase accessory motion into intermetatarsal joint plantar glide, using the second metatarsal as a reference point
- To increase range of motion at the intermetatarsal joints
- To decrease pain

Positioning
1. The patient is supine.
2. The foot is positioned in a neutral position.
3. The clinician is facing the dorsal surface of the patient's foot.
4. The stabilizing hand grips the midshaft of one metatarsal with the thumb on the dorsal surface and the index finger on the plantar surface.
5. The mobilizing/manipulating hand grips the midshaft of the other metatarsal with the thumb on the dorsal surface and the index finger on the plantar surface.

Procedure
1. The clinician applies a grade I traction to the joint.
2. The stabilizing hand holds one metatarsal in position.
3. The mobilizing/manipulating hand glides the first metatarsal in a plantar direction on the second metatarsal, the third metatarsal in a plantar direction on the second metatarsal, the fourth metatarsal in a plantar direction on the third metatarsal, and the fifth metatarsal in a plantar direction on the fourth metatarsal (see Figure 8-24).

Particulars
- This technique might be especially effective for increasing range of motion into increasing the transverse arch of the foot.

METATARSOPHALANGEAL JOINTS

Osteokinematic motions:
   Flexion/extension
   Abduction/adduction
Ligaments:
   Plantar ligaments
   Collateral ligaments
Joint orientation:
   Metatarsals: anterior
   Phalanges: posterior
Concave joint surface:
   Proximal phalanx
Type of joint:
   Synovial
Resting position:
   10 degrees of extension[5]
Close-packed position:
   First metatarsophalangeal joint: full extension
   Second through fifth metatarsophalangeal joints: full flexion[5]
Capsular pattern of restriction:
   First metatarsophalangeal joint: marked limitation in extension and slight limitation in flexion
   Second through fifth metatarsophalangeal joints: variable, but flexion is generally more limited than extension[6]

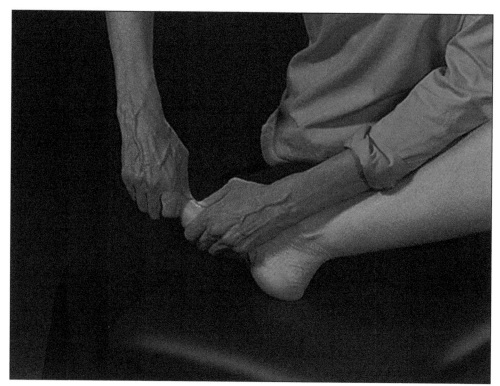

Figure 8-25 Distraction.

Distraction (Figure 8-25, Video 8-25)

Purpose

- To examine for metatarsophalangeal joint impairment
- To increase accessory motion into metatarsophalangeal joint distraction
- To increase range of motion at the metatarsophalangeal joints
- To decrease pain

Positioning

1. The patient is supine.
2. The metatarsophalangeal joint is positioned in the resting position if conservative techniques are indicated or approximating restricted range of motion if more aggressive techniques are indicated.
3. The clinician is facing the lateral surface of the patient's foot.
4. The stabilizing hand grips the head of the metatarsal with the thumb on the dorsal surface and the index finger on the plantar surface.
5. The mobilizing/manipulating hand grips the proximal end of the proximal phalanx with the thumb on the dorsal surface and the index finger on the plantar surface.

Procedure

1. The stabilizing hand holds the metatarsal in position.
2. The mobilizing/manipulating hand moves the proximal phalanx distally in a direction perpendicular to the joint surface of the proximal phalanx (see Figure 8-25).
3. The clinician could wear surgical gloves to reduce slippage against the patient's skin.

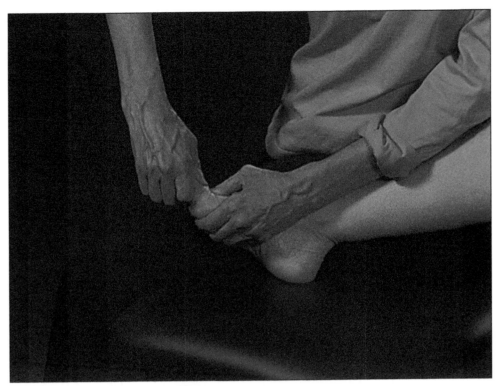

Figure 8-26 Dorsal glide.

Dorsal Glide (Figure 8-26, Video 8-26)

Purpose
- To examine for metatarsophalangeal joint impairment
- To increase accessory motion into metatarsophalangeal joint dorsal glide
- To increase range of motion at the metatarsophalangeal joint
- To decrease pain

Positioning
1. The patient is supine.
2. The metatarsophalangeal joint is positioned in the resting position if conservative techniques are indicated or approximating restricted range of motion if more aggressive techniques are indicated.
3. The clinician is facing the lateral surface of the patient's foot.
4. The stabilizing hand grips the head of the metatarsal with the thumb on the dorsal surface and the index finger on the plantar surface.
5. The mobilizing/manipulating hand grips the proximal end of the proximal phalanx with the thumb on the dorsal surface and the index finger on the plantar surface.

Procedure
1. The clinician applies a grade I traction to the joint.
2. The stabilizing hand holds the metatarsal in position.
3. The mobilizing/manipulating hand glides the proximal phalanx in a dorsal direction (see Figure 8-26).
4. The clinician could wear surgical gloves to reduce slippage against the patient's skin.

Particulars
- This technique might be especially effective for increasing range of motion into metatarsophalangeal joint extension.

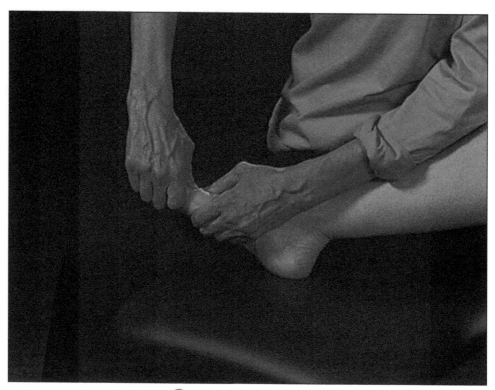

▶ **Figure 8-27** Plantar glide.

Plantar Glide (Figure 8-27, Video 8-27)

Purpose
- To examine for metatarsophalangeal joint impairment
- To increase accessory motion into metatarsophalangeal joint plantar glide
- To increase range of motion at the metatarsophalangeal joint
- To decrease pain

Positioning
1. The patient is supine.
2. The metatarsophalangeal joint is positioned in the resting position if conservative techniques are indicated or approximating restricted range of motion if more aggressive techniques are indicated.
3. The clinician is facing the lateral surface of the patient's foot.
4. The stabilizing hand grips the head of the metatarsal with the thumb on the dorsal surface and the index finger on the plantar surface.
5. The mobilizing/manipulating hand grips the proximal end of the proximal phalanx with the thumb on the dorsal surface and the index finger on the plantar surface.

Procedure
1. The clinician applies a grade I traction to the joint.
2. The stabilizing hand holds the metatarsal in position.
3. The mobilizing/manipulating hand glides the proximal phalanx in a plantar direction (see Figure 8-27).
4. The clinician could wear surgical gloves to reduce slippage against the patient's skin.

Particulars
- This technique might be especially effective for increasing range of motion into metatarsophalangeal joint flexion.

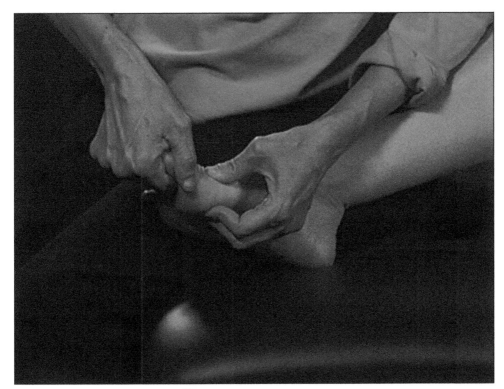

▶ **Figure 8-28** Medial glide.

Medial Glide (Figure 8-28, Video 8-28)

Purpose
- To examine for metatarsophalangeal joint impairment
- To increase accessory motion into metatarsophalangeal joint medial glide
- To increase range of motion at the metatarsophalangeal joint
- To decrease pain

Positioning
1. The patient is supine.
2. The metatarsophalangeal joint is positioned in the resting position if conservative techniques are indicated or approximating restricted range of motion if more aggressive techniques are indicated.
3. The clinician is facing the lateral surface of the patient's foot.
4. The stabilizing hand grips the head of the metatarsal with the thumb on the dorsal and medial surfaces and the index finger on the plantar and medial surfaces.
5. The mobilizing/manipulating hand grips the proximal end of the proximal phalanx on the lateral and medial surfaces.

Procedure
1. The clinician applies a grade I traction to the joint.
2. The stabilizing hand holds the metatarsal in position.
3. The mobilizing/manipulating hand glides the proximal phalanx in a medial direction (see Figure 8-28).
4. The clinician could wear surgical gloves to reduce slippage against the patient's skin.

Particulars
- This technique might be especially effective for increasing range of motion into metatarsophalangeal joint movement toward the midline of the body.

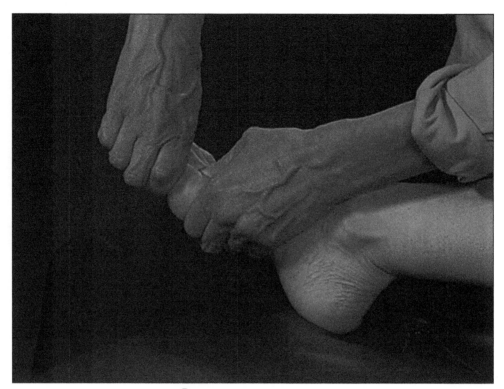

Figure 8-29 Lateral glide.

Lateral Glide (Figure 8-29, Video 8-29)

Purpose
- To examine for metatarsophalangeal joint impairment
- To increase accessory motion into metatarsophalangeal joint lateral glide
- To increase range of motion at the metatarsophalangeal joint
- To decrease pain

Positioning
1. The patient is supine.
2. The metatarsophalangeal joint is positioned in the resting position if conservative techniques are indicated or approximating restricted range of motion if more aggressive techniques are indicated.
3. The clinician is facing the lateral surface of the patient's foot.
4. The stabilizing hand grips the head of the metatarsal with the thumb on the dorsal and lateral surfaces and the index finger on the plantar and lateral surfaces.
5. The mobilizing/manipulating hand grips the proximal end of the proximal phalanx on the lateral and medial surfaces.

Procedure
1. The clinician applies a grade I traction to the joint.
2. The stabilizing hand holds the metatarsal in position.
3. The mobilizing/manipulating hand glides the proximal phalanx in a lateral direction (see Figure 8-29).
4. The clinician could wear surgical gloves to reduce slippage against the patient's skin.

Particulars
- This technique might be especially effective for increasing range of motion into metatarsophalangeal joint movement away from the midline of the body.

INTERPHALANGEAL JOINTS OF TOES ONE THROUGH FIVE

Osteokinematic motion:
  Flexion/extension
Ligaments:
  Medial collateral
  Lateral collateral
Joint orientation:
  Proximal phalanx: anterior (distal)
  Distal phalanx: posterior (proximal)
Concave joint surface:
  Distal phalanx
Type of joint:
  Synovial
Resting position:
  Slight flexion[5]
Close-packed position:
  Full extension[5]
Capsular pattern of restriction:
  Not described by Cyriax[6]

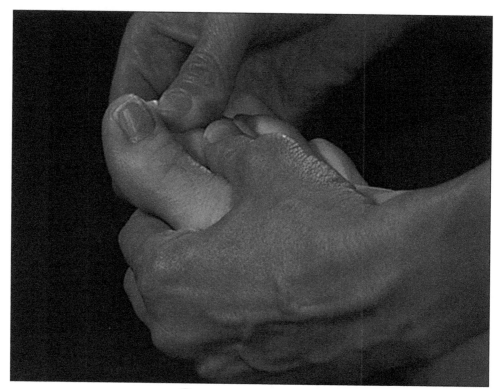

▶ **Figure 8-30** Distraction.

Distraction (Figure 8-30, Video 8-30)

Purpose
- To examine for toe interphalangeal joint impairment
- To increase accessory motion into toe interphalangeal joint distraction
- To increase range of motion at the toe interphalangeal joints
- To decrease pain

Positioning
1. The patient is supine.
2. The interphalangeal joint is positioned in the resting position if conservative techniques are indicated or approximating restricted range of motion if more aggressive techniques are indicated.
3. The clinician is facing the lateral of the patient's foot.
4. The stabilizing hand grips the distal end of the more proximal phalanx with the thumb on the dorsal surface and the index finger on the plantar surface.
5. The mobilizing/manipulating hand grips the proximal end of the more distal phalanx with the thumb on the dorsal surface and the index finger on the plantar surface.

Procedure
1. The stabilizing hand holds the more proximal phalanx in position.
2. The mobilizing/manipulating hand moves the more distal phalanx distally in a direction perpendicular to the joint surface of the distal phalanx (see Figure 8-30).
3. The clinician could wear surgical gloves to reduce slippage against the patient's skin.

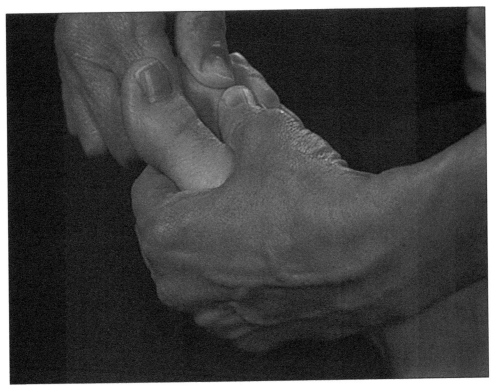

▶ **Figure 8-31** Dorsal glide.

Dorsal Glide (Figure 8-31, Video 8-31)

Purpose
- To examine for toe interphalangeal joint impairment
- To increase accessory motion into toe interphalangeal joint dorsal glide
- To increase range of motion at the interphalangeal joints
- To decrease pain

Positioning
1. The patient is supine.
2. The interphalangeal joint is positioned in the resting position if conservative techniques are indicated or approximating restricted range of motion if more aggressive techniques are indicated.
3. The clinician is facing the lateral surface of the patient's foot.
4. The stabilizing hand grips the distal end of the more proximal phalanx with the thumb on the dorsal surface and the index finger on the plantar surface.
5. The mobilizing/manipulating hand grips the proximal end of the more distal phalanx with the thumb on the dorsal surface and the index finger on the plantar surface.

Procedure
1. The clinician applies a grade I traction to the joint.
2. The stabilizing hand holds the more proximal phalanx in position.
3. The mobilizing/manipulating hand glides the more distal phalanx in a dorsal direction (see Figure 8-31).
4. The clinician could wear surgical gloves to reduce slippage against the patient's skin.

Particulars
- This technique might be especially effective for increasing range of motion into interphalangeal joint extension.

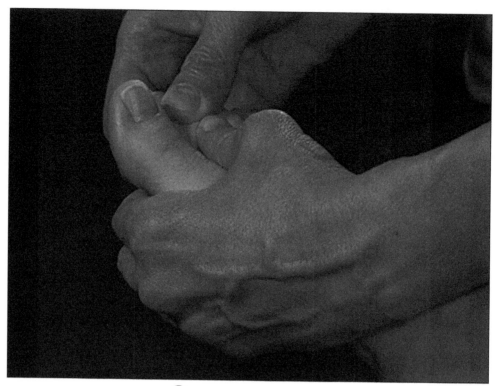

▶ **Figure 8-32** Plantar glide.

Plantar Glide (Figure 8-32, Video 8-32)

Purpose
- To examine for toe interphalangeal joint impairment
- To increase accessory motion into toe interphalangeal joint plantar glide
- To increase range of motion at the interphalangeal joints
- To decrease pain

Positioning
1. The patient is supine.
2. The interphalangeal joint is positioned in the resting position if conservative techniques are indicated or approximating restricted range of motion if more aggressive techniques are indicated.
3. The clinician is facing the lateral surface of the patient's foot.
4. The stabilizing hand grips the distal end of the more proximal phalanx with the thumb on the dorsal surface and the index finger on the plantar surface.
5. The mobilizing/manipulating hand grips the proximal end of the more distal phalanx with the thumb on the dorsal surface and the index finger on the plantar surface.

Procedure
1. The clinician applies a grade I traction to the joint.
2. The stabilizing hand holds the more proximal phalanx in position.
3. The mobilizing/manipulating hand glides the more distal phalanx in a plantar direction (see Figure 8-32).
4. The clinician could wear surgical gloves to reduce slippage against the patient's skin.

Particulars
- This technique might be especially effective for increasing range of motion into interphalangeal joint flexion.

REFERENCES

1. Loudon JK, Reiman MP, Sylvain J. The efficacy of manual joint mobilisation/manipulation in treatment of lateral ankle sprains: a systematic review. *Br J Sports Med*. 2014;48:365-370.

2. Martin RL, Davenport TE, Paulseth S, Wukich DK, Godges JJ. Ankle stability and movement coordination impairments: ankle ligament sprains clinical practice guidelines linked to the International Classification of Functioning, Disability and Health from the Orthopaedic Section of the American Physical Therapy Association. *J Orthop Sports Phys Ther*. 2013;43:A1-A40.

3. Kavanagh J. Is there a positional fault at the inferior tibiofibular joint in patients with acute or chronic ankle sprains compared to normals? *Man Ther*. 1999;4:19-24.

4. Beazell JR, Grindstaff TL, Sauer LD, et al. Effects of a proximal or distal tibiofibular joint manipulation on ankle range of motion and functional outcomes in individuals with chronic ankle instability. *J Orthop Sports Phys Ther*. 2012;42:125-1134.

5. Kaltenborn FM. *Manual Mobilization of the Joints: The Kaltenborn Method of Joint Examination and Treatment*, Vol I: The Extremities. 6th ed. Oslo, Norway: Norli; 2002.

6. Cyriax J. *Textbook of Orthopaedic Medicine*, Vol I: Diagnosis of Soft Tissue Lesions. 8th ed. London: Bailliere Tindall; 1982.

7. Reid A, Birmingham TB, Alcock G. Efficacy of mobilization with movement for patients with limited dorsiflexion after ankle sprain: a crossover trial. *Physiother Can*. 2007;59:166-172.

8. Collins N, Teys P, Vicenzino B. The initial effects of a Mulligan's mobilization with movement technique on dorsiflexion and pain in subacute ankle sprains. *Man Ther*. 2004;9:77-82.

9. Vicenzino B, Branjerdporn M, Teys P, Jordan K. Initial changes in posterior talar glide and dorsiflexion of the ankle after mobilization with movement in individuals with recurrent ankle sprain. *J Orthop Sports Phys Ther*. 2006;36:464-471.

10. Brantingham JW, Bonnefin D, Perle SM, et al. Manipulative therapy for lower extremity conditions: update of a literature review. *J Manipulative Physiol Ther*. 2012;35:127-166.

11. Jennings J, Davies GJ. Treatment of cuboid syndrome secondary to lateral ankle sprains: a case series. *J Orthop Sports Phys Therap*. 2005;35:409-415.

The Axillary Skeletal System

CHAPTER 9

Introduction to the Axillary Skeletal System

The axial skeletal system differs from the appendicular skeletal system in several important ways. One major difference is that movement in one joint is mechanically linked to movement at the same joint on the opposite side of the body. For example, with normal lower cervical forward bending, the facet joint surfaces on the left side and the right side of C2 glide up and forward simultaneously on the facet joint surfaces of C3. Additionally, most of the axial skeletal system shelters the spinal cord and spinal nerve roots, and contains multiple small muscles and joints that are located in close proximity to one another. These considerations render the axial skeletal system far more complex and more difficult to evaluate and treat than the appendicular skeletal system. The accessory motion examination and joint mobilization/manipulation intervention also differ in the axial skeletal system in several important ways and are described subsequently.

TERMINOLOGY

Vertebral motion at C2-3 through L5-S1 involves movement of the vertebral bodies and the paired facet joints. To differentiate movement of a vertebra from that of the articulation between two vertebrae, the latter is commonly referred to as a motion segment. By convention, movement at a motion segment is generally described as the movement of the more superior vertebral body on the more inferior vertebral body; this is the case regardless of which vertebra is actually moving. For example, if a patient is lying prone and lifts the left shoulder off the treatment table, T8 is rotating left on T9. Some clinicians simply would state that T8 is rotating left. If the prone patient lifts the right pelvis off the treatment table, motion is still described as T8 rotating left on T9, even though the actual movement is that of T9 rotating right on T8. The reference point for motion is the vertebral body and not the spinous processes, even though the clinician evaluating spinal movement from behind the patient observes or palpates the T8 spinous process moving to the right of midline when the patient moves into left rotation at T8 on T9.

In this description of joint movement, the assumption is made that vertebral motion occurs sequentially from the structure initiating the motion. In the case of the prone patient lifting the left shoulder off the treatment table, the assumption is that motion starts around T2 or T3 and when this motion segment has moved to end range, rotation begins at the adjacent motion segment below, and then sequentially moves down the spine one motion segment at a time.

COUPLED MOTION

Articular surfaces are not entirely congruent, and they are not consistently located in cardinal planes. Motion in one plane should therefore be accompanied by a specific pattern of motion in at least one other plane. This phenomenon is called coupled motion, and although it is most likely present in peripheral joints, principles of coupled motion are applied primarily in relation to the spine.

Many clinicians use information about specific patterns of spinal coupled motion to evaluate for joint hypomobility and to determine patient positioning and direction of glide mobilization/manipulation interventions. For example, assuming that side bending and rotation are coupled toward the same side in the lower cervical spine, when a person side bends to the left at C5-6, that person also would rotate simultaneously to the left at that motion segment. Based on knowledge of the pattern of coupled motion, the clinician might assume that if left side bending were hypomobile at C5-6, left rotation also would be hypomobile at that motion segment, and treatment directed at restoring motion into left rotation at C5-6 would also treat the hypomobility into left side bending at C5-6.

Normal and abnormal coupling in the thoracic and lumbar spine have been studied extensively. Some form of coupled motion is most likely present in these spinal joints; however, there is a great deal of disagreement in the literature regarding the nature of this coupled motion. Results from one critical review addressing thoracic spine coupled motion indicated that coupling patterns were inconsistent across different studies.[1] Similar conclusions were drawn in a critical review of lumbar spine coupled motion.[2] Furthermore, coupled motion has been shown to entail movements in the range of less than three degrees, too small to be detected with manual palpation techniques. Concepts related to coupled motion are therefore not likely to be helpful in evaluating and treating thoracic and lumbar spinal conditions.

Several studies have addressed coupling behavior in the cervical spine. In a 2007 systematic review, the authors concluded that side bending and rotation are likely coupled to the same side in the lower cervical joints. In relation to the upper cervical joints, coupling behavior was too variable to draw any conclusions about patterns of movement.[3]

PRECAUTIONS AND CONTRAINDICATIONS TO JOINT MOBILIZATION AND MANIPULATION RELATED SPECIFICALLY TO THE SPINE

Because spinal joints differ from peripheral joints, many additional concerns need to be considered when determining whether and how to perform spinal mobilization/manipulation techniques. These concerns are listed subsequently. Owing to the proximity of the central nervous system and cervical arteries, the potential adverse effects of mobilization/manipulation are more severe in the spine than in the extremities. All of the conditions listed should therefore be viewed more as contraindications than as precautions.

Precautions and Contraindications to Spinal Mobilization and Manipulation Interventions

1. Spinal cord involvement in the area being treated
2. Spondylolisthesis in the area being treated

3. Severe scoliosis in the area being treated
4. Suspected aneurysm in the area being treated
5. Positive neurologic signs if the spine or pelvis is being treated with grade V techniques

Precautions and Contraindications Specifically to Cervical Spine Mobilization and Manipulation Interventions

1. Any indication of cervical artery disease, such as reports of dizziness with neck movements, because cervical spine joint manipulation has been shown to produce cerebrovascular accidents
2. Any indication of ligamentous instability in the upper cervical spine because cervical spine joint manipulation has been shown to cause injury to the spinal cord. This includes traumatized upper cervical ligaments if there is any evidence that the trauma might have caused the upper cervical joints to become unstable; rheumatoid arthritis in the cervical spine because joint mobilization/manipulation might produce subluxation or dislocation of cervical spine joints; and genetic disorders affecting joint laxity in the spine, such as Down syndrome.

Precautions and Contraindications Specifically to Lumbar Spine and Pelvic Joint Mobilization and Manipulation Interventions

1. Cauda equina syndrome because mobilization/manipulation might exacerbate the condition

REFERENCES

1. Sizer PS, Brismée J-M, Cook C. Coupling behavior of the thoracic spine: a systematic review of the literature. *J Manipulative Physiol Ther.* 2007;30:390-399.
2. Legaspi O, Edmond SL. Does the evidence support the existence of lumbar spine coupled motion? A critical review of the literature. *J Orthop Sports Phys Ther.* 2007;37:169-178.
3. Cook C, Hegedus E, Showalter C, Sizer PS. Coupling behavior of the cervical spine: a systematic review of the literature. *J Manipulative Physiol Ther.* 2006;29: 570-575.

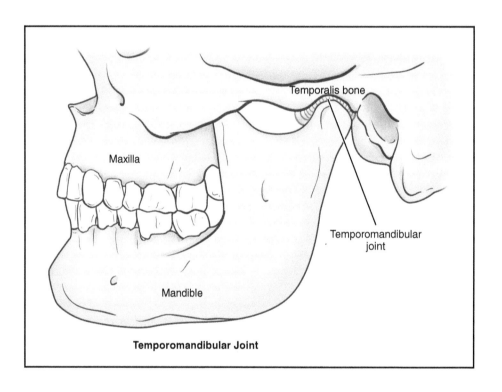

Maxilla

Temporalis bone

Temporomandibular
joint

Mandible

Temporomandibular Joint

CHAPTER 10

The Temporomandibular Joint

BASICS

The temporomandibular joints are an integral component of basic functional activities including eating and talking. For these activities an individual should be able to open the mouth wide enough at both temporomandibular joints to allow placement of two of the individual's knuckles or three of the individual's fingers between the teeth.

Temporomandibular Joints

Anatomically, the temporomandibular joints consist of the paired convex articular surface of the mandible, which articulates with the paired concave articular surface of the temporal bone. An intraarticular disc separates these joint surfaces. Motion at the temporomandibular joint includes opening and closing, protraction and retraction, and side gliding.

Jaw opening occurs as a result of a combination of temporomandibular rotation and gliding. Protraction and retraction occur via a gliding motion, with minimal, if any, rotation. Joint limitations in retraction are uncommon. With side gliding, the temporomandibular joint on the side to which the chin is moving rotates and shifts slightly laterally, and the temporomandibular joint on the opposite side glides forward, medially, and downward.

SPECIFIC PATHOLOGY AND TEMPOROMANDIBULAR JOINT MOBILIZATION/MANIPULATION

Temporomandibular Joint Disorders

In a 2013 systematic review of manual therapy and multimodal interventions for patients with upper-quadrant disorders, the investigators identified three studies addressing mobilization/manipulation for temporomandibular joint disorders. The authors concluded that there is a fair level of evidence to support the use of multiple interventions, including joint mobilization/manipulation to the kinetic chain including the temporomandibular joint, for treatment of temporomandibular disorders. Outcomes included pain, range of motion, and improvements in function, and persisted for up to 6 months posttreatment.[1]

A different 2013 systematic review specifically addressed joint mobilization/manipulation for treatment of temporomandibular disc displacement. The authors concluded that mobilization/manipulation, either alone or in conjunction with other manual therapy interventions, was no more effective than surgery or other conservative interventions in relation to pain, range of motion, or function for up to 5 years follow-up.[2]

TEMPOROMANDIBULAR JOINTS

Osteokinematic motions:
    Opening/closing
    Protraction/retraction
    Side gliding left and right
Ligaments:
    Temporomandibular ligament
    Sphenomandibular ligament
    Stylomandibular ligament
Joint orientation:
    Temporalis: inferior, anterior, lateral
    Mandible: superior, posterior, medial
Type of joint:
    Synovial
Concave joint surface:
    Temporalis
Resting position:
    Mouth slightly open[3]
Close-packed position:
    Mouth closed[3]
Capsular pattern of restriction:
    Limitation in mouth opening[4]

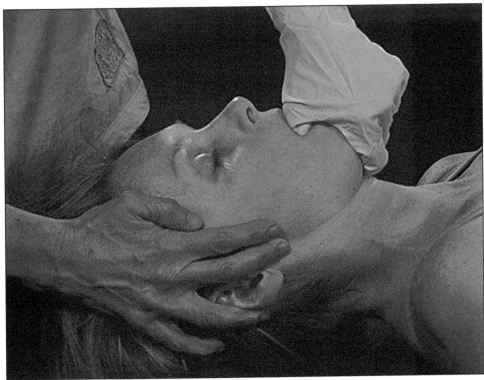

Figure 10-1 Distraction.

Distraction (Figure 10-1, Video 10-1)

Purpose
- To examine for temporomandibular joint impairment
- To increase accessory motion into temporomandibular joint distraction
- To increase range of motion at the temporomandibular joint
- To decrease pain

Positioning
1. The patient is supine.
2. The temporomandibular joint is positioned in the resting position if conservative techniques are indicated or approximating restricted range of motion if more aggressive techniques are indicated.
3. The clinician is at the head of the treatment table, facing the temporomandibular joint.
4. The clinician should wear surgical gloves to protect the clinician and patient from transmission of infection.
5. The stabilizing hand supports the head laterally on the same side as the joint being mobilized/manipulated.
6. The mobilizing/manipulating hand is positioned with the thumb over the lower molars and the fingers wrapped around the lateral lower jaw on the side to be mobilized/manipulated.

Procedure
1. The stabilizing hand holds the head in position.
2. The mobilizing/manipulating hand moves the mandible inferiorly in a direction perpendicular to the joint surface of the temporalis and guides this movement with the fingers (see Figure 10-1).

Particulars
- In the case of bilateral temporomandibular joint impairment, this technique can be performed on both temporomandibular joints simultaneously by positioning and moving both hands as if they were both mobilizing/manipulating hands.

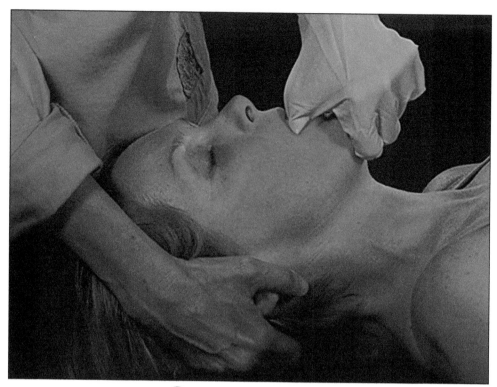

Figure 10-2 Anterior glide.

Anterior Glide (Figure 10-2, Video 10-2)

Purpose

- To examine for temporomandibular joint impairment
- To increase accessory motion into temporomandibular joint anterior glide
- To increase range of motion at the temporomandibular joint
- To decrease pain

Positioning

1. The patient is supine.
2. The temporomandibular joint is positioned in the resting position if conservative techniques are indicated or approximating restricted range of motion if more aggressive techniques are indicated.
3. The clinician is at the head of the treatment table, facing the temporomandibular joint.
4. The clinician should wear surgical gloves to protect the clinician and patient from transmission of infection.
5. The stabilizing hand supports the head laterally and anteriorly on the same side as the joint being mobilized/manipulated.
6. The mobilizing/manipulating hand is positioned with the thumb over the lower molars and the fingers wrapped around the lateral lower jaw on the side to be mobilized/manipulated.

Procedure

1. The clinician applies a grade I traction to the joint.
2. The stabilizing hand holds the head in position.
3. The mobilizing/manipulating hand glides the mandible in an anterior direction with the thumb and guides the movement with the fingers (see Figure 10-2).

Particulars

- This technique might be especially effective for increasing range of motion into temporomandibular joint protraction.

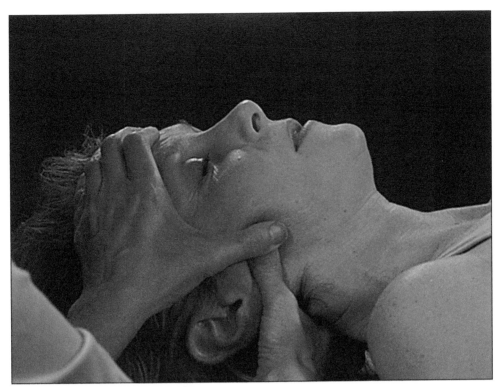

Figure 10-3 Medial glide.

Medial Glide (Figure 10-3, Video 10-3)

Purpose
- To examine for temporomandibular joint impairment
- To increase accessory motion into temporomandibular joint medial glide
- To increase range of motion at the temporomandibular joint
- To decrease pain

Positioning
1. The patient is supine.
2. The temporomandibular joint is positioned in the resting position if conservative techniques are indicated or approximating restricted range of motion if more aggressive techniques are indicated.
3. The clinician is at the side of the patient's head, facing the temporomandibular joint.
4. The mobilizing/manipulating hand is positioned with the thumb over the guiding hand.
5. The guiding hand is positioned with the thumb on the mandibular condyle.

Procedure
1. The mobilizing/manipulating hand glides the mandible in a medial direction with the thumb.
2. The guiding hand controls the position of the mobilizing/manipulating hand (see Figure 10-3).

Particulars
- This technique might be especially effective for increasing range of motion into temporomandibular joint side gliding to the side away from the side of the joint being treated.

REFERENCES

1. Brantingham JW, Cassa TK, Bonnefin D, et al. Manipulative and multimodal therapy for upper extremity and temporomandibular disorders: a systematic review. *J Manipulative Physiol Ther.* 2013;36:143-201.
2. Alves BMF, Macedo CR, Januzzi E, et al. Mandibular manipulation for the treatment of temporomandibular disorder. *J Craniofac Surg.* 2013;24:488-493.
3. Kaltenborn FM. *Manual Mobilization of the Joints: The Kaltenborn Method of Joint Examination and Treatment*, Vol 2. The Spine. 4th ed. OPTP; 2003.
4. Cyriax J. *Textbook of Orthopaedic Medicine*, Vol 1. Diagnosis of Soft Tissue Lesions. 8th ed. London: Bailliere Tindall; 1982.

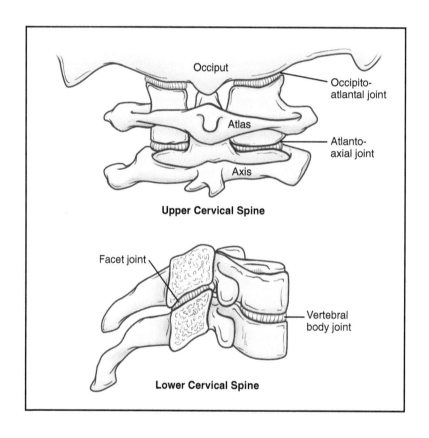

Upper Cervical Spine

Occiput

Occipito-atlantal joint

Atlas

Atlanto-axial joint

Axis

Lower Cervical Spine

Facet joint

Vertebral body joint

CHAPTER **11**

Cervical Spine

BASICS

The cervical spine is commonly divided into upper (occiput through C1-2) and lower (C2-3 and below) components. Most clinicians categorize the upper thoracic motion segments (T1-2 and T2-3) as if they were part of the lower cervical spine, because they resemble cervical vertebrae, with the notable exception of the attachment to ribs.

Upper Cervical Joints

Forward bending and backward bending are the primary motions occurring at the occipitoatlantal joint. This joint accounts for 15 degrees of motion in the sagittal plane. Rotation occurs primarily at the atlantoaxial joint, accounting for 45 degrees of rotation in each direction.

Lower Cervical and Upper Thoracic Joints

Motion into forward and backward bending is completed by the lower cervical spine. More movement occurs at the C5-6 motion segment than at any other lower cervical spine motion segment. Lower cervical spine motion is guided by the facet joints, which are angulated 45 degrees anteriorly from the frontal plane. Forward bending occurs as the inferior facet joints of the more superior vertebra glide up and forward on the superior facet joints of the more inferior vertebra. Backward bending is associated with a downward and backward gliding of the facets of the more superior vertebra on the facets of the more inferior vertebra.

The lower cervical spine is responsible for approximately 40 degrees of rotation in either direction, accounting for about 50% of total movement into rotation. More movement into lower cervical side bending and rotation occurs at the C5-6 motion segment than at any other lower cervical spine motion segment. As with forward bending, lower cervical side bending and rotation are guided by the angulation of the facet joints. Movement into side bending and rotation to the left is accompanied by an upward and forward glide of the right facet joints and a downward and backward glide of the left facet joints of the more superior vertebra and vice versa for movement into right side bending and rotation.

Although coupled motion most likely does not occur in a specific direction in any other spinal location, evidence suggests that there is coupling in the lower cervical spine such that rotation and side bending occur to the same side.[1] This coupling pattern has the following implications: a patient with joint hypomobility into side bending left at a specific motion segment would be expected to have hypomobility into ipsilateral rotation at that segment. Similarly, by placing a motion segment at end range into side bending left, the clinician can assume that rotation left is also at end range. Finally, the clinician can expect that when treating a hypomobility impairment into left side bending, that treatment would also address a left rotation hypomobility impairment. A decrease in upward gliding motion of a right cervical facet joint would therefore result in a decrease in left rotation and side-bending range of motion, whereas a decrease in downward gliding motion of a right cervical facet joint would result in a decrease in right rotation and side-bending range of motion. Similarly, restoring rotation range of motion at a motion segment should result in a corresponding increase in side-bending range of motion.

RISKS OF CERVICAL SPINE MOBILIZATION/MANIPULATION

The cervical spine is comprised of a high concentration of vascular and nervous tissue, rendering it more susceptible to adverse events than most other joints. In a 2010 systematic review, the authors reported a small but significant increase in transient neurologic symptoms and neck pain following cervical spine mobilization and manipulation interventions among patients with neck pain.[2] Severe adverse events, including cervical artery dissection and joint subluxation, although rare,[3] are of far greater concern.

Most of the clinical literature has focused on the risk of cervical manipulation interventions. Risks associated with cervical manipulation vary and have been reported to be between one in 50,000 and one in 5,850,000 manipulations.[4,5] Cervical artery dissections have been reported as being the most common significant adverse event, followed by disc herniations, cerebral vascular accidents, and vertebral dislocations or fractures.[6] In 2012, Puentedura et al.[6] investigated the extent to which significant adverse events could be prevented with appropriate screening, concluding that fully 44% were preventable. They recommended screening for the following conditions before performing any cervical spine manipulation technique:

- Acute fracture
- Dislocation
- Ligamentous rupture
- Instability
- Tumor
- Infection
- Acute myelopathy
- Surgery
- Acute soft tissue injury
- Osteoporosis
- Ankylosing spondylitis
- Rheumatoid arthritis
- Vascular disease
- Vertebral artery abnormalities
- Connective tissue disease
- Anticoagulation therapy
- Vertebrobasilar insufficiency
- Facial or intraoral anesthesia or paraesthesia
- Visual disturbances
- Dizziness/vertigo
- Blurred vision
- Diplopia
- Nausea
- Tinnitus
- Drop attacks
- Dysarthria
- Dysphagia
- Any symptom listed above aggravated by position or movement of the neck
- No change or worsening of symptoms after multiple manipulations

One basic tenet of manual therapy is to choose the least aggressive intervention that will result in achieving preestablished therapeutic goals. The issue of whether cervical manipulation is more effective than cervical mobilization is therefore paramount in making this determination. In a 2010 systematic review, investigators concluded that, based on moderate evidence, manipulation and mobilization resulted in similar pain, function, and patient satisfaction outcomes. This was the case primarily for follow-ups of intermediate length.[7]

Similarly, clinicians might need to decide between performing thoracic manipulation or cervical mobilization or manipulation techniques. In a 2013 systematic review, the investigators reported that thoracic spine manipulation might benefit some patients with neck pain; however, there is no evidence to suggest that it is more effective for reducing pain or improving function than other interventions commonly administered to patients with neck pain, such as cervical mobilization, cervical manipulation, and exercise.[8] Evidently, joint mobilization/manipulation techniques targeting the thoracic or cervical spine are equally beneficial, suggesting that some patients with neck pain might benefit from interventions to both areas.

SPECIFIC PATHOLOGY AND CERVICAL SPINE JOINT MOBILIZATION/MANIPULATION

Nonspecific Neck Pain

Several systematic reviews addressing the efficacy of mobilization/manipulation of the cervical spine for treatment of neck pain have been published. Some of the conclusions drawn from these systematic reviews addressed the efficacy of manual therapy, which includes joint mobilization/manipulation as well as soft tissue techniques. The authors' conclusions were similar in relation to manual therapy in general and specifically joint mobilization/manipulation, and are summarized as follows:

- Mobilization/manipulation[7] and manual therapy[9] are effective in reducing neck pain immediately after treatment. Furthermore, manual therapy has been shown to be more effective than exercise in reducing pain short term.[9]
- Mobilization/manipulation do not result in long-term benefits for patients with neck pain.[7,9] Similarly, the evidence for the long-term efficacy of manual therapy is limited, irrespective of the chronicity of the pain.[9,10]
- Adding exercises to manual therapy of the cervical spine is more effective than manual therapy alone.[9,10] This is especially the case in relation to reducing pain and improving function and quality of life among patients with chronic neck pain.[9] These findings are supported by a 2008 clinical practice guideline for patients with neck pain, in which the authors concluded, based on strong evidence, that combining cervical mobilization/manipulation and exercise is more effective for reducing neck pain and disability than mobilization/manipulation alone.[11]

Headache

In a 2012 systematic review of six studies addressing the efficacy of cervical manipulation, the authors concluded that, based on weak evidence, cervical manipulation in combination with other interventions commonly performed by physical therapists might be an effective treatment in the management of cervicogenic headache.[12] These findings were echoed in a different 2012 systematic review, in which the authors concluded that the evidence for cervical manipulation interventions for tension type headache is "encouraging but inconclusive."[13]

These findings were supported by a 2008 clinical practice guideline for patients with headache, in which the authors concluded that combining cervical mobilization/manipulation and exercise is more effective for reducing headache and disability than manipulation and mobilization alone. These latter findings supporting the efficacy of a combination of interventions were based on strong evidence.[11]

Temporomandibular Joint Disorders

In a 2013 systematic review, the authors concluded that there is fair evidence to support the use of cervical spine manipulation when implemented in conjunction with other interventions, including exercise and manipulation to other joints within the kinematic chain.[14]

A 2015 systematic review supported this conclusion. Based on low to high evidence, the authors reported that upper cervical mobilization or manipulation techniques are more effective in addressing pain and limitations in range of motion than control groups.[15]

Lateral Epicondylalgia

In a 2013 systemic review addressing conservative interventions for patients with lateral epicondylalgia, the authors reported moderate evidence supporting the use of cervical and thoracic manipulation as an adjunct to a regimen of stretching and strengthening exercises and wrist and forearm mobilization.[16]

UPPER CERVICAL JOINTS (OCCIPUT THROUGH C2)

Osteokinematic motions: occipitoatlantal joint:
  Forward/backward bending
  Side bending
  Rotation
Osteokinematic motions: atlantoaxial joint:
  Rotation
  Forward/backward bending
  Side bending
Ligaments:
  Tectorial membrane
  Ligamentum nuchae
  Alar ligaments
  Transverse ligaments
  Apical ligament
  Interspinous ligament
  Supraspinous ligament
  Anterior longitudinal ligament
  Posterior longitudinal ligament
Joint orientation:
  Occiput: inferior
  Atlas superior surface: superior
  Atlas inferior facet: inferior, medial
  Axis superior facet: superior, lateral
  Atlas also encircles the odontoid process of the axis
Type of joint:
  Synovial
Concave joint surface:
  None, these are plane joints
Resting position:
  Not described by Kaltenborn
Close-packed position:
  Not described by Kaltenborn
Capsular pattern of restriction:
  For the entire cervical spine, side bending and rotation are equally limited and extension is more limited than flexion.[17]

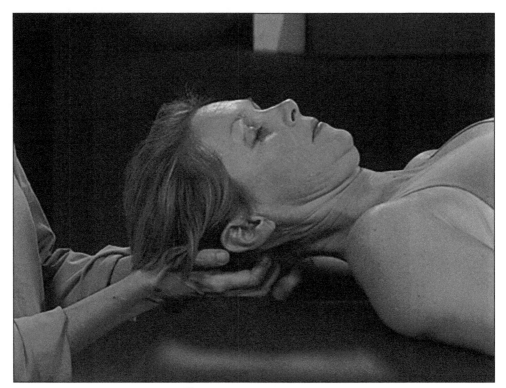

▶ **Figure 11-1** Distraction.

Distraction (Figure 11-1, Video 11-1)

Purpose
- To examine for upper cervical spine joint impairment
- To increase accessory motion into upper cervical joint distraction
- To increase range of motion at the upper cervical spine
- To decrease pain

Positioning
1. The patient is supine.
2. The cervical spine is positioned in midrange in relation to forward/backward bending, side bending, and rotation.
3. The clinician is at the patient's head, facing the patient.
4. Both hands are positioned with the fingertips inferior to the base of the occiput and the hands on the posterior surface of the skull.

Procedure
1. Testing for signs and symptoms of a potential adverse response to cervical movement should be performed before executing this or any other mobilization/manipulation technique involving cervical spine movement.
2. Both fingers move the occiput superiorly in a direction perpendicular to the joint surface of the suboccipital joint by lifting the skull away from the clinician's palms and allowing the weight of the head to distract the occiput from the cervical spine.
3. This position can be maintained for several minutes to stretch suboccipital tissue (see Figure 11-1).

Particulars
- This is not a grade V manipulation technique.
- This technique also stretches the suboccipital musculature.

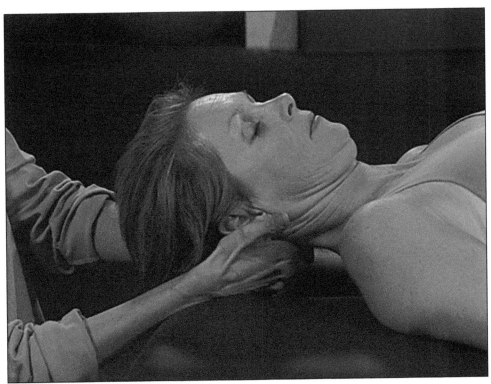

Figure 11-2 Forward-bending glide.

Forward-Bending Glide (Figure 11-2, Video 11-2)

Purpose
- To examine for upper cervical spine joint impairment
- To increase accessory motion into upper cervical spine forward bending
- To increase range of motion at the upper cervical spine
- To decrease pain

Positioning
1. The patient is supine.
2. The cervical spine is positioned in midrange in relation to forward/backward bending, side bending, and rotation.
3. The clinician is at the patient's head, facing the patient.
4. The stabilizing hand holds the axis in position by placing the lateral (radial) border of the index finger on the superior surface of the spinous process of the axis.
5. The mobilizing hand grips the occiput posteriorly with the web space.

Procedure
1. Testing for signs and symptoms of a potential adverse response to cervical movement should be performed before executing this or any other mobilization/manipulation technique involving cervical spine movement.
2. The stabilizing hand holds the axis in position.
3. The mobilizing hand glides the occiput superiorly, allowing the head to move into forward bending (see Figure 11-2).

Particulars
- This is not a grade V manipulation technique.
- This technique might be especially effective for increasing range of motion into upper cervical spine forward bending.

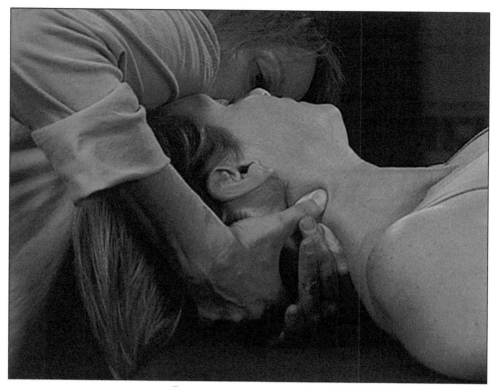

Figure 11-3 Rotation glide.

Rotation Glide (Figure 11-3, Video 11-3)

Purpose
- To examine for upper cervical spine joint impairment
- To increase accessory motion into upper cervical spine rotation
- To increase range of motion at the upper cervical spine
- To decrease pain

Positioning
1. The patient is supine.
2. The cervical spine is positioned in midrange in relation to forward/backward bending, side bending, and rotation.
3. The clinician is at the patient's head, facing the patient with the clinician's anterior shoulder (the shoulder on the same side as the mobilizing/manipulating hand) positioned on the patient's forehead.
4. The stabilizing hand grips the axis posteriorly with the web space and laterally with the fingers and thumb.
5. The mobilizing/manipulating hand grips the occiput posteriorly.

Procedure
1. Testing for signs and symptoms of a potential adverse response to cervical movement should be performed before executing this or any other mobilization/manipulation technique involving cervical spine movement.
2. The clinician applies a grade I traction to the joints.
3. The stabilizing hand holds the axis.
4. The mobilizing/manipulating hand glides the occiput into rotation as the shoulder guides the motion (see Figure 11-3).

Particulars
- This technique might be especially effective for increasing range of motion into upper cervical spine rotation in the direction of vertebral body movement.

LOWER CERVICAL JOINTS (C3-4 THROUGH T2-3)

Osteokinematic motions:
    Forward/backward bending
    Side bending
    Rotation
Ligaments:
    Anterior longitudinal ligament
    Posterior longitudinal ligament
    Supraspinous ligament
    Interspinous ligament
    Ligamentum flavum
    Intertransverse ligaments
Joint orientation:
    Inferior facet of superior vertebra: inferior, anterior, lateral
    Superior facet of inferior vertebra: superior, posterior, medial
    Superior vertebral body: inferior
    Inferior vertebral body: superior
Type of joint:
    Facets: synovial
    Disc: amphiarthrodial
Concave joint surface:
    None, these are plane joints
Resting position:
    Not described by Kaltenborn
Close-packed position:
    Not described by Kaltenborn
Capsular pattern of restriction:
    For the entire cervical spine, side bending and rotation are equally limited and extension is more limited than flexion[17]

Distraction (Figure 11-4, Video 11-4)

Purpose

- To examine for cervical spine joint impairment
- To increase accessory motion into cervical vertebral body distraction
- To increase range of motion at the cervical spine
- To decrease pain

Positioning

1. The patient is supine.
2. The cervical spine is positioned in midrange in relation to forward/backward bending, side bending, and rotation.
3. The clinician is at the patient's head, facing the patient.
4. The mobilizing/manipulating hand grips the occiput posteriorly with the web space.
5. The guiding hand gently grips the chin.

Procedure

1. Testing for signs and symptoms of a potential adverse response to cervical movement should be performed before executing this or any other mobilization/manipulation technique involving cervical spine movement.
2. The clinician leans backward, moving the head in a superior direction and distracting the vertebral bodies from one another.
3. Most of the force exerted by the clinician should be directed to the occiput because excessive pressure on the chin might cause the patient to develop temporomandibular joint problems (see Figure 11-4).

Particulars

- It is important to screen for temporomandibular joint impairments before performing this technique.

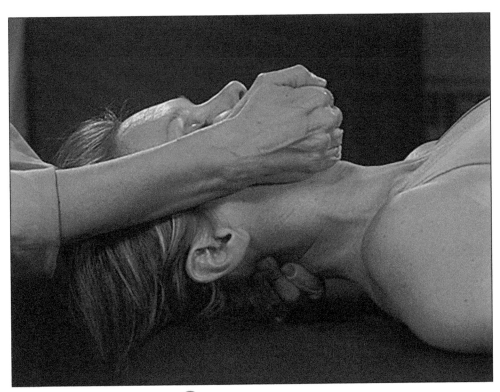

Figure 11-4 Distraction.

Anterior Glide Using the Spinous Processes (Figure 11-5, Video 11-5)

Purpose

- To examine for lower cervical spine joint impairment
- To increase accessory motion into lower cervical joint anterior glide
- To increase range of motion at the lower cervical spine
- To decrease pain

Positioning

1. The patient is supine or prone.
2. The cervical spine is positioned in midrange in relation to forward/backward bending, side bending, and rotation.
3. The clinician is at the patient's head, facing the lower cervical spine.
4. The mobilizing/manipulating hand is positioned with the thumb over the thumb of the guiding hand.
5. The guiding hand is positioned with the thumb over the spinous process being mobilized/manipulated.

Procedure

1. The mobilizing/manipulating hand glides the spinous process anteriorly.
2. The guiding hand controls the position of the mobilizing/manipulating hand (see Figure 11-5).

Particulars

- When performed with the patient prone, this technique also is called springing. If it is being performed as an examination technique, the term *spring testing* is used.
- This technique is commonly performed using a grade V manipulation.

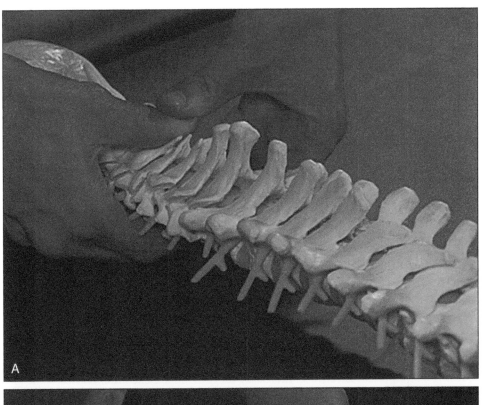

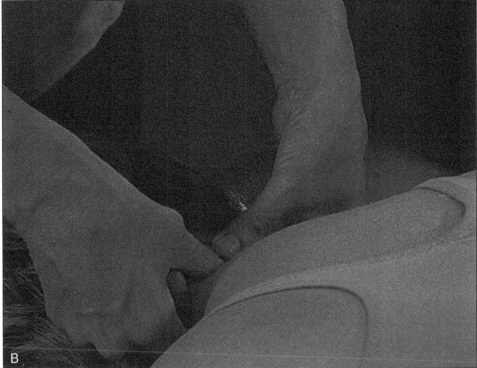

Figure 11-5 **A** and **B,** Anterior glide using the spinous processes.

Anterior/Superior Glide Using the Spinous Processes: First Technique (Figure 11-6, Video 11-6)

Purpose
- To examine for lower cervical spine joint impairment
- To increase accessory motion into lower cervical joint anterior/superior glide
- To increase range of motion at the lower cervical spine
- To decrease pain

Positioning
1. The patient is supine or prone.
2. The cervical spine is positioned in midrange in relation to forward/backward bending, side bending, and rotation.
3. The clinician is at the patient's head, facing the lower cervical spine.
4. The stabilizing hand is positioned with the middle finger or the thumb on the spinous process of the more inferior vertebra.
5. The mobilizing/manipulating hand is positioned with the middle finger or the thumb over the most inferior surface of the spinous process of the more superior vertebra.

Procedure
1. The stabilizing hand holds the more inferior vertebra in position.
2. The mobilizing/manipulating hand glides the spinous process of the more superior vertebra anteriorly and superiorly (see Figure 11-6).

Particulars
- This technique might be especially effective for increasing range of motion into lower cervical spine forward bending.

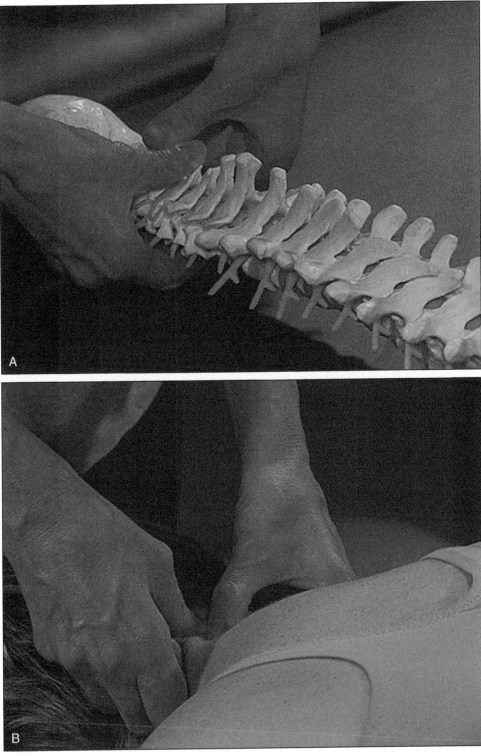

Figure 11-6 **A** and **B,** Anterior/superior glide using the spinous processes: first technique.

Anterior/Superior Glide Using the Spinous Processes: Second Technique (Figure 11-7, Video 11-7)

Purpose
- To examine for lower cervical spine joint impairment
- To increase accessory motion into lower cervical joint anterior/superior glide
- To increase range of motion at the lower cervical spine
- To decrease pain

Positioning
1. The patient is supine or prone.
2. The cervical spine is positioned in midrange in relation to forward/backward bending, side bending, and rotation.
3. The clinician is at the patient's head, facing the lower cervical spine.
4. The stabilizing hand is positioned with the middle finger or the thumb on the spinous process of the more superior vertebra.
5. The mobilizing/manipulating hand is positioned with the middle finger or the thumb over the most inferior surface of the spinous process of the more inferior vertebra.

Procedure
1. The stabilizing hand holds the more superior vertebra in position.
2. The mobilizing/manipulating hand glides the spinous process of the more inferior vertebra anteriorly and superiorly (see Figure 11-7).

Particulars
- This technique might be especially effective for increasing range of motion into lower cervical spine backward bending.

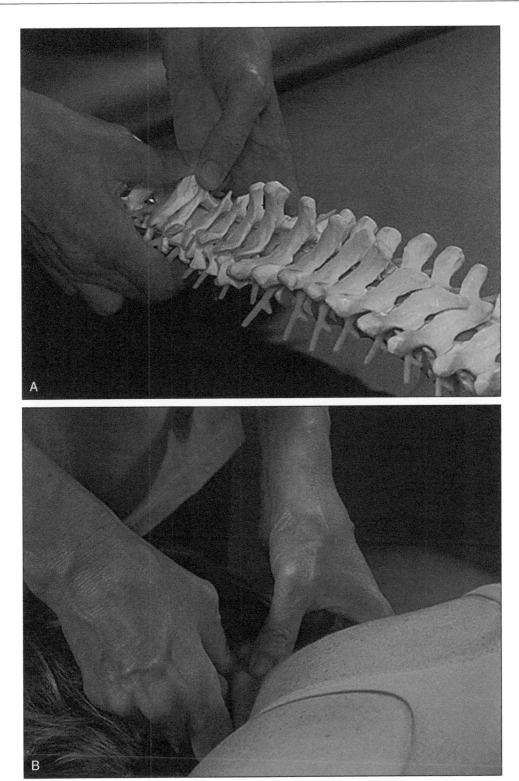

Figure 11-7 **A** and **B,** Anterior/superior glide using the spinous processes: second technique.

Lateral Glide Using the Spinous Processes (Figure 11-8, Video 11-8)

Purpose
- To examine for lower cervical spine joint impairment
- To increase accessory motion into lower cervical vertebral body rotation and into facet joint distraction on the side toward which the vertebral body is rotating
- To increase range of motion at the lower cervical spine
- To decrease pain

Positioning
1. The patient is supine or prone.
2. The cervical spine is positioned in midrange in relation to forward/backward bending, side bending, and rotation.
3. The clinician is at the patient's head, facing the lower cervical spine.
4. The stabilizing hand is positioned with the tip of the middle finger or the thumb on the lateral surface of the spinous process of the more inferior vertebra.
5. The mobilizing/manipulating hand is positioned with the tip of the middle finger or the thumb on the lateral surface of the spinous process of the more superior vertebra opposite the side of the stabilizing hand.

Procedure
1. The stabilizing hand holds the more inferior vertebra in position.
2. The mobilizing/manipulating hand glides the more superior spinous process toward the contralateral side (see Figure 11-8).

Particulars
- This technique might be especially effective for increasing range of motion into lower cervical spine rotation in the direction of vertebral body movement (in the direction opposite the movement of the spinous process).

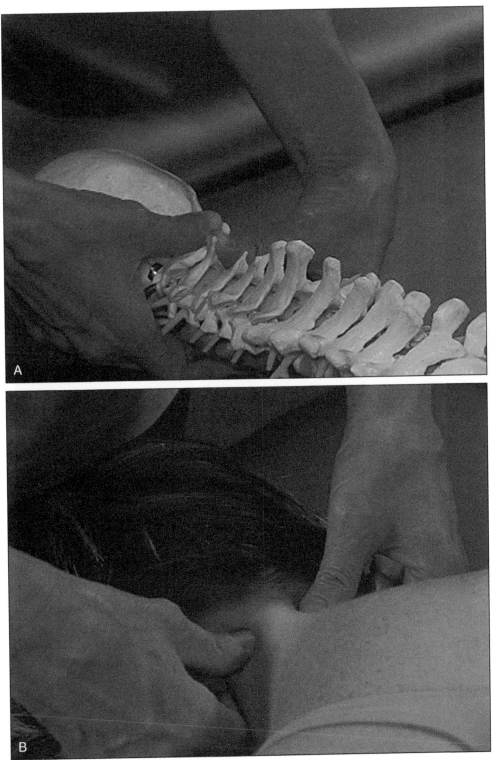

Figure 11-8 **A** and **B,** Lateral glide using the spinous processes.

Anterior Glide Using the Facet Joints: First Technique (Figure 11-9, Video 11-9)

Purpose

- To examine for lower cervical spine joint impairment
- To increase accessory motion into lower cervical anterior glide
- To increase range of motion at the lower cervical spine
- To decrease pain

Positioning

1. The patient is supine or prone.
2. The cervical spine is positioned in midrange in relation to forward/backward bending, side bending, and rotation.
3. The clinician is at the patient's head, facing the lower cervical spine.
4. One hand is positioned with the tip of the middle finger or the thumb on the facet articular pillar of one vertebra.
5. The other hand is positioned with the tip of the middle finger or the thumb on the opposite facet articular pillar of the same vertebra.

Procedure

1. Both hands simultaneously glide the facet articular pillars anteriorly (see Figure 11-9).

Particulars

- This technique is commonly performed using a grade V manipulation.

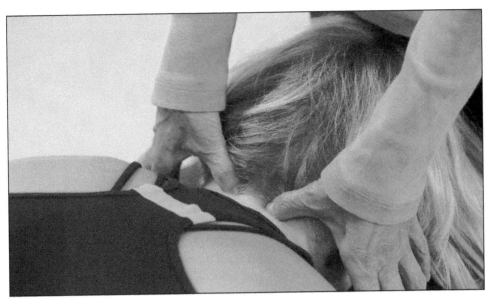

Figure 11-9 Anterior glide using the facet joints: first technique.

Anterior Glide Using the Facet Joints: Second Technique (Figure 11-10, Video 11-10)

Purpose
- To examine for lower cervical spine joint impairment
- To increase accessory motion into lower cervical vertebral body rotation and into facet joint distraction on the side toward which the vertebral body is rotating
- To increase range of motion at the lower cervical spine
- To decrease pain

Positioning
1. The patient is supine or prone.
2. The cervical spine is positioned in midrange in relation to forward/backward bending, side bending, and rotation.
3. The clinician is at the patient's head, facing the lower cervical spine.
4. The stabilizing hand is positioned with the tip of the middle finger or the thumb on the facet articular pillar of the more inferior vertebra.
5. The mobilizing/manipulating hand is positioned with the tip of the middle finger or the thumb on the facet articular pillar of the more superior vertebra opposite the side of the stabilizing hand.

Procedure
1. The stabilizing hand holds the more inferior vertebra in position.
2. The mobilizing/manipulating hand glides the more superior facet in an anterior and superior direction (see Figure 11-10).

Particulars
- This technique might be especially effective for increasing range of motion into lower cervical spine rotation in the direction of vertebral body movement.
- This technique is commonly performed using a grade V manipulation.

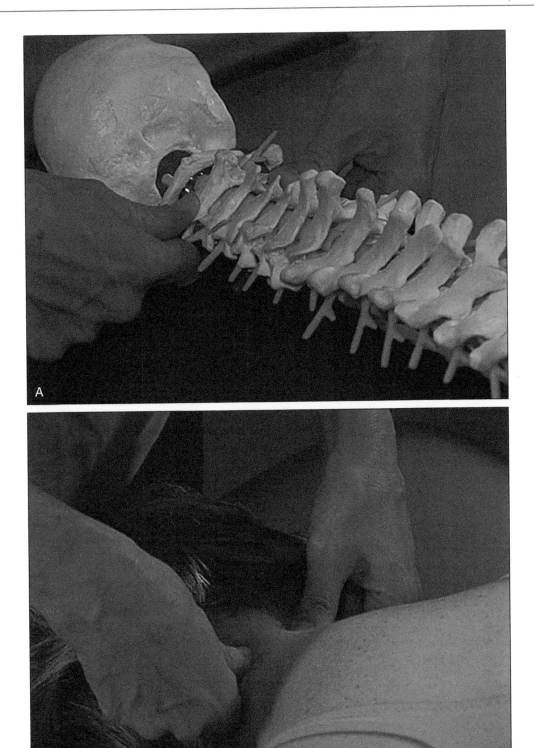

Figure 11-10 **A** and **B,** Anterior glide using the facet joints: second technique.

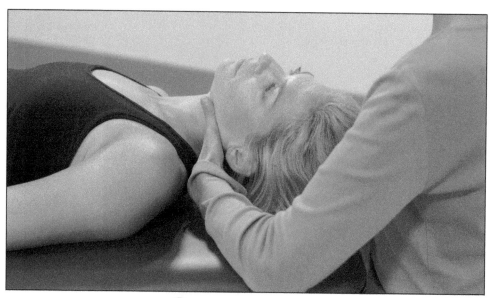

▶ **Figure 11-11** Side glide.

Side Glide (Figure 11-11, Video 11-11)
Purpose
- To examine for lower cervical spine joint impairment
- To increase accessory motion into lower cervical joint side glide
- To increase range of motion at the lower cervical spine
- To decrease pain

Position
1. The patient is supine.
2. The cervical spine is positioned in midrange in relation to forward/backward bending, side bending, and rotation.
3. The clinician is at the patient's head, facing the lower cervical spine.
4. The stabilizing hand is positioned with the second metacarpophalangeal joint over the posterolateral facet joint of the more superior vertebra of the motion segment being mobilized/manipulated and the palm of the hand or forearm cradling the head.
5. The mobilizing/manipulating hand is positioned with the second metacarpophalangeal joint over the contralateral posterolateral facet joint of the more inferior vertebra of the motion segment being mobilized/manipulated.
6. The clinician locks the more superior vertebra of the motion segment being mobilized/manipulated by side bending the patient's neck toward the mobilizing hand to the extent that the motion segment above the one being mobilized/manipulated is fully side bent, but the motion segment being mobilized/manipulated has not yet moved.

Procedure
1. Testing for signs and symptoms of a potential adverse response to cervical movement should be performed before executing this or any other mobilization/manipulation technique involving cervical spine movement.
2. The stabilizing hand supports the more superior vertebra.
3. The mobilizing/manipulating hand glides the more inferior vertebra toward the patient's contralateral eye, thereby gliding the vertebra in the plane of the facet joint (see Figure 11-11).

Particulars
- This technique is commonly performed using a grade V manipulation.

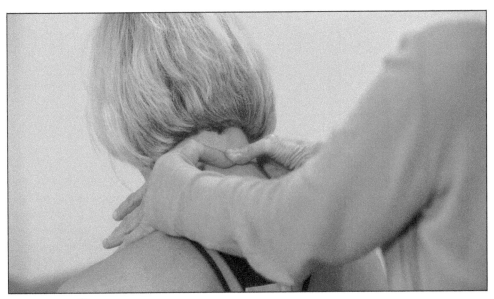

▶ **Figure 11-12** Forward-bending glide mobilization with movement.

Forward-Bending Glide Mobilization with Movement (Figure 11-12, Video 11-12)

Purpose
- To decrease pain
- To increase pain-free range of motion into cervical forward bending

Positioning
1. The patient is sitting with the head in neutral.
2. The clinician is standing behind the patient with the medial/ulnar border of the guiding thumb on the patient's spinous process and the mobilizing thumb on top of the guiding thumb.

Procedure
1. The clinician performs an anterior and superior glide to the patient's spinous process in the plane of the facet joint.
2. While maintaining an anterior and superior glide, the clinician instructs the patient to forward bend the neck as far as possible as long as the movement is pain free.
3. The clinician maintains the anterior and superior glide while the patient moves the neck to the starting position.
4. The clinician continually adjusts his or her position in relation to the treatment plane, to maintain the joint mobilization force during joint movement (see Figure 11-12).

Particulars
- This technique are indicated only if they can be performed without reproducing the patient's pain/symptoms.
- This technique should result in an immediate increase in range of motion and/or a decrease in pain.
- If effective (the technique results in an immediate increase in range of motion and/or decrease in pain), these techniques should be repeated (~2 to 3 times).

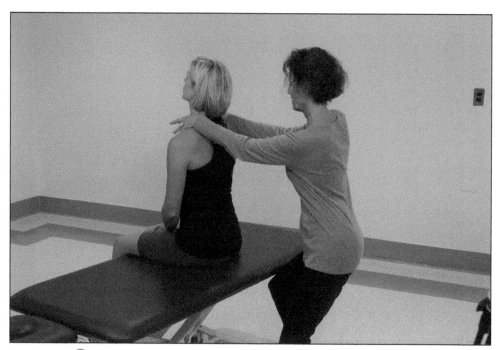

▶ **Figure 11-13** Backward-bending glide mobilization with movement.

Backward-Bending Glide Mobilization with Movement (Figure 11-13, Video 11-13)

Purpose
- To decrease pain
- To increase pain-free range of motion into cervical backward bending

Positioning
1. The patient is sitting with the head in neutral.
2. The clinician is standing behind the patient with the medial/ulnar border of the guiding thumb on the patient's spinous process and the mobilizing thumb on top of the guiding thumb.

Procedure
1. The clinician performs an anterior and superior glide to the patient's spinous process.
2. While maintaining an anterior and superior glide in the plane of the facet joint, the clinician instructs the patient to backward bend the neck as far as possible as long as the movement is pain free.
3. The clinician maintains the anterior and superior glide while the patient moves the neck to the starting position.
4. The clinician continually adjusts his or her own position in relation to the treatment plane to maintain the joint mobilization force during joint movement. Adjusting to the change in facet joint plane is necessary to complement the osteokinematic changes accompanying normal physiologic movement (see Figure 11-13).

Particulars
- This technique are indicated only if they can be performed without reproducing the patient's pain/symptoms.
- This technique should result in an immediate increase in range of motion and/or a decrease in pain.
- If effective (the technique results in an immediate increase in range of motion and/or decrease in pain), these techniques should be repeated (~2 to 3 times).

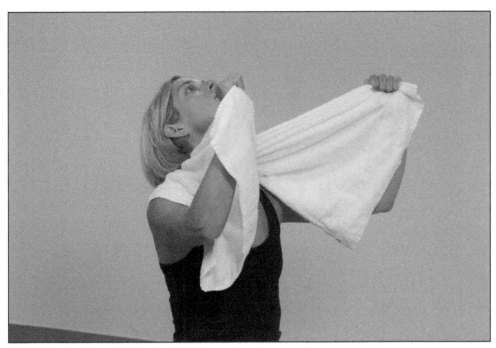

Figure 11-14 Backward-bending glide self-mobilization with movement.

Backward-Bending Glide Self-Mobilization with Movement (Figure 11-14, Video 11-14)

Purpose
- To decrease pain
- To increase pain-free range of motion into cervical backward bending
- To reinforce gains in range of motion into backward bending achieved during treatment

Positioning
1. The patient is sitting with the head in neutral.
2. The patient places the selvedge of the middle of a towel on the spinous processes of the motion segment being targeted.
3. The patient grasps the edges of the towel with both hands and pulls anterior and superior in the plane of the facet joint.

Procedure
1. The patient pulls on the towel with both hands, thereby applying an anterior and superior glide to the targeted motion segment.
2. The patient then backward bends the neck as far as possible as long as the movement is pain free, making minor adjustments to the towel as needed to accommodate for changes in the treatment plane.
3. The patient maintains the anterior and superior glide while returning the neck to the neutral position (see Figure 11-14).

Particulars
- This technique can be performed by the patient as part of a home program.
- This technique are indicated only if they can be performed without reproducing the patient's pain/symptoms.
- This technique should result in an immediate increase in range of motion and/or a decrease in pain.
- If effective (the technique results in an immediate increase in range of motion and/or decrease in pain), these techniques should be repeated (~2 to 3 times).

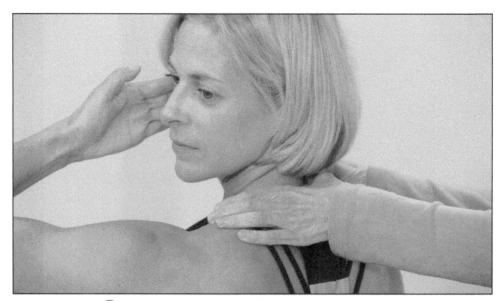

▶ Figure 11-15 Rotation glide mobilization with movement.

Rotation Glide Mobilization with Movement (Figure 11-15, Video 11-15)

Purpose
- To decrease pain
- To increase pain-free range of motion into cervical rotation

Positioning
1. The patient is sitting with the head in neutral.
2. The clinician is standing behind the patient with the medial/ulnar border of the guiding thumb on one of the patient's facet articular pillars and the mobilizing thumb on top of the guiding thumb.

Procedure
1. The clinician performs an anterior and superior glide to the patient's facet joint.
2. While maintaining an anterior and superior glide, the clinician instructs the patient to rotate the neck as far as possible as long as the movement is painfree.
3. If pain free at end range, the clinician instructs the patient to apply overpressure into rotation by placing the hand on the opposite cheekbone and turning the head.
4. The clinician maintains the anterior and superior glide while the patient moves the neck to the starting position.
5. The clinician continually adjusts his or her own position in relation to the treatment plane to maintain the joint mobilization force during joint movement (see Figure 11-15).

Particulars
- The mobilization force is typically applied on the side of pain; the direction of patient movement should occur toward the side of the restriction in range of motion or the direction that produces the patient's pain.
- This technique are indicated only if they can be performed without reproducing the patient's pain/symptoms.
- This technique should result in an immediate increase in range of motion and/or a decrease in pain.
- If effective (the technique results in an immediate increase in range of motion and/or decrease in pain), these techniques should be repeated (~6 to 10 times).
- Typically 3 sets of 10 repetitions are applied, but clinical decision making is imperative based on the patient's irritability.
- In a study performed on patients with cervicogenic dizziness, subjects were randomly assigned to receive a mobilization with movement technique which included self mobilization with movement techniques, a Maitland posteroanterior glide and exercise, or placebo. Subjects randomized to the mobilization with movement group were treated with this rotation mobilization with movement technique at C2 into the direction that reproduced dizziness if dizziness was reproduced with rotation. At 12 weeks follow-up, both groups demonstrated similar improvements in frequency and intensity of dizziness, and these improvements were greater than those experienced by the placebo group.[18]

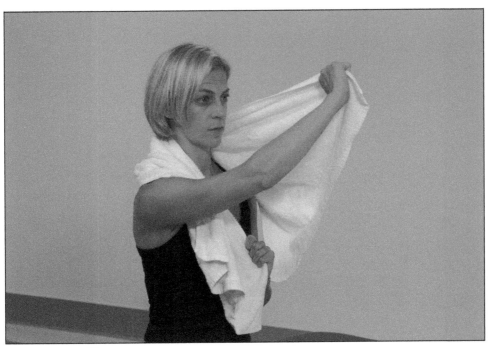

▶ **Figure 11-16** Rotation glide self-mobilization with movement.

Rotation Glide Self-Mobilization with Movement (Figure 11-16, Video 11-16)

Purpose
- To decrease pain
- To increase pain-free range of motion into cervical rotation
- To reinforce gains in range of motion into rotation achieved during treatment with a home program

Positioning
1. The patient is sitting with the head in neutral.
2. The patient places the selvedge of the middle of a towel on the motion segment being targeted.
3. The patient reaches across the chest with the hand opposite the side of cervical rotation and holds this end of the towel inferiorly on the chest.
4. The patient reaches across the chest with the other hand and holds the other end of the towel at the level of the eyes in the plane of the facet.

Procedure
1. The patient pulls gently on the towel with both hands, thereby making the towel taught and then pulls on the towel with the hand located at eye level, applying an anterior and superior glide to the targeted facet joint.
2. The patient then rotates the neck as far as possible as long as the movement is pain free while maintaining the tension on the towel.
3. The patient maintains the anterior and superior glide while returning the neck to the neutral position (see Figure 11-16).

Particulars
- This technique can be performed by the patient as part of a home program.
- This technique are indicated only if they can be performed without reproducing the patient's pain/symptoms.
- This technique should result in an immediate increase in range of motion and/or a decrease in pain.
- If effective (the technique results in an immediate increase in range of motion and/or decrease in pain), these techniques should be repeated (up to 3 sets of 3 to 6 repetitions, with a reassessment after one set).
- During subsequent sessions, when successful, 3 sets of 6–10 repetitions can be performed with instructions on applying overpressure at the end of range.

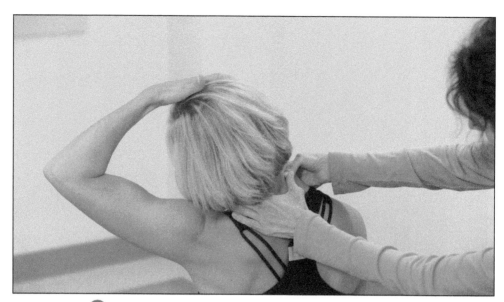

Figure 11-17 Side-bending glide mobilization with movement.

Side-Bending Glide Mobilization with Movement (Figure 11-17, Video 11-17)

Purpose
- To decrease pain
- To increase pain-free range of motion into cervical side bending

Positioning
1. The patient is sitting with the head in neutral.
2. The clinician is standing behind the patient with the medial/ulnar border of the guiding thumb on the patient's facet articular pillar and the mobilizing thumb on top of the guiding thumb.

Procedure
1. The clinician performs an anterior and superior glide to the patient's facet joint.
2. While maintaining an anterior and superior glide, the clinician instructs the patient to side bend the neck as far as possible as long as the movement is pain free.
3. If pain free at end range, the clinician instructs the patient to apply overpressure into side bending by placing the hand on the opposite parietal area and tipping the head.
4. The clinician maintains the anterior and superior glide while the patient moves the neck to the starting position.
5. The clinician continually adjusts his or her own position in relation to the treatment plane to maintain the joint mobilization force during joint movement (see Figure 11-17).

Particulars
- The mobilization force is typically applied on the side of pain; the direction of patient movement should occur toward the side of the restriction in range of motion or the direction that produces the patient's pain.
- This technique are indicated only if they can be performed without reproducing the patient's pain/symptoms.
- This technique should result in an immediate increase in range of motion and/or a decrease in pain.
- If effective (the technique results in an immediate increase in range of motion and/or decrease in pain), these techniques should be repeated (~2 to 3 times).

REFERENCES

1. Cook C, Hegedus E, Showalter C, Sizer PS. Coupling behavior of the cervical spine: a systematic review of the literature. *J Manipulative Physiol Ther*. 2006;29: 570-575.

2. Carlesso LC, Gross AR, Santaguida L, et al. Adverse events associated with the use of cervical manipulation and mobilization for the treatment of neck pain in adults: a systematic review. *Man Ther*. 2010;15: 434-444.

3. Thiel HW, Bolton JE, Docherty S, Portlock JC. Safety of chiropractic manipulation of the cervical spine: a prospective national survey. *Spine*. 2007;32: 2375-2378.

4. Haldeman S, Carey P, Townsend M, Papadopoulos C. Arterial dissections following cervical manipulation: the chiropractic experience. *CMAJ*. 2001;165: 905-906.

5. Magarey ME, Rebbeck T, Coughlan B, et al. Premanipulative testing of the cervical spine review, revision and new clinical guidelines. *Man Ther*. 2004;9:95-108.

6. Puentedura EJ, March J, Anders J, et al. Safety of cervical spine manipulation: are adverse events preventable and are manipulations being performed appropriately? A review of 134 case reports. *J Man Manip Ther*. 2012;20:66-74.

7. Gross A, Miller J, D'Sylva J, et al. Manipulation or mobilisation for neck pain: a Cochrane review. *Man Ther*. 2010;15:315-333.

8. Huisman PA, Speksnijder CM, de Wijer A. The effect of thoracic spine manipulation on pain and disability in patients with non-specific neck pain: a systematic review. *Disabil Rehabil*. 2013;35:1677-1685.

9. Miller J, Gross A, D'Sylva J, et al. Manual therapy and exercise for neck pain: a systematic review. *Man Ther*. 2010;15:334-354.

10. Vincent K, Maigne J-Y, Fischhoff C, Lanlo O, Dagenais S. Systematic review of manual therapies for nonspecific neck pain. *Joint Bone Spine*. 2013;80: 508-515.

11. Childs JD, Cleland JA, Elliott JM, et al. Neck pain: clinical practice guidelines linked to the International Classification of Functioning, Disability, and Health from the Orthopaedic Section of the American Physical Therapy Association. *J Orthop Sports Phys Ther*. 2008;38:A1-A34.

12. Chaibi A, Russell MB. Manual therapies for cervicogenic headache: a systematic review. *J Headache Pain*. 2012;13:351-359.

13. Posadzki P, Ernst E. Spinal manipulations for tension-type headaches: a systematic review of randomized controlled trials (review). *Complement Ther Med*. 2012;20:232-239.

14. Brantingham JW, Cassa TK, Bonnefin D, et al. Manipulative and multimodal therapy for upper extremity and temporomandibular disorders: a systematic review. *J Manipulative Physiol Ther*. 2013;36: 143-201.

15. Calixtre LB, Moreira RFC, Franchini GH, Alburquerque-Sendin F, Oliveira AB. Manual therapy for the management of pain and limited range of motion in subjects with signs and symptoms of temporomandibular disorder: a systematic review of randomized controlled trials. *J Oral Rehabil*. 2015;1-15. doi: 10.1111/joor.12321.

16. Hoogvliet P, Randsdorp MS, Dingemanse R, Koes BW, Huisstede BMA. Does effectiveness of exercise therapy and mobilisation techniques offer guidance for the treatment of lateral and medial epicondylitis? A systematic review. *Br J Sports Med*. 2013;47: 1112-1119.

17. Cyriax J. *Textbook of Orthopaedic Medicine*. Vol 1. 8th ed. Diagnosis of Soft Tissue Lesions. London: Bailliere Tindall; 1982.

18. Reid SA, Callister R, Katekar MG, Rvett DA. Effects of cervical spine manual therapy on range of motion, head repositioning, and balance in participants with cervicogenic dizziness: a randomized controlled trial. *Arch Phys Med Rehabil*. 2014;95: 1603-1612.

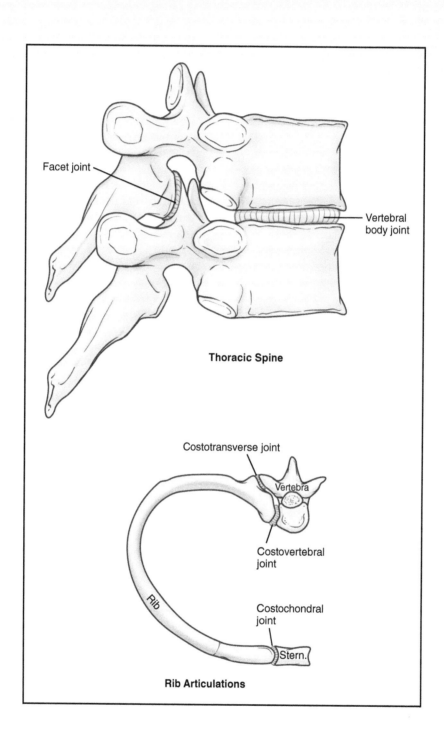

Thoracic Spine

Facet joint

Vertebral body joint

Rib Articulations

Costotransverse joint

Vertebra

Costovertebral joint

Costochondral joint

Rib

Stern.

CHAPTER 12

The Thoracic Spine and Ribs

BASICS

One major role related specifically to the thoracic spine and ribs is the protection of vital organs. The thoracic spine also provides stability in the upright position. The ribs assist in this role by blocking thoracic spine motion. Despite its function as a supporting structure, the thoracic spine accounts for 25% of the total movement in the spine.

Thoracic Joints

The spinous processes in the thoracic spine are positioned inferior to the motion segment. They can be used as a lever to move the vertebral bodies, theoretically resulting in a gliding of the facet articulations that corresponds to the physiologic movement that occurs with forward and backward bending in the thoracic spine.

The facet joints in the thoracic spine are oriented in a similar manner to the facet joints of the cervical spine except that they are aligned more vertically, almost parallel with the frontal plane. Similar to the lower cervical spine, osteokinematic movement at the thoracic spine is accompanied by a gliding motion between the two facet articulations, although with less movement in an anterior direction.

Rib Joints

Thoracic spine motion is restricted primarily by the ribs. The ribs attach to the vertebral bodies and to the vertebral transverse processes of the thoracic spine. Rib movement is guided by thoracic spine motion and the act of breathing.

The first rib is capable of only a small amount of motion because it is fused anteriorly to the sternum. Ribs two through five move primarily in an anterior and superior direction with inspiration and in a posterior and inferior direction with expiration; this is called pump-handle motion. Ribs seven through ten move primarily laterally and superiorly with inspiration and medially and inferiorly with expiration; this is called bucket-handle motion. Ribs five through seven are transitional ribs and exhibit characteristics of both types of movements. All of these motions are accompanied by rotation of the ribs around their longitudinal axes. Ribs 11 and 12 are capable of movement but generally are held in a relative position of expiration posteriorly by the quadratus lumborum muscle. When they do move, it is in a lateral direction with inspiration and in a medial direction with expiration; this is called caliper motion.

SPECIFIC PATHOLOGY AND THORACIC SPINE AND RIB JOINT MOBILIZATION/MANIPULATION

Midback Pain

There is a paucity of research addressing the efficacy of mobilization/manipulation for patients with thoracic spine pain and none that specifically addresses this intervention in relation to the ribs. In an early study of thoracic spine pain, 30 subjects with mechanical midback pain were randomly assigned to receive grade V manipulation to hypomobile thoracic segments or detuned ultrasound for a maximum of six treatment sessions.[1] Subjects receiving manipulation showed a significant reduction in pain at follow-up compared with the placebo group. These changes were maintained at 1-month follow-up.

Neck Pain

Numerous studies have evaluated the effectiveness of performing a thoracic spine manipulation for treatment of patients with neck pain. Four systemic reviews have summarized these findings. In the earliest of these reviews, published in 2010, the authors concluded that thoracic spine manipulation results in improvements in pain and function in patients with acute neck pain and an immediate reduction in pain in patients with chronic neck pain.[2] These conclusions were corroborated in a second systemic review, published in 2011, which stated that thoracic spine manipulation produces short-term improvements in pain, function, and range of motion in patients with acute or subacute neck pain.[3] The authors of a more recent systematic review, published in 2013, reported moderate short-term effects in patients with acute neck pain and limited effects for those with chronic neck pain.[4] These findings in relation to thoracic spine thrust manipulation were preempted by a 2008 clinical practice guideline, in which the authors recommended this intervention for treatment of disability and pain in patients with neck and neck-related arm pain.[10]

In the final, 2013 systematic review, the authors drew conclusions regarding the relative efficacy of spinal manipulation. They reported that thoracic spine manipulation might benefit some patients with neck pain; however there is no evidence to suggest that it is more effective for reducing pain or improving function than other interventions commonly administered to patients with neck pain, such as spinal mobilization, cervical manipulation, and exercise.[5] In relation to cervical manipulation, because this intervention poses a greater risk of harm to patients than thoracic manipulation these findings suggest that thoracic manipulation might offer a safer, yet equally effective treatment option.

Lateral Epicondylalgia

In a systemic review addressing conservative interventions for patients with lateral epicondylalgia, the authors reported moderate evidence supporting the use of cervical and thoracic manipulation as an adjunct to a regimen of stretching and strengthening exercises and wrist and forearm mobilization.[6]

Osteoporosis

In one study, the investigators concluded that 3 months of treatment with joint mobilization resulted in a decrease in kyphotic curvature in older female subjects with osteoporosis.[8]

THORACIC JOINTS (T3-4 THROUGH T12-L1)

Osteokinematic motions:
   Forward/backward bending
   Side bending
   Rotation
Ligaments:
   Anterior longitudinal ligament
   Posterior longitudinal ligament
   Supraspinous ligament
   Interspinous ligament
   Ligamentum flavum
   Intertransverse ligaments
Joint orientation:
   Inferior facet of superior vertebra: anterior, inferior, medial
   Superior facet of inferior vertebra: posterior, superior, lateral
   Superior vertebral body: inferior
   Inferior vertebral body: superior
Type of joint:
   Facets: synovial
   Disc: amphiarthrodial
Concave joint surface:
   None, these are plane joints
Resting position:
   Not described by Kaltenborn
Close-packed position:
   Not described by Kaltenborn
Capsular pattern of restriction:
   Difficult to determine[7]

Anterior Glide Using the Spinous Processes: First Technique (Figure 12-1, Video 12-1)

Purpose

- To examine for thoracic spine joint impairment
- To increase accessory motion into thoracic joint anterior glide
- To increase range of motion at the thoracic spine
- To decrease pain

Positioning

1. The patient is prone.
2. The thoracic spine is placed in midrange in relation to forward/backward bending, side bending, and rotation.
3. The clinician is at the patient's side, facing the thoracic spine.
4. The mobilizing/manipulating hand is positioned with the heel of the hand or the thumb over the guiding hand.
5. The guiding hand is positioned with the thumb over the spinous process being mobilized/manipulated.

Procedure

1. The mobilizing/manipulating hand glides the spinous process anteriorly as the patient exhales.
2. The guiding hand controls the position of the mobilizing/manipulating hand (see Figure 12-1).

Particulars

- This technique also is called springing. If it is being performed as an examination technique, the term *spring testing* is used.
- This technique is commonly performed using a grade V manipulation.

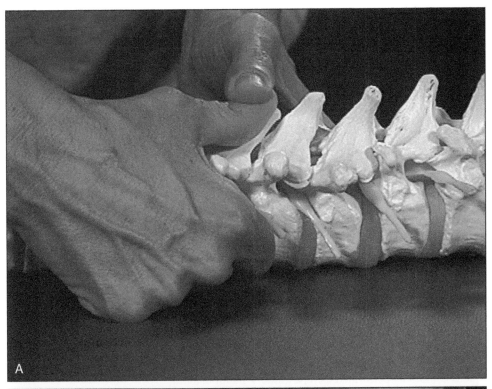

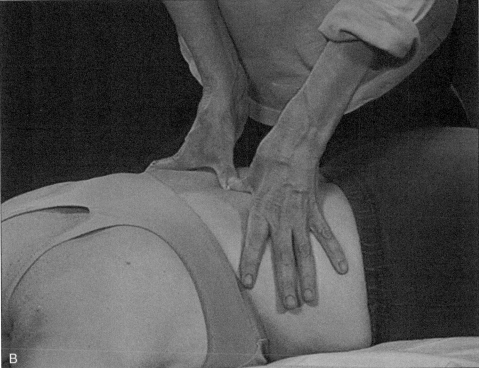

Figure 12-1 **A** and **B,** Anterior glide using the spinous processes: first technique.

Anterior Glide Using the Spinous Processes: Second Technique (Figure 12-2, Video 12-2)

Purpose

- To examine for thoracic spine joint impairment
- To increase accessory motion into thoracic joint anterior glide
- To increase range of motion at the thoracic spine
- To decrease pain

Positioning

1. The patient is prone.
2. The thoracic spine is placed in midrange in relation to forward/backward bending, side bending, and rotation.
3. The clinician is at the patient's side, facing the thoracic spine.
4. The stabilizing hand is positioned with the thumb or the anterior surface of the pisiform on the spinous process of the more inferior vertebra.
5. The mobilizing/manipulating hand is positioned with the thumb or the medial (ulnar) surface of the pisiform over the spinous process of the more superior vertebra.

Procedure

1. The stabilizing hand holds the vertebra in position.
2. The mobilizing/manipulating hand glides the spinous process anteriorly as the patient exhales (see Figure 12-2).

Particulars

- This technique might be especially effective for increasing range of motion into thoracic spine backward bending.
- This technique is commonly performed using a grade V manipulation.

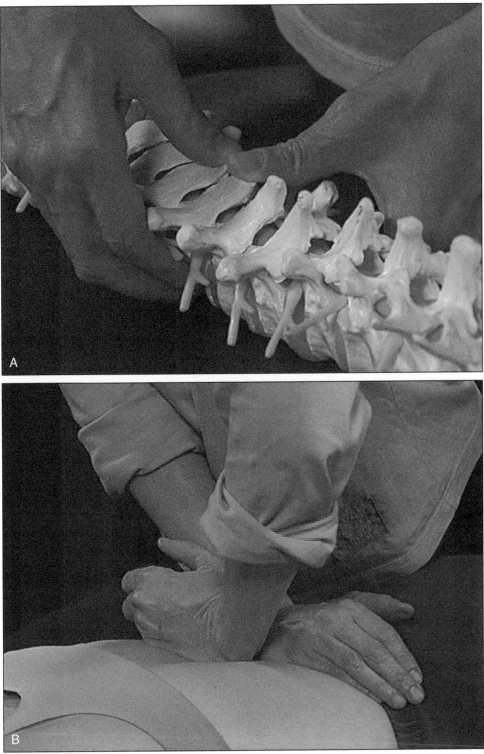

Figure 12-2 **A** and **B,** Anterior glide using the spinous processes: second technique.

Anterior Glide Using the Spinous Processes: Third Technique (Figure 12-3, Video 12-3)

Purpose
- To examine for thoracic spine joint impairment
- To increase accessory motion into thoracic joint anterior glide
- To increase range of motion at the thoracic spine
- To decrease pain

Positioning
1. The patient is prone.
2. The thoracic spine is placed in midrange in relation to forward/backward bending, side bending, and rotation.
3. The clinician is at the patient's side, facing the thoracic spine.
4. The stabilizing hand is positioned with the thumb or the medial (ulnar) surface of the pisiform on the spinous process of the more superior vertebra.
5. The mobilizing/manipulating hand is positioned with the thumb or the anterior surface of the pisiform over the spinous process of the more inferior vertebra.

Procedure
1. The stabilizing hand holds the vertebra in position.
2. The mobilizing/manipulating hand glides the spinous process anteriorly as the patient exhales (see Figure 12-3).

Particulars
- This technique might be especially effective for increasing range of motion into thoracic spine forward bending.
- This technique is commonly performed using a grade V manipulation.

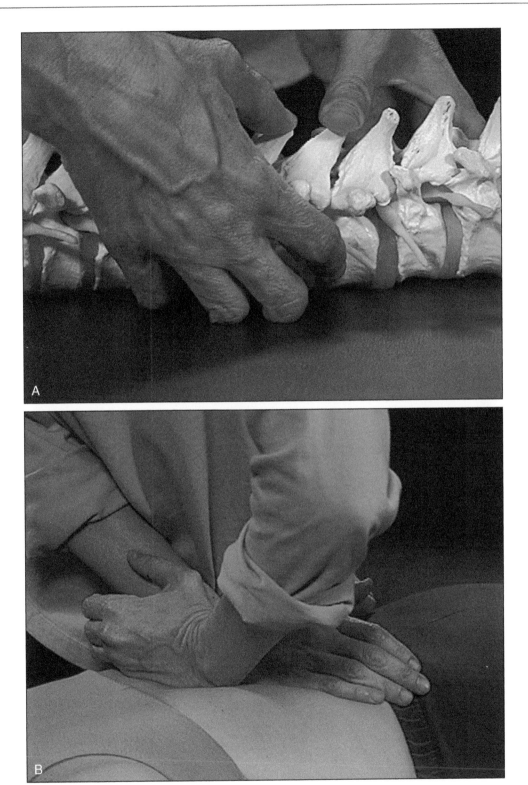

Figure 12-3 **A** and **B,** Anterior glide using the spinous processes: third technique.

Lateral Glide Using the Spinous Processes (Figure 12-4, Video 12-4)

Purpose
- To examine for thoracic spine joint impairment
- To increase accessory motion into thoracic vertebral body rotation and into facet joint distraction on the side toward which the vertebral body is rotating
- To increase range of motion at the thoracic spine
- To decrease pain

Positioning
1. The patient is prone.
2. The thoracic spine is placed in midrange in relation to forward/backward bending, side bending, and rotation.
3. The clinician is at the patient's side, facing the thoracic spine.
4. The stabilizing hand is positioned with the thumb or the anterior surface of the pisiform on the lateral surface of the spinous process of the more inferior vertebra.
5. The mobilizing/manipulating hand is positioned with the thumb or the anterior surface of the pisiform on the lateral surface of the spinous process of the more superior vertebra opposite the side of the stabilizing hand.

Procedure
1. The stabilizing hand holds the more inferior vertebra in position.
2. The mobilizing/manipulating hand glides the more superior spinous process toward the contralateral side as the patient exhales (see Figure 12-4).

Particulars
- This technique might be especially effective for increasing range of motion into thoracic spine rotation in the direction of vertebral body movement (in the direction opposite the movement of the spinous processes).
- This technique is commonly performed using a grade V manipulation.

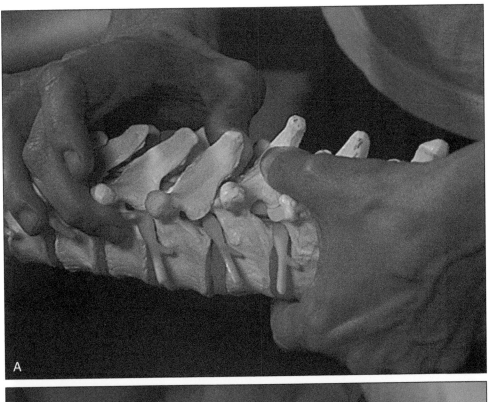

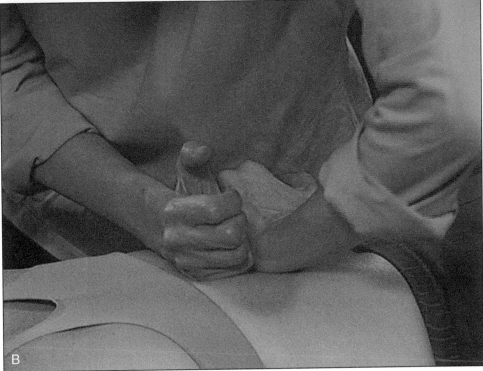

Figure 12-4 **A** and **B,** Lateral glide using the spinous processes.

Anterior Glide Using the Transverse Processes: First Technique (Figure 12-5, Video 12-5)

Purpose
- To examine for thoracic spine joint impairment
- To increase accessory motion into thoracic joint anterior glide
- To increase range of motion at the thoracic spine
- To decrease pain

Positioning
1. The patient is prone.
2. The thoracic spine is positioned in midrange in relation to forward/backward bending, side bending, and rotation.
3. The clinician is at the patient's side, facing the thoracic spine.
4. One hand is positioned with the anterior surface of the pisiform on the transverse process of one vertebra.
5. The other hand is positioned with the anterior surface of the pisiform on the opposite transverse process of the same vertebra.
6. The clinician rotates each hand around the pisiform to aid in maintaining the position of the pisiform on the transverse process.

Procedure
1. Both hands simultaneously glide the transverse processes anteriorly as the patient exhales (see Figure 12-5).

Particulars
- This technique is commonly performed using a grade V manipulation.

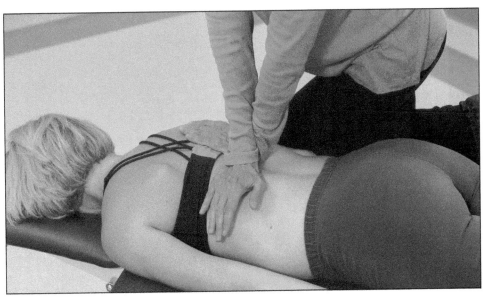

Figure 12-5 Anterior Glide using the transverse process: first technique.

Anterior Glide Using the Transverse Processes: Second Technique (Figure 12-6, Video 12-6)

Purpose
- To examine for thoracic spine joint impairment
- To increase accessory motion into thoracic vertebral body rotation and into facet joint distraction on the side toward which the vertebral body is rotating
- To increase range of motion at the thoracic spine
- To decrease pain

Positioning
1. The patient is prone.
2. The thoracic spine is positioned in midrange in relation to forward/backward bending, side bending, and rotation.
3. The clinician is at the patient's side, facing the thoracic spine.
4. The stabilizing hand is positioned with the thumb or the anterior surface of the pisiform on the transverse process of the more inferior vertebra.
5. The mobilizing/manipulating hand is positioned with the thumb or the anterior surface of the pisiform on the transverse process of the more superior vertebra opposite the side of the stabilizing hand.

Procedure
1. The stabilizing hand holds the more inferior vertebra in position.
2. The mobilizing/manipulating hand glides the more superior transverse process in an anterior direction as the patient exhales (see Figure 12-6).

Particulars
- This technique might be especially effective for increasing range of motion into thoracic spine rotation in the direction of vertebral body movement.
- This technique is commonly performed using a grade V manipulation.

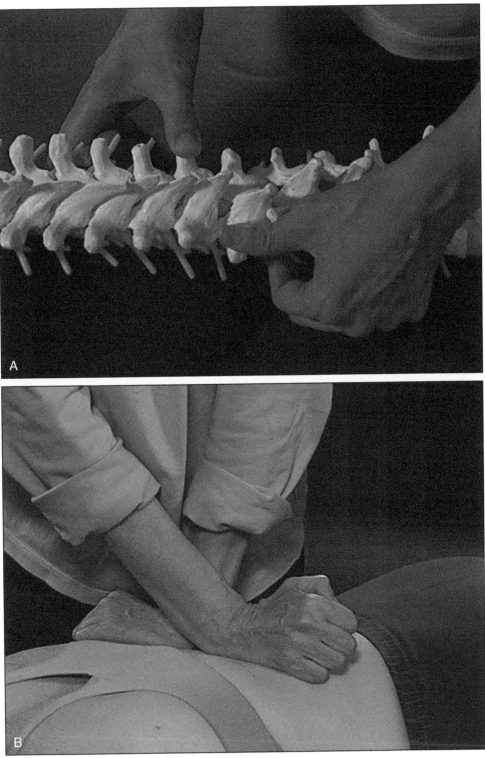

Figure 12-6 **A** and **B,** Anterior glide using the transverse processes.

Backward-Bending Glide (Figure 12-7, Video 12-7)

Purpose
- To increase accessory motion into thoracic backward bending
- To increase range of motion at the thoracic spine
- To decrease pain

Positioning
1. The patient is sitting with the arms positioned across the chest.
2. The thoracic spine is positioned in midrange in relation to forward/backward bending, side bending, and rotation.
3. The clinician is at the patient's side, facing the patient with the clinician's arms across the patient's chest and the clinician's anterior shoulder and hand supporting the patient's shoulders.
4. The clinician locks the more superior vertebrae by backward bending the trunk to the extent that the motion segment above the one being mobilized/manipulated is fully backward bent but the motion segment being mobilized/manipulated has not yet moved.
5. The stabilizing hand is positioned with the thumb or pisiform on the inferior tip of the more inferior spinous process of intended vertebral body motion.

Procedure
1. The stabilizing hand holds the inferior vertebra in position.
2. The mobilizing/manipulating hand backward bends the patient's trunk (see Figure 12-7).

Particulars
- To examine for joint mobility, the patient is positioned sitting with arms across the chest. The clinician is facing the side of the patient's trunk with one shoulder positioned in front of the patient's shoulder, the arm reaching across the patient's anterior trunk, and the hand positioned on the contralateral shoulder. The clinician palpates the T3-4 motion segment by placing the palpating finger between the T3 and T4 spinous processes, backward bends the patient until the clinician feels motion between T3 and T4, and grades the amount of motion that occurred into backward bending. After grading the motion, the clinician restores slack to the T3-4 motion segment by moving the spine slightly back toward neutral and moves the palpating finger to the T4-5 motion segment. This process is repeated until motion into backward bending at all thoracic vertebral motion segments is graded.
- The intervention technique might be especially effective for increasing range of motion into thoracic spine backward bending.
- In a randomized controlled trial of postmenopausal women with thoracic kyphosis, the investigators compared a 3-month physical therapy regimen consisting of joint mobilization techniques performed similar to this technique, exercises to address posture, and taping with a control group. Subjects assigned to the treatment group demonstrated significant improvements in their kyphotic curvature compared with the control group, although there were no differences in changes in pain or quality of life across these two groups.[8]

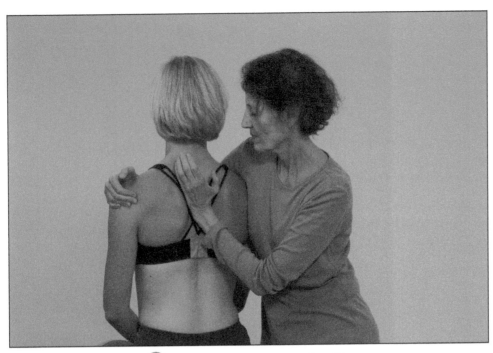

Figure 12-7 Backward-bending glide.

Distraction Manipulation (Figure 12-8, Video 12-8)

Purpose

- To increase accessory motion in thoracic spine joints
- To increase range of motion at the thoracic spine
- To decrease pain

Positioning

1. The patient is seated on the treatment table with arms across the chest.
2. The clinician can place a rolled towel horizontally along the patient's spine.
3. The clinician stands behind the patient, reaches around the patient, and grips the patient's elbows while interlocking the fingers.
4. The clinician places the sternum on the patient's midthoracic spine.
5. The clinician steps or leans backward, thereby taking up tissue resistance.

Procedure

1. The clinician performs a grade V manipulation manipulation by quickly moving the patient's trunk upward and backward (see Figure 12-8).

Particulars

- The examination procedure for determining whether this treatment technique is indicated is unclear. Many clinicians would consider pain the indication for treatment. Nevertheless, an evaluation of joint mobility is prudent to determine whether any hypermobility is present and to identify specific areas of hypomobility. To examine for joint mobility, the patient is positioned sitting with arms across the chest. The clinician is facing the side of the patient's trunk with one shoulder positioned in front of the patient's shoulder, the arm reaching across the patient's anterior trunk, and the hand positioned on the contralateral shoulder. The clinician palpates the T3-4 motion segment by placing the palpating finger between the T3 and T4 spinous processes, forward bends the patient until the clinician feels motion between T3 and T4, and grades the amount of motion that occurred into forward bending. This process is repeated until motion into forward bending at all thoracic vertebral motion segments is graded. It is repeated for backward-bending motion.
- This intervention technique should be performed using a grade V manipulation.
- This technique might be an effective intervention for reducing pain and improving function in patients with neck pain.
- In a study in which subjects served as their own controls, this technique, when combined with a manipulation procedure targeted at the cervicothoracic junction and a rib manipulation technique performed only if indicated, resulted in improvements in disability and pain in subjects with shoulder impingement syndrome 48 hours after the interventions were administered.[9]

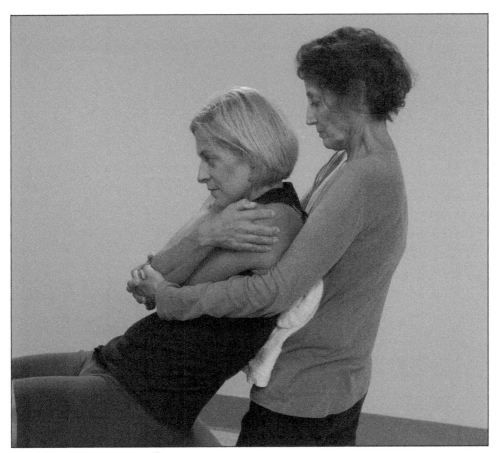

Figure 12-8 Distraction manipulation.

Posterior-Superior Manipulation (Figure 12-9, Video 12-9)

Purpose
- To increase accessory motion in thoracic spine joints
- To increase range of motion at the thoracic spine
- To decrease pain

Positioning
1. The patient is supine with the fingers laced together at the base of the neck and the elbows touching.
2. The thoracic spine is positioned in midrange in relation to forward/backward bending, side bending, and rotation.
3. The clinician is at the patient's side.
4. A pillow can be used to separate the patient's chest from the clinician.
5. The clinician lifts the patient's contralateral shoulder, rotating the patient toward the clinician, and reaches across the front of the patient's trunk to position the stabilizing hand on the patient's thoracic spine.
6. The stabilizing hand is positioned on the more inferior vertebra such that the hand is opened (this is a more comfortable position for the clinician) or closed, the metacarpophalangeal joint of the index finger is on the patient's transverse process closest to the clinician, the thenar eminence is on the patient's transverse process farthest away from the clinician, and the thumb is along the side of the patient's spinous processes above the motion segment being stabilized (Figure 12-9A).
7. The clinician repositions the patient in supine position and then slides the stabilizing hand down the spine slightly, thereby decreasing movement of the clinician's hand on the patient's skin.
8. The clinician locks the more superior vertebrae by forward bending the spine using the patient's arms as a fulcrum to the extent that the clinician feels the weight of the patient's thorax on the clinician's hand more than in any other position.
9. The manipulating hand grips the patient's elbows.

Procedure
1. The stabilizing hand holds the more inferior vertebra in position.
2. The manipulating hand glides the more superior vertebra posteriorly by thrusting the patient's elbows in a posterior direction as the patient exhales, directing the force through the long axis of the patient's upper arms. The clinician should use body weight to assist in directing this force (see Figure 12-9B).

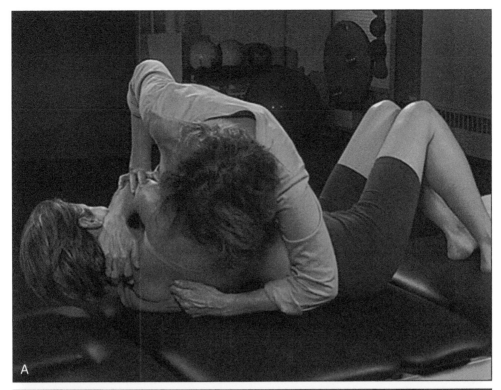

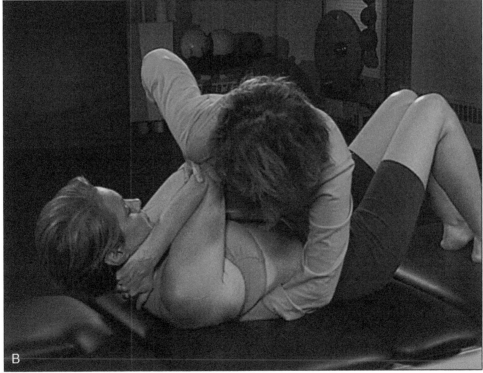

Figure 12-9 **A** and **B,** Posterior superior Manipulation.

Particulars
- The examination procedure for determining whether this treatment technique is indicated is unclear. Many clinicians would consider pain the indication for treatment. Nevertheless, an evaluation of joint mobility is prudent, to determine whether any hypermobility is present and to identify specific areas of hypomobility. To examine for joint mobility, the patient is positioned sitting with arms across the chest. The clinician is facing the side of the patient's trunk with one shoulder positioned in front of the patient's shoulder, the arm reaching across the patient's anterior trunk, and the hand positioned on the contralateral shoulder. The clinician palpates the T3-4 motion segment by placing the palpating finger between the T3 and T4 spinous processes, forward bends the patient until the clinician feels motion between T3 and T4, and grades the amount of motion that occurred into forward bending. This process is repeated until motion into forward bending at all thoracic vertebral motion segments is graded. It is repeated for backward-bending motion.
- This intervention technique should be performed using a grade V manipulation.
- This technique can be modified to target the upper thoracic spine by instructing the patient to perform a bridge to the extent that the clinician feels the weight of the patient's thorax on the clinician's hand more than in any other position.
- This technique is sometimes called the Chicago technique.
- This technique might be an effective intervention for reducing pain and improving function in patients with neck pain.

RIB JOINTS

Osteokinematic motions:
    Anterior/posterior
    Lateral/medial
    Superior/inferior
    Rotation
Ligaments: costovertebral joints:
    Capsular ligament
    Radiate ligament
    Intraarticular ligament
Ligaments: costotransverse joints:
    Capsular ligament
    Costotransverse ligament
Joint orientation:
    Vertebral body: posterior, lateral
    Rib at costovertebral joint: anterior, medial
    Vertebral transverse process: anterior, lateral
    Rib at costotransverse joint: posterior, medial
    Sternum: lateral, inferior
    Rib at costochondral joint: medial, superior
Type of joint:
    Costovertebral joint: synovial
    Costotransverse joint: synovial
    Costochondral joint: synchondrosis
Concave joint surface:
    None, these are plane joints
Resting position:
    Not described by Kaltenborn
Close-packed position:
    Not described by Kaltenborn
Capsular pattern of restriction:
    Not described by Cyriax

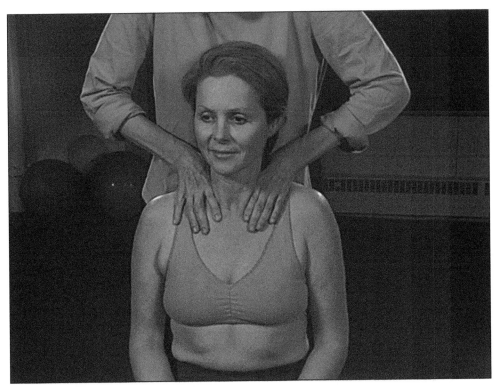

Figure 12-10 Inferior glide of the first rib/passive accessory motion.

Inferior Glide of the First Rib (Figure 12-10, Video 12-10)

Purpose
- To examine for first rib joint impairment
- To increase accessory motion in the articulations at the first rib
- To increase range of motion at the first rib
- To decrease pain

Positioning
1. The patient is sitting.
2. The trunk is positioned in midrange in relation to forward/backward bending, side bending, and rotation.
3. The clinician is behind the patient, facing the patient's trunk.
4. The stabilizing hand is positioned on the superior surface of the first rib on the side that is not being mobilized/manipulated.
5. The mobilizing hand is positioned on the superior surface of the first rib on the side being mobilized/manipulated.

Procedure
1. The stabilizing hand holds the rib in position.
2. The mobilizing/manipulating hand glides the rib in an inferior direction as the patient exhales (see Figure 12-10).

Particulars
- This technique might be effective in correcting a first rib joint inspiration positional fault or chronic positioning of the first rib into elevation, such as in patients with chronic obstructive pulmonary disease who breathe primarily using the apical musculature. This positional fault might be a contributing factor to the onset of thoracic outlet syndrome.
- This technique is commonly performed using a grade V manipulation.

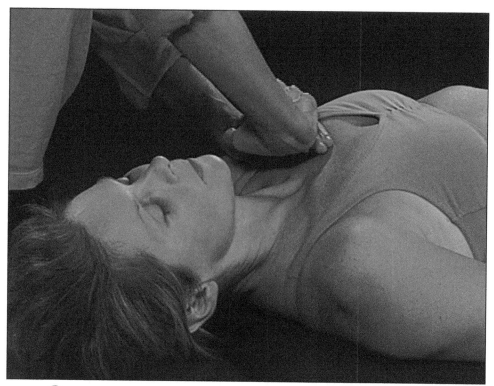

▶ **Figure 12-11** Expiration glide of ribs 2 through 7/passive physiologic motion.

Expiration Glide of Ribs Two through Seven (Figure 12-11, Video 12-11)
Purpose
- To examine for rib joint impairment
- To increase accessory motion in the articulations at ribs 2 through 7
- To increase range of motion at ribs two through seven
- To decrease pain

Positioning
1. The patient is supine.
2. The trunk is positioned in midrange in relation to forward/backward bending, side bending, and rotation.
3. The clinician is at the patient's side, facing the patient's trunk.
4. The mobilizing hand is positioned on the anterior or anterolateral surface of the trunk with the medial (ulnar) border of the hand between the rib being mobilized and the one above it.
5. The guiding hand is positioned over the mobilizing hand.

Procedure
1. The mobilizing hand guides the rib in a posterior and inferior direction as the patient exhales and resists anterior and superior motion as the patient inhales.
2. The guiding hand controls the position of the mobilizing hand (see Figure 12-11).

Particulars
- This is not a grade V manipulation technique.
- This technique might be especially effective for increasing range of motion into pump-handle expiration at ribs 2 through 7.

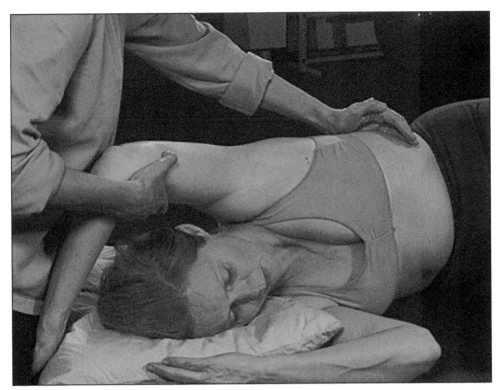

Figure 12-12 Expiration glide of ribs 5 through 11/passive physiologic motion.

Expiration Glide of Ribs 5 through 11 (Figure 12-12, Video 12-12)

Purpose
- To examine for rib joint impairment
- To increase accessory motion in the articulations at ribs 5 through 11
- To increase range of motion at ribs 5 through 11
- To decrease pain

Positioning
1. The patient is side lying with the arm positioned over the head.
2. The trunk is positioned in midrange in relation to forward/backward bending, side bending, and rotation.
3. The clinician is at the patient's head, facing the patient's trunk.
4. The mobilizing hand is positioned on the lateral surface of the trunk with the medial (ulnar) border of the hand between the rib being mobilized and the one above it.
5. The guiding hand holds the patient's arm.

Procedure
1. The mobilizing hand guides the rib in a medial and inferior direction as the patient exhales and resists lateral and superior motion as the patient inhales.
2. The guiding hand controls the position of the patient's arm (see Figure 12-12).

Particulars
- This is not a grade V manipulation technique.
- This technique might be especially effective for increasing range of motion into bucket-handle expiration at ribs 5 through 11.

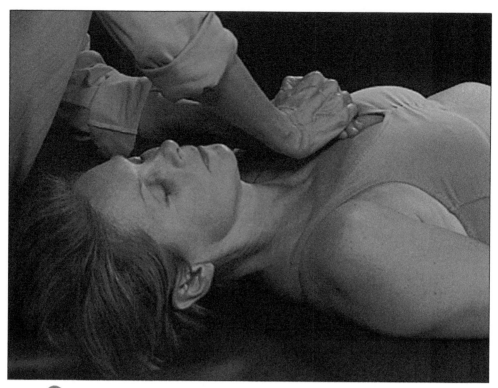

Figure 12-13 Inspiration glide of ribs 2 through 7/passive physiologic motion.

Inspiration Glide of Ribs Two through Seven (Figure 12-13, Video 12-13)

Purpose

- To examine for rib joint impairment
- To increase accessory motion in the articulations at ribs 2 through 7
- To increase range of motion at ribs 2 through 7
- To decrease pain

Positioning

1. The patient is supine.
2. The trunk is positioned in midrange in relation to forward/backward bending, side bending, and rotation.
3. The clinician is at the patient's side, facing the patient's trunk.
4. The mobilizing hand is positioned on the anterior or anterolateral surface of the trunk with the medial (ulnar) border of the hand between the rib being mobilized and the one below it.
5. The guiding hand is positioned over the mobilizing hand.

Procedure

1. The mobilizing hand guides the rib in an anterior and superior direction as the patient inhales and resists posterior and inferior motion as the patient exhales.
2. The guiding hand controls the position of the mobilizing hand (see Figure 12-13).

Particulars

- This is not a grade V manipulation technique.
- This technique might be especially effective for increasing range of motion into bucket-handle inspiration at ribs 2 through 7.

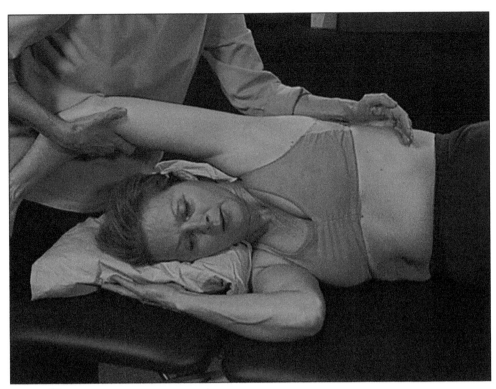

Figure 12-14 Inspiration glide of ribs 5 through 11/passive physiologic motion.

Inspiration Glide of Ribs 5 through 11 (Figure 12-14, Video 12-14)

Purpose
- To examine for rib joint impairment
- To increase accessory motion in the articulations at ribs 5 through 11
- To increase range of motion at ribs 5 through 11
- To decrease pain

Positioning
1. The patient is side lying with the arm positioned over the head.
2. The trunk is positioned in midrange in relation to forward/backward bending, side bending, and rotation.
3. The clinician is at the patient's head, facing the patient's trunk.
4. The mobilizing hand is positioned on the lateral surface of the trunk with the medial (ulnar) border of the hand between the rib being mobilized and the one below it.
5. The guiding hand holds the patient's arm.

Procedure
1. The mobilizing hand guides the rib in a lateral and superior direction as the patient inhales and resists medial and inferior motion as the patient exhales.
2. The guiding hand controls the position of the patient's arm (see Figure 12-14).

Particulars
- This is not a grade V manipulation technique.
- This technique might be especially effective for increasing range of motion into bucket-handle inspiration at ribs 5 through 11.

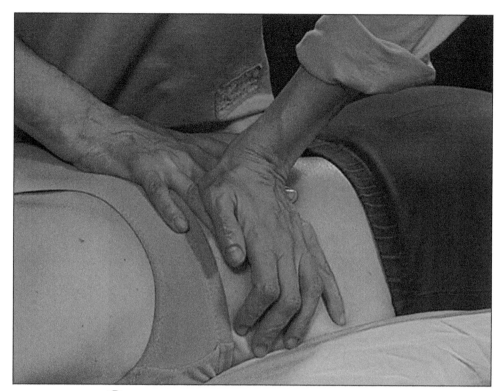

▶ **Figure 12-15** Anterior glide/passive accessory motion.

Anterior Glide of the Ribs (Figure 12-15, Video 12-15)

Purpose
- To examine for rib joint impairment
- To increase accessory motion in the rib articulations
- To increase range of motion at the ribs
- To decrease pain

Positioning
1. The patient is prone.
2. The trunk is positioned in midrange in relation to forward/backward bending, side bending, and rotation.
3. The clinician is at the patient's side, facing the patient's trunk.
4. The mobilizing/manipulating hand is positioned with the palm of the hand over the guiding hand.
5. The guiding hand is positioned with the anterior surface of the middle or index finger on the rib being mobilized/manipulated.

Procedure
1. The mobilizing/manipulating hand glides the rib anteriorly as the patient exhales.
2. The guiding hand controls the position of the mobilizing/manipulating hand (see Figure 12-15).

REFERENCES

1. Schiller L. Effectiveness of spinal manipulative therapy in the treatment of mechanical thoracic spine pain: a pilot randomized clinical trial. *J Manipulative Physiol Ther.* 2001;24:394-401.

2. Gross A, Miller J, D'Sylva J, et al. Manipulation or mobilisation for neck pain. *Cochrane Database Syst Rev.* 2010;(1):CD004249.

3. Cross KM, Kuenze C, Grindstaff T, Hertel J. Thoracic spine thrust manipulation improve pain, range of motion, and self-reported function in patients with mechanical neck pain: a systematic review. *J Orthop Sports Phys Ther.* 2011;41:633-642.

4. Vincent K, Maigne JY, Fischhoff C, Lanlo O, Dagenais S. Systematic review of manual therapies for nonspecific neck pain. *Joint Bone Spine.* 2013;80:508-515.

5. Huisman PA, Speksnijder CM, de Wijer A. The effect of thoracic spine manipulation on pain and disability in patients with non-specific neck pain: a systematic review. *Disabil Rehabil.* 2013;35:1677-1685.

6. Hoogvliet P, Randsdorp MS, Dingemanse R, Koes BW, Huisstede BMA. Does effectiveness of exercise therapy and mobilisation techniques offer guidance for the treatment of lateral and medial epicondylitis? A systematic review. *Br J Sports Med.* 2013;47:1112-1119.

7. Cyriax J. *Textbook of Orthopaedic Medicine*, Vol. 1. 8th ed. Diagnosis of Soft Tissue Lesions. London: Bailliere Tindall; 1982.

8. Bautmans I, Van Arken J, Van Mackelenberg M, Mets T. Rehabilitation using manual mobilization for thoracic kyphosis in elderly postmenopausal patients with osteoporosis. *J Rehabil Med.* 2010;42:129-135.

9. Boyles RE, Ritland BM, Miracle BM, et al. The short-term effects of thoracic spine thrust manipulation on patients with shoulder impingement syndrome. *Man Ther.* 2009;14:375-380.

10. Childs JD, Cleland JA, Elliott JM, et al. Neck pain: Clinical practice guidelines linked to the International Classification of Functioning, Disability, and Health from the Orthopedic Section of the American Physical Therapy Association. *J Orthop Sports Phys Ther.* 2008;38:A1-A34.

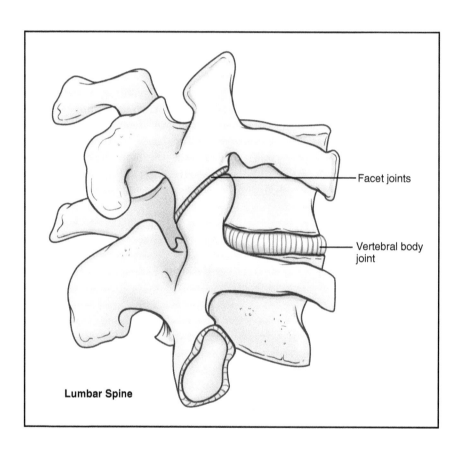

Facet joints

Vertebral body
joint

Lumbar Spine

CHAPTER 13

The Lumbar Spine

BASICS

Lumbar Joints

A greater amount of motion exists in the lumbar spine than in the thoracic spine because of the absence of ribs. As is the case in the thoracic and lower cervical joints, the degree and direction of movement in the lumbar spine are dictated by the orientation of the facet joints. The facet joints for the L1 through L4 motion segments are located in the sagittal plane, whereas the L4-5 and L5-S1 facets are aligned closely with the frontal plane. As a result, more forward and backward bending occur in the lower lumbar spine than in the upper lumbar spine. With forward bending, both facets on the more superior lumbar vertebra glide upward, whereas with backward bending they glide downward.

RISKS OF LUMBAR SPINE MOBILIZATION/MANIPULATION

Risk of serious injury from lumbar spinal manipulation is rare and seems to be limited to cauda equina syndrome. In a 2004 systematic review the risk of this injury was reported to be less than one in 3.7 million manipulations.[1]

SPECIFIC PATHOLOGY AND LUMBAR SPINE MOBILIZATION/MANIPULATION

Nonspecific Low Back Pain

A vast majority of studies addressing mobilization/ manipulation interventions for patients with low back pain have specifically addressed grade V manipulations, possibly because of the focus by chiropractors on this technique. Studies evaluating the efficacy of lumbar manipulation for the treatment of patients with low back pain abound, numerous enough to warrant an update of a systematic review of systematic reviews.[2] The authors of this manuscript included seven systematic reviews, stating that three of these reported positive results, three reported negative results, and one yielded an inconclusive result.

Two systematic reviews were published by the Cochrane Collaboration, a highly regarded independent, nonprofit, nongovernmental organization formed to organize medical research information to facilitate the choices that health professionals, patients, policy makers,

and others face in health interventions according to the principles of evidence-based medicine.[3] One of these systematic reviews, published in 2013, addressed the efficacy of manipulation for patients with acute low back pain and the other, published in 2011, addressed patients with chronic low back pain.

The authors of the Cochrane review addressing patients with acute low back pain based their results on 20 randomized clinical trials that met the criteria for inclusion in their review. They concluded that there is no difference in changes in function or pain outcomes when manipulation was compared with inert or placebo interventions for all follow-up time periods. Furthermore, including manipulation with other conservative interventions for acute low back pain did not improve these outcomes. The authors based these conclusions on low-quality to very low-quality evidence. They also reported, based on very low to moderate evidence, that there was no difference in the effect of manipulation compared with other conservative interventions.[4]

In the Cochrane systematic review addressing the efficacy of lumbar spine manipulation for patients with chronic low back pain, the authors included 26 randomized clinical trials. They concluded that there is high-quality evidence demonstrating a small, statistically significant but not clinically relevant short-term improvement in function and pain compared with other conservative interventions. When lumbar manipulation interventions are added to other conservative treatments for low back pain, there is also a statistically significant short-term positive effect on function and pain. These latter findings were based on quality of evidence ranging from low to high. The investigators concluded that long-term outcomes were not well studied.[5]

In a 2012 clinical practice guideline addressing physical therapy interventions for patients with low back pain, the authors reported on the efficacy of manual therapy. They recommended using manipulation in patients with acute low back and low back related buttock or thigh pain to improve function and decrease pain. In relation to subacute and chronic low back and low back related leg pain, both mobilization/manipulation and soft tissue techniques were recommended to reduce disability and pain and to improve range of motion. They based these recommendations on strong evidence.[6]

Discrepancies in these recommendations could be due in part to differences in the effects of manipulation versus manual therapy. Irrespective of these potential differences, however, larger effect sizes might have occurred if the investigators had subclassified patients with low back pain to optimize outcomes, because one possible reason for the small effect sizes is that these studies included heterogeneous groups of patients, some of whom will benefit from manipulation and some of whom will not. Identifying subgroups of patients who are more likely to respond positively to joint mobilization/manipulation would inform the choice of interventions and enhance outcomes.

In response to the need to subclassify patients with low back pain to maximize outcomes with lumbar spine manipulation, two separate studies identified and validated a clinical prediction rule to classify patients who are likely to experience dramatic improvements with this intervention.[7,8] The following five variables were predictive of a positive outcome after manipulation: (1) duration of symptoms was less than 16 days, (2) at least one hip had more than 35 degrees of medial rotation, (3) one or more lumbar spine levels were hypomobile, (4) there were no symptoms distal to the knee, and (5) Fear Avoidance Behavior Questionnaire work score was less than 19 (indicating low levels of fear avoidance beliefs). The presence of four of these five variables increased the probability of successful outcome after manipulation from 45% to between 92% and 95%.

This clinical prediction rule was evaluated in two subsequent randomized clinical trials. In the first of these studies, patients who met the clinical prediction rule and received lumbar manipulations experienced less disability at follow-up than those who were not matched in relation to the rule and the manipulation intervention.[9] In the second of these studies, the clinical prediction rule performed no better than chance in identifying patients with acute, nonspecific low back pain who benefited from lumbar spine manipulation interventions.[10] These studies suggest that, although promising, this clinical prediction rule for spinal manipulation needs refinement.

Lumbar Radiculopathy

In a 2011 systematic review, the authors addressed the efficacy of lumbar manipulation for patients with lumbar radiculopathy. They concluded that manipulation is more effective than placebo for acute radiculopathy. In relation to chronic radiculopathy, the authors similarly concluded that manipulation was beneficial, but based this conclusion on weak evidence.[11]

LUMBAR JOINTS

Osteokinematic motions:
  Forward/backward bending
  Side bending
  Rotation
Ligaments:
  Anterior longitudinal ligament
  Posterior longitudinal ligament
  Supraspinous ligament
  Interspinous ligament
  Ligamentum flavum
  Intertransverse ligaments
Joint orientation:
  Inferior facet of superior vertebra through L3-4: anterior, lateral
  Superior facet of inferior vertebra through L3-4: posterior, medial
  Inferior facet of L4-5 and L5-S1: anterior
  Superior facet of L4-5 and L5-S1: posterior
  Superior vertebral body: inferior
  Inferior vertebral body: superior
Type of joint:
  Facets: synovial
  Disc: amphiarthrodial
Concave joint surface:
  None, these are plane joints
Resting position:
  Not described by Kaltenborn
Close-packed position:
  Not described by Kaltenborn
Capsular pattern of restriction:
  Difficult to determine[12]

Anterior Glide Using Spinous Processes (Figure 13-1, Video 13-1)

Purpose
- To examine for lumbar spine joint impairment
- To increase accessory motion into lumbar joint anterior glide
- To increase range of motion at the lumbar spine
- To decrease pain

Positioning
1. The patient is prone.
2. The lumbar spine is positioned in midrange in relation to forward/backward bending, side bending, and rotation.
3. The clinician is at the patient's side, facing the lumbar spine.
4. The mobilizing/manipulating hand is positioned with the heel of the hand or the thumb over the guiding hand.
5. The guiding hand is positioned with the thumb or the middle finger over the spinous process being mobilized/manipulated.

Procedure
1. The mobilizing/manipulating hand glides the spinous process anteriorly as the patient exhales.
2. The guiding hand controls the position of the mobilizing/manipulating hand (see Figure 13-1).

Particulars
- This technique also is called springing. If it is being performed as an examination technique, the term *spring testing* is used.
- This technique is commonly performed using a grade V manipulation.

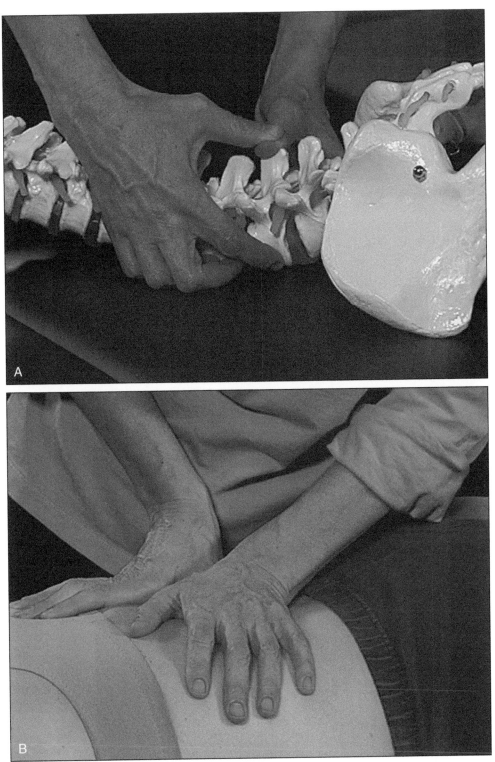

Figure 13-1 **A** and **B,** Anterior glide using the spinous processes.

Superior Glide Using the Spinous Processes: First Technique (Figure 13-2, Video 13-2)

Purpose
- To examine for lumbar spine joint impairment
- To increase accessory motion into lumbar joint superior glide
- To increase range of motion at the lumbar spine
- To decrease pain

Positioning
1. The patient is prone.
2. The lumbar spine is positioned in midrange in relation to forward/backward bending, side bending, and rotation.
3. The clinician is at the patient's side, facing the lumbar spine.
4. The stabilizing hand is positioned with the thumb or the medial (ulnar) surface of the pisiform on the spinous process of the more superior vertebra.
5. The mobilizing/manipulating hand is positioned with the thumb or the anterior surface of the pisiform on the most inferior surface of the spinous process of the more inferior vertebra.

Procedure
1. The stabilizing hand holds the vertebra in position.
2. The mobilizing/manipulating hand glides the spinous process superiorly as the patient exhales (see Figure 13-2).

Particulars
- This technique might be especially effective for increasing range of motion into lumbar spine backward bending.

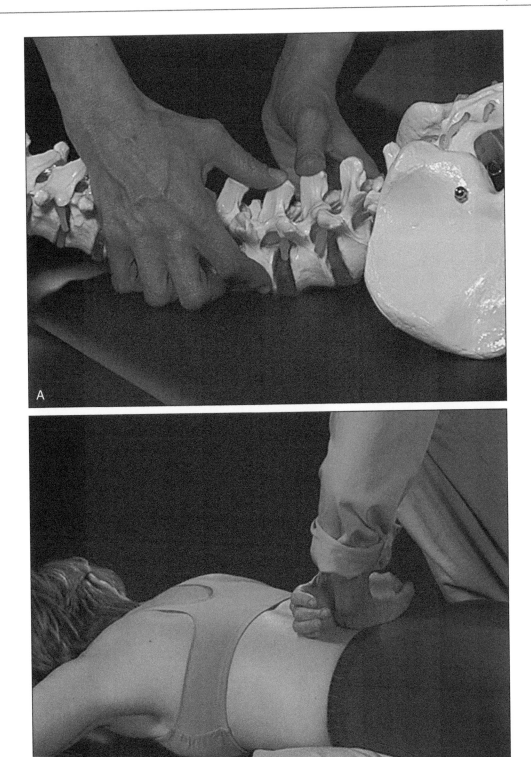

Figure 13-2 A and **B,** Superior glide using the spinous processes: first technique.

Superior Glide Using the Spinous Processes: Second Technique (Figure 13-3, Video 13-3)

Purpose
- To examine for lumbar spine joint impairment
- To increase accessory motion into lumbar joint superior glide
- To increase range of motion at the lumbar spine
- To decrease pain

Positioning
1. The patient is prone.
2. The lumbar spine is positioned in midrange in relation to forward/backward bending, side bending, and rotation.
3. The clinician is at the patient's side, facing the lumbar spine.
4. The stabilizing hand is positioned with the thumb or the anterior surface of the pisiform on the spinous process of the more inferior vertebra.
5. The mobilizing/manipulating hand is positioned with the thumb or the medial (ulnar) surface of the pisiform on the most inferior surface of the spinous process of the more superior vertebra.

Procedure
1. The stabilizing hand holds the vertebra in position.
2. The mobilizing/manipulating hand glides the spinous process superiorly as the patient exhales (see Figure 13-3).

Particulars
- This technique might be especially effective for increasing range of motion into lumbar spine forward bending.

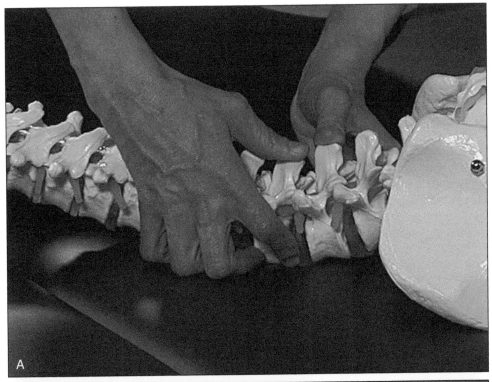

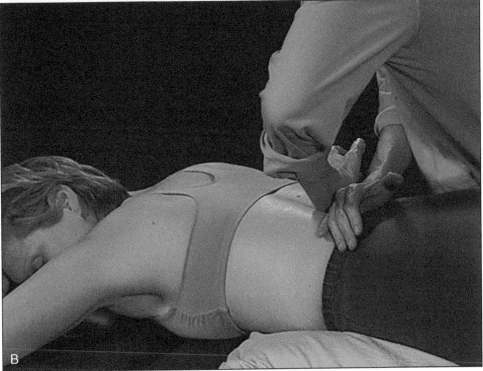

Figure 13-3 **A** and **B,** Superior glide using the spinous processes: second technique.

Lateral Glide Using the Spinous Processes (Figure 13-4, Video 13-4)

Purpose

- To examine for lumbar spine joint impairment
- To increase accessory motion into lumbar vertebral body rotation and into facet joint distraction on the side toward which the vertebral body is rotating
- To increase range of motion at the lumbar spine
- To decrease pain

Positioning

1. The patient is prone.
2. The lumbar spine is positioned in midrange in relation to forward/backward bending, side bending, and rotation.
3. The clinician is at the patient's side, facing the lumbar spine.
4. The stabilizing hand is positioned with the thumb or the anterior surface of the pisiform on the lateral surface of the spinous process of the more inferior vertebra.
5. The mobilizing/manipulating hand is positioned with the thumb on the medial (ulnar) surface of the pisiform on the lateral surface of the spinous process of the more superior vertebra opposite the side of the stabilizing hand.

Procedure

1. The stabilizing hand holds the more inferior vertebra in position.
2. The mobilizing/manipulating hand glides the more superior spinous process toward the contralateral side as the patient exhales (see Figure 13-4).

Particulars

- This technique might be especially effective for increasing range of motion into lumbar spine rotation in the direction of vertebral body movement (in the direction opposite the movement of the spinous processes).

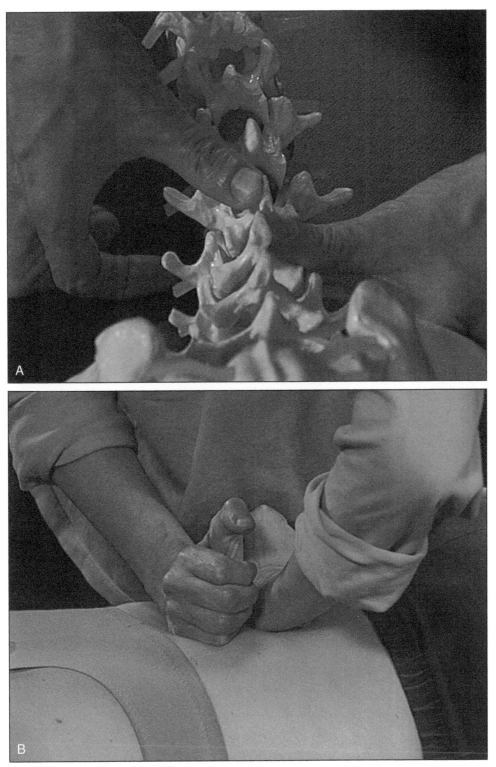

Figure 13-4 **A** and **B,** Lateral glide using the spinous processes.

Anterior Glide Using the Transverse Processes: First Technique (Figure 13-5, Video 13-5)

Purpose
- To examine for lumbar spine joint impairment
- To increase accessory motion into lumbar joint anterior glide
- To increase range of motion at the lumbar spine
- To decrease pain

Positioning
1. The patient is prone.
2. The lumbar spine is positioned in midrange in relation to forward/backward bending, side bending, and rotation.
3. The clinician is at the patient's side, facing the lumbar spine.
4. One hand is positioned with the anterior surface of the pisiform on the transverse process of one vertebra.
5. The other hand is positioned with the anterior surface of the pisiform on the opposite transverse process of the same vertebra.
6. The clinician rotates each hand around the pisiform to aid in maintaining the position of the pisiform on the transverse process.

Procedure
1. Both hands simultaneously glide the transverse processes anteriorly as the patient exhales (see Figure 13-5).

Particulars
- The L5-S1 motion segment cannot be treated with this technique because the iliac crests obscures the transverse processes.
- This technique is commonly performed using a grade V manipulation.

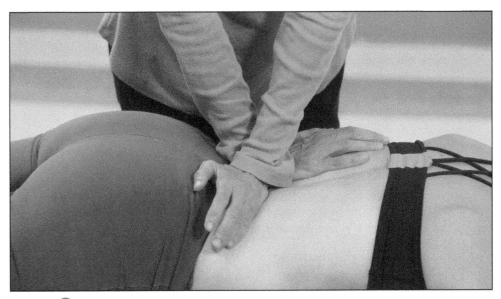

Figure 13-5 Anterior glide using the transverse processes: first technique.

Anterior Glide Using the Transverse Processes: Second Technique (Figure 13-6, Video 13-6)

Purpose
- To examine for lumbar spine joint impairment
- To increase accessory motion into lumbar vertebral body rotation and into facet joint distraction on the side toward which the vertebral body is rotating
- To increase range of motion at the lumbar spine
- To decrease pain

Positioning
1. The patient is prone.
2. The lumbar spine is positioned in midrange in relation to forward/backward bending, side bending, and rotation.
3. The clinician is at the patient's side, facing the lumbar spine.
4. The stabilizing hand is positioned with the thumb or the anterior surface of the pisiform on the transverse process of the more inferior vertebra.
5. The mobilizing/manipulating hand is positioned with the thumb or the anterior surface of the pisiform on the transverse process of the more superior vertebra opposite the side of the stabilizing hand.

Procedure
1. The stabilizing hand holds the more inferior vertebra in position.
2. The mobilizing/manipulating hand glides the more superior transverse process in an anterior direction as the patient exhales (see Figure 13-6).

Particulars
- The L5-S1 motion segment cannot be treated with this technique because the iliac crests obscures the transverse processes.
- This technique might be especially effective for increasing range of motion into lumbar spine rotation in the direction of vertebral body movement.
- This technique is commonly performed using a grade V manipulation.

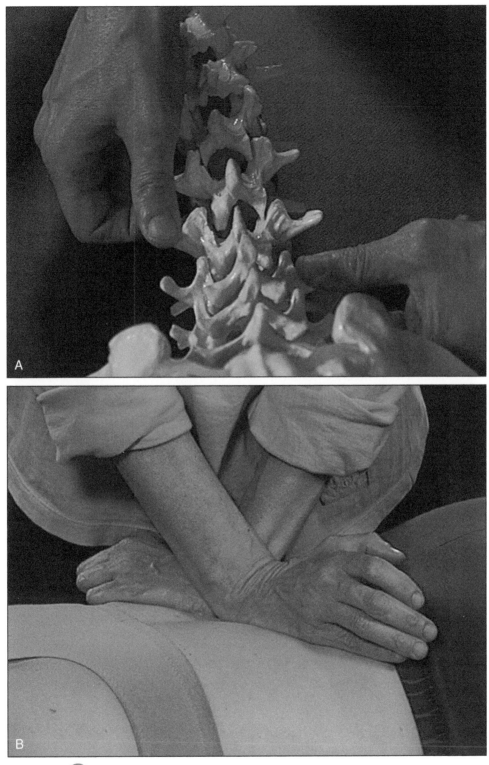

Figure 13-6 **A** and **B,** Anterior glide using the transverse processes.

Rotation Glide (Figure 13-7, Video 13-7)

Purpose

- To increase accessory motion into lumbar vertebral body rotation and into facet joint distraction on the side toward which the patient is rotating
- To increase range of motion at the lumbar spine
- To decrease pain

Positioning

1. The patient is lying on the side not being treated with the arm resting over the clinician's mobilizing/manipulating arm.
2. The lumbar spine is positioned in midrange in relation to forward/backward bending, side bending, and rotation.
3. The clinician is at the side of the treatment table, facing the patient's anterior trunk.
4. A pillow can be used to separate the patient's chest from the clinician.
5. The clinician locks the more inferior vertebrae by bringing the patient's knees toward the chest to the extent that the motion segment below the one being mobilized/manipulated is fully flexed, but the motion segment being mobilized/manipulated has not yet moved.
6. The clinician next locks the more superior vertebrae by rotating the upper trunk away from the clinician (and in the direction of the intended vertebral body motion) to the extent that the motion segment above the one being mobilized/manipulated is fully rotated, but the motion segment being mobilized/manipulated has not yet moved.
7. One hand is positioned with the middle finger on the lower lateral surface of the spinous process (the side of the spinous process closest to the treatment table) of the more inferior vertebra and the forearm on the patient's pelvis.
8. The other hand is positioned with the thumb on the upper lateral surface of the spinous process (the side of the spinous process farthest away from the treatment table) of the more superior vertebra and the forearm or elbow anterior and medial to the patient's shoulder.

Procedure

1. The clinician's hand on the more inferior vertebra glides the spinous process upward as the forearm rotates the pelvis forward and the patient exhales.
2. The clinician's hand on the more superior vertebra simultaneously glides the spinous process downward as the forearm rotates the upper trunk backward (see Figure 13-7, B).

Particulars

- The examination procedure for this technique differs from the intervention procedure. To examine for joint mobility into rotation, the patient is positioned prone with both knees bent to 90 degrees. The clinician is facing the side of the patient's trunk and holds the patient's legs in position at the ankles. The clinician palpates the L5-S1 motion segment by placing the palpating finger between the L5 and S1 spinous processes. With the patient's knees bent, the clinician moves the patient's ankles toward the clinician, keeping the knees bent and rotating the lumbar spine in the same direction in which the ankles are moving. The clinician palpates for motion between L5 and S1 and grades the amount of motion into rotation that occurred. After grading the motion, the clinician restores slack to the L5-S1 motion segment by moving the ankles slightly back toward midline and moves the palpating finger to the L4-5 motion segment. This process is repeated until motion into rotation at all lumbar vertebral motion segments is graded. Mobility into left and right rotation is graded (see Figure 13-7, A).
- The intervention technique might be especially effective for increasing range of motion into lumbar spine rotation in the direction of vertebral body movement.
- Because this intervention technique also produces distraction of the facet joints, it might also be effective in increasing range of motion into lumbar forward/backward bending and side bending.
- This intervention technique is commonly performed using a grade V manipulation.
- The clinician can direct most of the mobilizing/manipulating force to the spinous processes if it is important for the motion to be localized to the motion segment being treated or the clinician can direct most of the mobilizing/manipulating force through the pelvis and trunk if it is not as important for the motion to be localized to the motion segment being treated.
- Alternatively, if this intervention is appropriate for all the lumbar joints, the clinician can direct the force exclusively through the pelvis and trunk.

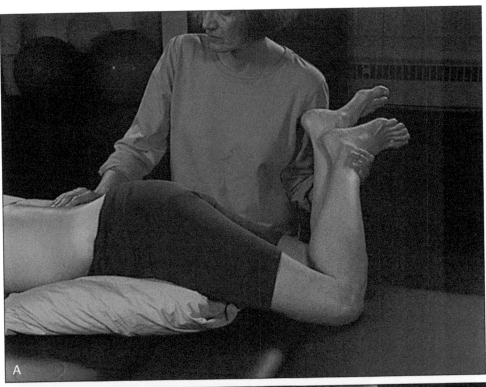

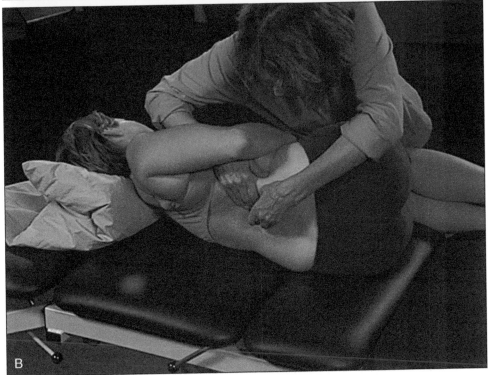

Figure 13-7 Rotation glide. **A,** Examination, **B,** Mobilization/manipulation.

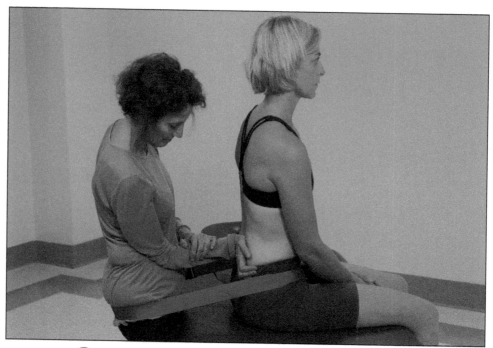

▶ Figure 13-8 Forward-bending glide mobilization with movement.

Forward-Bending Glide Mobilization with Movement (performed on L4 and above) (Figure 13-8, Video 13-8)

Purpose
- To decrease pain
- To increase pain-free range of motion into lumbar forward bending

Positioning
1. The patient is short sitting on the treatment table.
2. The clinician stands in a straddle position behind the patient.
3. The clinician places a stabilization belt around the patient's and the clinician's pelvis to stabilize the patient's pelvis.
4. The clinician places the hypothenar eminence of the mobilizing hand on the distal tip of the patient's spinous process by supinating the forearm and extending the wrist.
5. The clinician braces the elbow of the mobilizing hand against the clinician's pelvis for support.

Procedure
1. The clinician imparts a superior glide to the vertebra, taking the joint up to tissue resistance.
2. While maintaining the superior glide, the clinician instructs the patient to bend forward as far as possible as long as the movement is painfree. The patient is permitted to hold on to the treatment table to decrease the apprehension of falling forward with the forward-bending movement.
3. The clinician maintains the superior glide while the patient moves to the starting position.
4. The clinician continually adjusts his or her own position in relation to the treatment plane to maintain the joint mobilization force during joint movement (see Figure 13-8).

Particulars
- This technique are indicated only if they can be performed without reproducing the patient's pain/symptoms.
- This technique should result in an immediate increase in range of motion and/or a decrease in pain.
- If effective (the technique results in an immediate increase in range of motion and/or decrease in pain), these techniques should be repeated (~2 to 3 times).
- In a study of subjects with low back pain in which these subjects were their own controls, this mobilization with movement technique produced an immediate increase in spinal mobility but no decrease in self-reported pain.[13]

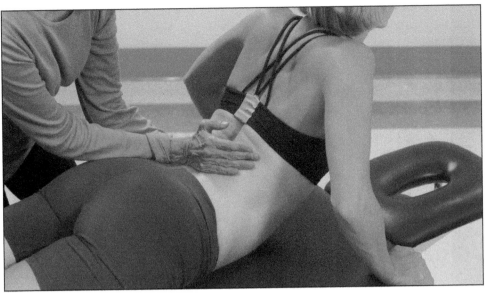

Figure 13-9 Backward-bending glide mobilization with movement.

Backward-Bending Glide Mobilization with Movement (Figure 13-9, Video 13-9)

Purpose
- To decrease pain
- To increase pain-free range of motion into lumbar backward bending

Positioning
1. The patient is prone on the treatment table.
2. The clinician stands at the patient's side.
3. The clinician places the hypothenar eminence of the mobilizing hand on the distal tip of the patient's spinous process.
4. The clinician places the guiding hand on the patient's anterior inferior ribs for support.

Procedure
1. The clinician imparts a superior glide to the vertebra, taking the joint up to tissue resistance.
2. While maintaining the superior glide, the clinician instructs the patient to bend backward as far as possible as long as the movement is painfree by performing a push-up while keeping the pelvis on the treatment table.
3. The patient momentarily sustains overpressure to the joint once the patient completes movement into backward bending.
4. The clinician maintains the superior glide while the patient moves to the starting position.
5. The clinician continually adjusts his or her own position in relation to the treatment plane to maintain the joint mobilization force during joint movement (see Figure 13-9).

Particulars
- This technique are indicated only if they can be performed without reproducing the patient's pain/symptoms.
- This technique should result in an immediate increase in range of motion and/or a decrease in pain.
- If effective (the technique results in an immediate increase in range of motion and/or decrease in pain), these techniques should be repeated (~2 to 3 times).

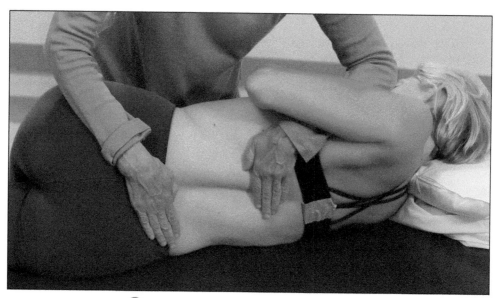

Figure 13-10 Lumbar rotation manipulation.

Lumbar Rotation Manipulation (Figure 13-10, Video 13-10)
Purpose
* To decrease pain in the lumbar region

Positioning
1. The patient is side lying close to the edge of the treatment table.
2. The lumbar spine is positioned in midrange in relation to forward/backward bending, side bending, and rotation.
3. The clinician is at the side of the treatment table, facing the patient's anterior trunk.
4. The clinician positions the forearm or elbow anterior and medial to the patient's shoulder and the hand in the area of the thoracolumbar junction.
5. The clinician places the other hand on the patient's lumbosacral area and rotates the pelvis toward the clinician.

Procedure
1. The clinician takes up tissue resistance into rotation by moving the top of the pelvis toward the clinician.
2. The clinician then performs a grade V manipulation into rotation by dropping both arms toward the floor (see Figure 13-10).

Particulars
* This technique might be especially effective if at least four of the following five criteria are met:
  Pain has been present for <16 days.
  The patient does not have pain below the knee.
  The patient has at least one hypomobile segment with lumbar posteroanterior glides.
  Fear Avoidance Behavior Questionnaire work subscale score is <19.
  Internal rotation in at least one hip is at least 35 degrees.

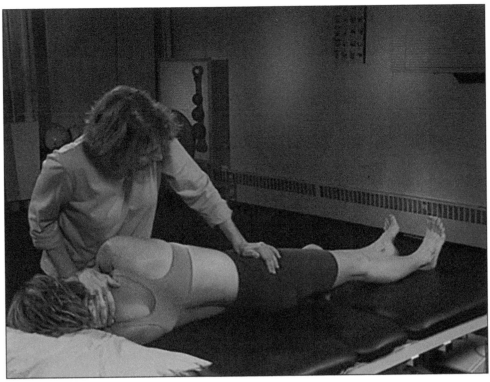

▶ **Figure 13-11** Lumbosacral rotation manipulation.

Lumbosacral Rotation Manipulation (Figure 13-11, Video 13-11)

Purpose
- To decrease pain in the sacroiliac and lumbar regions

Positioning
1. The patient is supine with the fingers laced together at the base of the neck and the elbows touching.
2. The spine and pelvis are positioned in midrange in relation to forward/backward bending, side bending, and rotation.
3. The clinician is at the patient's symptomatic side, facing the pelvis.
4. The clinician side bends the patient's lumbar spine by moving the patient's feet and then the patient's shoulders toward the side of the treatment table.
5. The clinician moves to the opposite side of the treatment table and rotates the patient's trunk toward the opposite direction of the side bending by using the patient's arms as a fulcrum.
6. The stabilizing hand is positioned on the patient's thoracolumbar spine.
7. The manipulating hand is positioned on the patient's anterior superior iliac spine.

Procedure
1. The stabilizing hand holds the upper trunk in position.
2. The manipulating hand thrusts the anterior superior iliac spine in a posterior, lateral, and inferior direction (see Figure 13-11).

Particulars
- This technique should be performed using grade V manipulations.
- This technique might be especially effective if at least four of the following five criteria are met:
  Pain has been present for <16 days.
  The patient does not have pain below the knee.
  The patient has at least one hypomobile segment with lumbar posteroanterior glides.
  Fear Avoidance Behavior Questionnaire work subscale score is <19.
  Internal rotation in at least one hip is at least 35 degrees.

REFERENCES

1. Oliphant D. Safety of spinal manipulation in the treatment of lumbar disk herniations: a systematic review and risk assessment. *J Manipulative Physiol Ther.* 2004;27:197-210.

2. Posadzki P, Ernst E. Spinal manipulation: an update of a systematic review of systematic reviews. *N Z Med J.* 2011;124:55-71.

3. Cochrane Community. Available at: <http://community.cochrane.org>; Accessed 5/2015.

4. Rubinstein SM, Terwee CB, Assendelft WJJ, de Boer MR, van Tulder MW. Spinal manipulative therapy for acute low back pain. An update of the Cochrane Review. *Spine.* 2013;38:E158-E177.

5. Rubinstein SM, van Middelkoop M, Assendelft WJJ, de Boer MR, van Tulder MW. Spinal manipulative therapy for chronic low-back pain: an update of a Cochrane review. *Spine.* 2011;36:E825-E846.

6. Delitto A, George SZ, Van Dillen L, et al. Low back pain clinical practice guidelines linked to the International Classification of Functioning, Disability, and Health from the Orthopaedic Section of the American Physical Therapy Association. *J Orthop Sports Phys Ther.* 2012;42:A1-A57.

7. Flynn T, Fritz J, Whitman J, et al. A clinical prediction rule for classifying patients with low back pain who demonstrate short-term improvement with spinal manipulation. *Spine.* 2002;27:2835-2843.

8. Childs JD, Fritz JM, Flynn TW, et al. A clinical prediction rule to identify patients with low back pain most likely to benefit from spinal manipulation: a validation study. *Ann Intern Med.* 2004;141:920-928.

9. Brennan GP, Fritz JM, Hunter SJ, et al. Identifying subgroups of patients with acute/subacute "nonspecific" low back pain: results of a randomized clinical trial. *Spine.* 2006;31:623-631.

10. Hancock MJ, Maher CG, Latimer J, et al. Independent evaluation of a clinical prediction rule for spinal manipulative therapy: a randomised controlled trial. *Eur Spine J.* 2008;17:936-943.

11. Leininger B, Bronfort G, Evans R, Reiter T. Spinal manipulation or mobilization for radiculopathy: a systematic review. *Phys Med Rehabil Clin N Am.* 2011;22:105-125.

12. Cyriax J. *Textbook of Orthopaedic Medicine.* Vol 1. 8th ed. Diagnosis of Soft Tissue Lesions. London: Bailliere Tindall; 1982.

13. Konstantinou K, Foster N, Rushton A, et al. Flexion mobilizations with movement techniques: the immediate effects on range of movement and pain in subjects with low back pain. *J Manipulative Physiol Ther.* 2007;30:178-185.

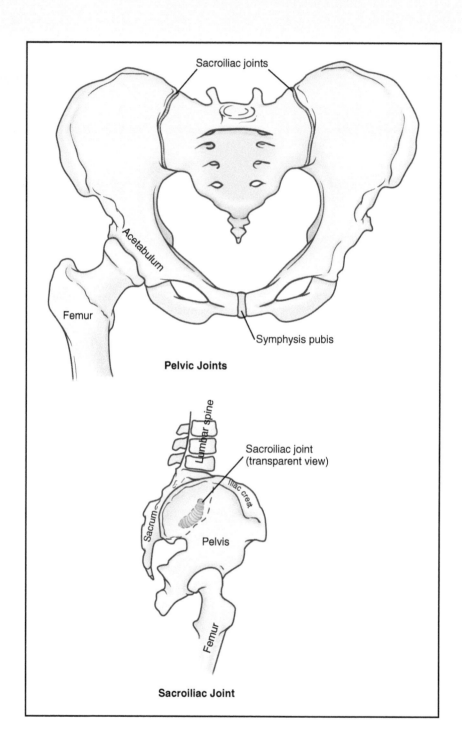

Pelvic Joints

Sacroiliac joints

Acetabulum

Femur

Symphysis pubis

Sacroiliac Joint

Lumbar spine

Sacroiliac joint
(transparent view)

Iliac crest

Sacrum

Pelvis

Femur

CHAPTER 14

Pelvic Joints

BASICS

The pelvis consists of three joints: two sacroiliac joints and one pubic joint. Because these joints are configured in the formation of a ring, impairment at one joint could theoretically cause pain at one or both of the other pelvic joints. Movement at these three joints is minimal and does not depend on muscular control.

Sacroiliac Joints

Motion at the sacroiliac joints is greater in women and decreases with age in both sexes. The decrease in motion occurs from progressive roughening of the iliac articular surfaces.

Despite the fact that clinicians have recognized that low back pain can originate from the sacroiliac joint for over 50 years, and that the prevalence of low back pain arising from the sacroiliac joint is estimated to be up to 30% of all patients with low back pain,[1] treatment of sacroiliac joint pain, especially in relation to joint mobilization/manipulation, remains enigmatic. Only one systematic review, published in 2012, was identified that addressed joint mobilization/manipulation interventions. The investigators simply stated that conservative measures can be used to address the underlying cause of sacroiliac joint pain and that exercise and manipulation are effective interventions when the cause is faulty movement patterns arising from posture and gait.[2] To date, there are no published studies that adequately address the indications for treatment or outcomes related to specific sacroiliac joint mobilization/manipulation techniques.

The lack of a unifying approach for evaluating and treating patients with sacroiliac joint conditions likely arises from a number of factors. First, pinpointing the anatomic location of the source of low back pain is difficult, and specific tests to identify sacroiliac joint conditions are not highly reliable or valid. Furthermore, because motion at the pelvic joints is minimal, identifying limitations in osteokinematic range of motion is not useful for determining appropriate interventions or evaluating the effects of specific treatments.

One approach to informing specific mobilization/manipulation interventions involves identifying mobility impairments at the pelvic joints and treating those joints identified as being hypomobile with mobilization/manipulation interventions to restore mobility. In the case of hypermobile pelvic joints, interventions would focus on treatments that stabilize the affected joint(s). The caveat to this approach for treating hypermobile joints is that if the hypermobility caused a positional fault to occur at the sacroiliac joint, then the joint would behave as if it was hypomobile and the intervention would theoretically entail a mobilization/manipulation technique to correct the positional fault, not to restore normal mobility to the joint. These issues are compounded by the difficulty in identifying position and mobility impairments at these joints and issues related to the efficacy of treating positional faults.

Another approach to treating pain arising from the sacroiliac joint is to perform nonspecific mobilization/manipulation techniques. Although they eliminate the need to identify a specific direction of mobilization/manipulation intervention, this approach is still dependent on obtaining an accurate assessment that the source of pain is arising from the sacroiliac joint.

Movement at the sacroiliac joint appears to consist of a combination of rotation and translation.[2] Nevertheless, when describing movement of the ilium on the sacrum, motion is commonly referred to as anterior or posterior rotation (referring to the direction of movement of the iliac crest). When describing movement of the sacrum on the ilium, motion is referred to as nutation or sacral flexion (anterior movement of the superior surface of the sacrum) or counternutation, or sacral extension (posterior movement of the superior surface of the sacrum). Although the presence of different terminology would suggest otherwise, ilial anterior torsion entails the same joint movement as sacral counternutation and ilial posterior torsion entails the same joint movement as sacral nutation.

Symphysis Pubis

The pubic symphysis is not well referenced in the clinical literature. Nevertheless, sacroiliac joint movement is believed to produce motion at the symphysis pubis. This motion is most often described as a gliding movement in a superior/inferior direction.

SPECIFIC PATHOLOGY AND SACROILIAC JOINT MOBILIZATION/ MANIPULATION

Hip Pain

In a study of 20 runners with reports of hip pain and evidence of sacroiliac joint impairment, subjects were randomly assigned to receive inferior glide mobilization to the hip or manipulation to the sacroiliac joint. At follow-up, subjects receiving the sacroiliac joint manipulation had significantly less pain than the group receiving hip mobilization.[3]

SACROILIAC JOINTS

Osteokinematic motions:
  Ilium: anterior/posterior rotation
  Sacrum: extension/flexion
Ligaments:
  Posterior sacroiliac ligaments (transverse, oblique, longitudinal)
  Anterior sacroiliac ligament
  Iliolumbar ligament
  Sacrospinous ligament
  Sacrotuberous ligament
Joint orientation:
  Sacrum: lateral, posterior
  Ilia: medial, anterior
Type of joint:
  Part synovial, part syndesmotic
Concave joint surface:
  None, this is a plane joint
Resting position:
  Not described by Kaltenborn
Close-packed position:
  Not described by Kaltenborn
Capsular pattern of restriction:
  Pain when the joints are stressed[4]

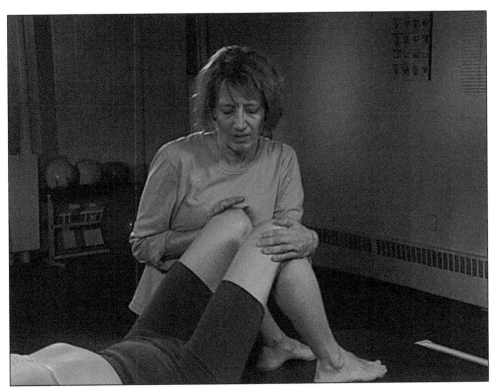

▶ **Figure 14-1** Distraction of the sacroiliac joint muscle energy.

Distraction of the Sacroiliac Joint Muscle Energy (Figure 14-1, Video 14-1)

Purpose
- To increase accessory motion in the sacroiliac joint
- To decrease pain

Positioning
1. The patient is supine with the knees bent, feet flat on the treatment table and hips abducted.
2. The spine and pelvis are positioned in midrange in relation to forward/backward bending, side bending, and rotation.
3. The clinician is at the patient's side, facing the pelvis.
4. Both hands are positioned such that each hand is on the lateral surface of each of the patient's knees.

Procedure
1. The clinician instructs the patient to perform an isometric contraction of the abductors by resisting a force provided by the clinician into hip adduction, thus distracting the iliac joint surfaces away from the sacrum as the abductors contract and pull on their attachments to the iliac crest.
2. This contraction is held for approximately 5 seconds.
3. The clinician brings the hips into more adduction.
4. This procedure can be repeated several times (see Figure 14-1).

Particulars
- This technique might be effective in correcting a sacroiliac joint positional fault.

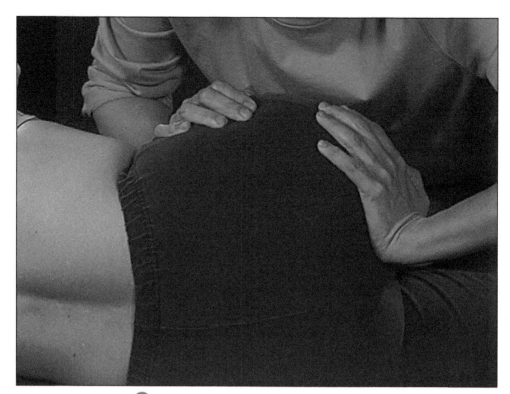

▶ **Figure 14-2** Posterior glide of the iliac crest.

Posterior Glide of the Iliac Crest (Figure 14-2, Video 14-2)

Purpose
- To increase accessory motion in the sacroiliac joint
- To decrease pain

Positioning
1. The patient is lying on the unaffected side, with the hip on the side to be mobilized/manipulated in flexion and the contralateral hip in extension.
2. The sacroiliac joint is approximating the restricted range into posterior rotation.
3. The clinician is at the patient's side, facing the anterior pelvis.
4. The mobilizing/manipulating hand is on the patient's anterior superior iliac spine and the anterior surface of the iliac crest.
5. The guiding hand is on the patient's ischium.

Procedure
1. The clinician applies a grade I traction to the joint by lifting the pelvis slightly with the arms of the mobilizing/manipulating and guiding hands.
2. The mobilizing/manipulating hand glides the anterior superior iliac spine and the anterior surface of the iliac crest in a posterior direction.
3. The guiding hand guides the ischium anteriorly (see Figure 14-2).

Particulars
- This technique might be effective in correcting a sacroiliac joint anterior rotation positional fault.

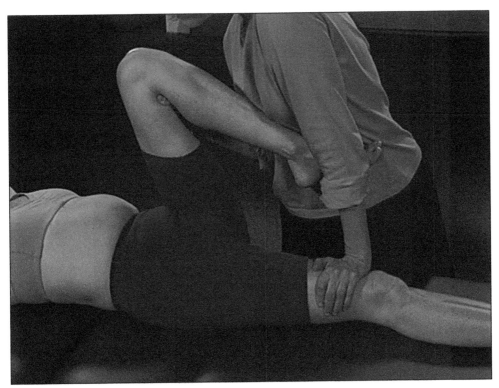

▶ **Figure 14-3** Posterior glide muscle energy.

Posterior Glide Muscle Energy (Figure 14-3, Video 14-3)

Purpose
- To increase accessory motion in the sacroiliac joint
- To decrease pain

Positioning
1. The patient is supine, with the side to be mobilized positioned with the hip flexed to the end of the available range and the unaffected side positioned with the hip extended.
2. The unaffected side can be positioned with the knee flexed off the edge of the treatment table.
3. The sacroiliac joint is approximating the restricted range into posterior rotation.
4. The clinician is at the patient's knee, facing the pelvis.
5. The stabilizing hand is positioned on the anterior surface of the distal thigh on the unaffected side.
6. The mobilizing hand is positioned on the posterior surface of the distal thigh on the affected side, with the clinician's trunk reinforcing the hand position.

Procedure
1. The clinician instructs the patient to perform an isometric contraction of the gluteus maximus by resisting a force provided by the clinician into hip flexion, thus gliding the pelvis into posterior rotation as the gluteus maximus contracts and pulls on its attachment to the posterior surface of the ilium.
2. This contraction is held for approximately 5 seconds.
3. The clinician brings the hip into more flexion until an increase in resistance is met.
4. This procedure can be repeated several times (see Figure 14-3).

Particulars
- The patient can be taught to perform this technique as part of a home program.
- This technique might be effective in correcting a sacroiliac joint anterior rotation positional fault.

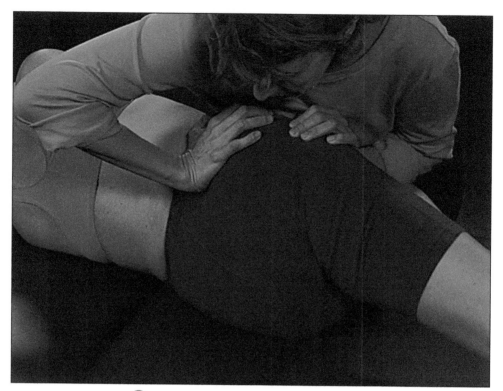

▶ **Figure 14-4** Anterior glide of the iliac crest.

Anterior Glide of the Iliac Crest (Figure 14-4, Video 14-4)

Purpose
- To increase accessory motion in the sacroiliac joint
- To decrease pain

Positioning
1. The patient is lying on the unaffected side, with the hip on the side to be mobilized/manipulated in extension and the contralateral hip in flexion.
2. The sacroiliac joint is approximating the restricted range into anterior rotation.
3. The clinician is at the patient's side, facing the anterior pelvis.
4. The mobilizing/manipulating hand is positioned over the posterior surface of the iliac crest.
5. The guiding hand is on the anterior and lateral surface of the pelvis distal to the anterior superior iliac spine.

Procedure
1. The clinician applies a grade I traction to the joint by lifting the pelvis slightly with the arms of the mobilizing/manipulating and guiding hands.
2. The mobilizing/manipulating hand glides the iliac crest anteriorly.
3. The guiding hand guides the anterior and lateral surface of the pelvis posteriorly (see Figure 14-4).

Particulars
- This technique might be effective in correcting a posterior rotation positional fault.

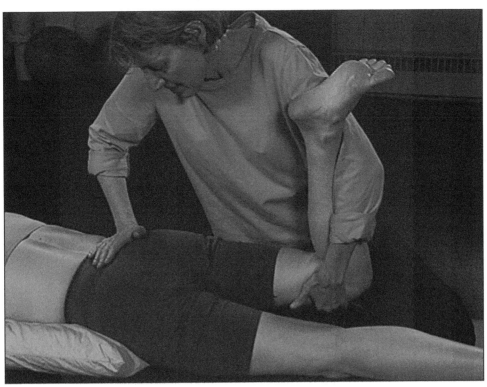

Figure 14-5 Anterior glide muscle energy.

Anterior Glide Muscle Energy (Figure 14-5, Video 14-5)

Purpose
- To increase accessory motion in the sacroiliac joint
- To decrease pain

Positioning
1. The patient is prone, with the side to be mobilized positioned with the hip extended and the knee flexed. The unaffected side can be positioned with the hip flexed off the edge of the treatment table.
2. The sacroiliac joint is approximating the restricted range into anterior rotation.
3. The clinician is at the patient's knee, facing the pelvis.
4. The guiding hand is positioned over the posterior surface of the iliac crest.
5. The mobilizing hand is on the anterior surface of the distal thigh with the clinician's arm or trunk supporting the patient's lower leg.

Procedure
1. The clinician lifts the thigh off of the treatment table and instructs the patient to perform an isometric contraction of the rectus femoris by resisting a force provided by the clinician into hip extension and knee flexion, thus gliding the pelvis into anterior rotation as the rectus femoris contracts and pulls on its attachment to the anterior inferior iliac spine.
2. This contraction is held for approximately 5 seconds.
3. The clinician brings the hip into more extension and the knee into more flexion until an increase in resistance is met.
4. This procedure can be repeated several times (see Figure 14-5).

Particulars
- This technique might be effective in correcting a sacroiliac joint posterior rotation positional fault.

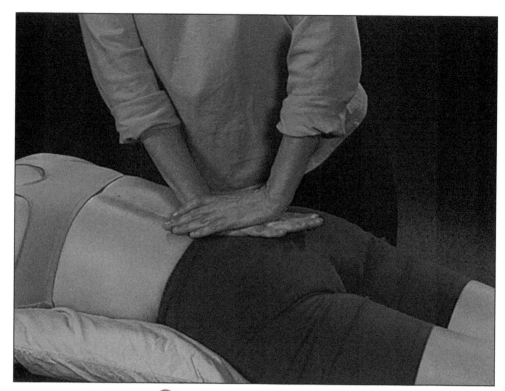

▶ **Figure 14-6** Sacral anterior glide.

Sacral Anterior Glide (Figure 14-6, Video 14-6)

Purpose

- To increase accessory motion in the sacroiliac joint
- To decrease pain

Positioning

1. The patient is prone.
2. The spine and pelvis are positioned in midrange in relation to forward/backward bending, side bending, and rotation.
3. The clinician is at the patient's side, facing the pelvis.
4. The heel of the mobilizing/manipulating hand is positioned over the superior surface of the sacrum.
5. The guiding hand is positioned over the mobilizing/manipulating hand.

Procedure

1. The mobilizing/manipulating hand glides the superior surface of the sacrum anteriorly, directing the sacrum into flexion (nutation).
2. The guiding hand controls the position of the mobilizing/manipulating hand (see Figure 14-6).

Particulars

- This technique might be effective in correcting a sacroiliac joint counternutation positional fault.

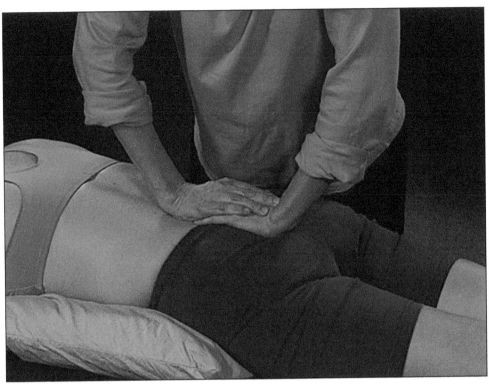

Figure 14-7 Sacral posterior glide.

Sacral Posterior Glide (Figure 14-7, Video 14-7)

Purpose
- To increase accessory motion in the sacroiliac joint
- To decrease pain

Positioning
1. The patient is prone.
2. The spine and pelvis are positioned in midrange in relation to forward/backward bending, side bending, and rotation.
3. The clinician is at the patient's side, facing the pelvis.
4. The heel of the mobilizing/manipulating hand is positioned over the inferior surface of the sacrum.
5. The guiding hand is positioned over the mobilizing/manipulating hand.

Procedure
1. The mobilizing/manipulating hand glides the inferior surface of the sacrum anteriorly, directing the sacrum into extension (counternutation).
2. The guiding hand controls the position of the mobilizing/manipulating hand (see Figure 14-7).

Particulars
- This technique might be effective in correcting a sacroiliac joint nutation positional fault.

SYMPHYSIS PUBIS

Osteokinematic motion:
  None
Ligament:
  Arcuate ligament
Joint orientation:
  Both pubic bones: medial
Type of joint:
  Syndesmotic
Concave joint surface:
  None, this is a plane joint
Resting position:
  Not described by Kaltenborn
Close-packed position:
  Not described by Kaltenborn
Capsular pattern of restriction:
  Pain when the joints are stressed[4]

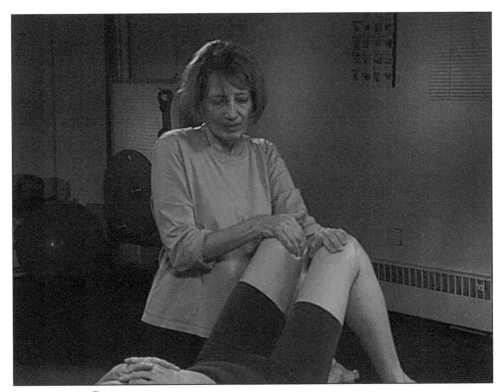

▶ **Figure 14-8** Distraction of the symphysis pubis muscle energy.

Distraction of the Symphysis Pubis Muscle Energy (Figure 14-8, Video 14-8)

Purpose
- To increase accessory motion in the symphysis pubis
- To decrease pain

Positioning

1. The patient is supine with the knees bent, feet flat on the treatment table, and hips adducted.
2. The spine and pelvis are positioned in midrange in relation to forward/backward bending, side bending, and rotation.
3. The clinician is at the patient's side, facing the pelvis.
4. Both hands are positioned such that each hand is on the medial surface of each of the patient's knees.

Procedure

1. The clinician instructs the patient to perform an isometric contraction of the adductors by resisting a force provided by the clinician into hip abduction, thus distracting the symphysis pubis joint surfaces away from one another as the adductors contract and pull on their attachments to the pubic rami.
2. This contraction is held for approximately 5 seconds.
3. The clinician brings the hips into more abduction until an increase in resistance is met.
4. This procedure can be repeated several times (see Figure 14-8).

Particulars

- This technique might be effective in correcting a symphysis pubis positional fault.

REFERENCES

1. Vanelderen P, Szadek K, Cohen SP, et al. Sacroiliac joint pain. *Pain Pract*. 2010;10:470-480.
2. Vleeming A, Schuenke MD, Masi AT, et al. The sacroiliac joint: an overview of its anatomy, function and potential clinical implications. *J Anat*. 2012;221: 537-567.
3. Cibulka MT, Delitto A. A comparison of two different methods to treat hip pain in runners. *J Orthop Sports Phys Ther*. 1993;17:172-176.
4. Cyriax J. *Textbook of Orthopaedic Medicine*. Vol 1. 8th ed. Diagnosis of Soft Tissue Lesions. London: Bailliere Tindall; 1982.

Index

Page numbers followed by "*f*" indicate figures, and "*t*" indicate tables.

A

Accessory motion
  and capsular patterns, 18-20
  convex-concave rules in, 15-18, 15*f*-18*f*, 19*t*
  defined, 6
  end feels, 14-15
  examination and evaluation of, 11
  pain with, 14, 22
  and positional faults, 20
Acromioclavicular joint, 28*f*, 29, 55-57
  anterior glide of, 57, 57*f*
  capsular pattern of restriction of, 55
  close-packed position of, 55
  concave surface of, 55
  convex-concave rules for, 19*t*
  ligaments of, 55
  orientation of, 55
  osteokinematic motions of, 55
  posterior glide of, 56, 56*f*
Actual resting position, 11
Adhesions, of joint capsule, 6
Adhesive capsulitis, of shoulder joint, 29
Ankle joint(s), 170-215
  anatomic terminology for, 171
  pronation and supination of, 171
  range of motion of, 171
  subtalar, 170*f*, 171, 190-195
    distraction of, 191, 191*f*
    lateral glide of, 193, 193*f*
    lateral tilt of, 195, 195*f*
    medial glide of, 192, 192*f*
    medial tilt of, 194, 194*f*
  talocrural, 170*f*, 171, 180-188
    anterior glide of talus on tibia and fibula of,
      183-184, 183*f*, 185*f*
    distraction of, 181, 181*f*
    posterior glide of, 182, 182*f*
  triplanar motion of, 171
Ankle sprains, lateral, 171-172
Anterior glide
  of acromioclavicular joint, 57, 57*f*
  of clavicle on sternum, 54, 54*f*
  of distal fibula, 177, 177*f*
  of distal radius, 80, 80*f*
  of distal row carpal joints, 112, 112*f*
  of glenohumeral joint
    first technique, 36, 37*f*
    second technique, 38, 39*f*

Anterior glide *(Continued)*
  of hip joint, 144-145, 144*f*-145*f*
  of humeroradial joint, 74, 74*f*
  of iliac crest, 320, 320*f*
  of intermetacarpal joints two through five, 121, 121*f*
  of interphalangeal joints, 135, 135*f*
  of lower cervical spine
    using facet joints of
      first technique, 248, 249*f*
      second technique, 250, 251*f*
    using spinous processes of, 240, 241*f*
  of lumbar joint
    using spinous processes, 294, 295*f*
    using transverse processes, 302, 303*f*, 304, 305*f*
  of metacarpophalangeal joints two through five, 129,
    129*f*
  of midcarpal joints, 103, 103*f*
    specific mobilizations/manipulations for, 108, 109*f*
  of proximal fibula, 174, 174*f*
  of proximal radius, 77, 77*f*
  of proximal row carpal, 96, 97*f*
  of radiocarpal joint, 87, 87*f*
    specific mobilizations/manipulations for, 90, 91*f*
  of ribs, 288, 288*f*
  sacral, 322, 322*f*
  of sacroiliac joint, 321, 321*f*
  of talus mobilization with movement, 186, 187*f*
  of talus on tibia and fibula, 183-184, 183*f*, 185*f*
  of temporomandibular joint, 226, 226*f*
  of thoracic joints
    grade V manipulation, 280-282, 281*f*
    using spinous processes/passive accessory vertebral
      motion, 264, 265*f*, 266, 267*f*, 268, 269*f*
    using transverse processes, 272, 274, 275*f*
  of tibia on femur, 155-157, 155*f*-157*f*
  of trapeziometacarpal joint, 116, 116*f*
Anterior/superior glide, of lower cervical spine, using
    spinous processes
  first technique, 242, 243*f*
  second technique, 244, 245*f*
Appendicular skeletal system, axillary *vs.*, 219
Arthrokinematic motion, 6
  convex-concave rules for, 19*t*
Atlantoaxial joint, 230*f*
  osteokinematic motions of, 233
Axillary skeletal system, 219-220
  appendicular *vs.*, 219
  coupled motion in, 219-220

Axillary skeletal system *(Continued)*
    precautions and contraindications to joint
        mobilization and manipulation of, 220
    terminology for, 219

B

Back pain
    low, 291-292
    mid, 261
Backward-bending glide
    of lower cervical spine
        mobilization with movement, 254, 254*f*
        self mobilization with movement, 255, 255*f*
    of lumbar spine, mobilization with movement, 309,
        309*f*
    of thoracic joints, 276
Bony end feels, 14-15
Breaking point, on stress-strain curve, 13, 13*f*

C

Calcaneocuboid joint, 170*f*, 171, 196
    convex-concave rules for, 19*t*
    cuboid in
        dorsal glide of, 199, 199*f*
        plantar glide of, 200, 200*f*
        whip/manipulation of, 201, 201*f*
Capsular patterns, examination and evaluation of,
    18-20
Capsule, joint, adhesions of, 6
Capsulitis, adhesive, of shoulder joint, 29
Carpal joints
    distal row
        anterior glide of, 112, 112*f*
        posterior glide of, 110, 111*f*
    proximal row
        anterior glide of, 96, 97*f*
        posterior glide of, 94, 95*f*
Carpal tunnel syndrome, 83
Carpometacarpal joint(s), 82*f*
    of thumb, convex-concave rules for, 19*t*
Cavitation, joint, 23
Cervical joint(s), 230-259
    coupled motion of, 219
    lower, 230*f*, 231, 237-258
        backward-bending glide
            mobilization with movement, 254, 254*f*
            self mobilization with movement, 255, 255*f*
        capsular pattern of restriction of, 237
        distraction of, 238, 239*f*
        facet, anterior glide of
            first technique, 248, 249*f*
            second technique, 250, 251*f*
        forward-bending glide mobilization of, with
            movement, 253, 253*f*
        ligaments of, 237
        orientation of, 237
        osteokinematic motions of, 237

Cervical joint(s) *(Continued)*
        rotation glide of
            mobilization with movement, 256, 256*f*
            self mobilization with movement, 257, 257*f*
            side-bending glide mobilization with movement of,
                258, 258*f*
            side glide of, 252, 252*f*
        spinous processes of
            anterior glide using, 240, 241*f*
            anterior/superior glide using, first technique,
                242, 243*f*
            anterior/superior glide using, second technique,
                244, 245*f*
            lateral glide using, 246, 247*f*
    mobilization/manipulation of
        for headache, 232
        for lateral epicondylalgia, 233
        for nonspecific neck pain, 232
        risk of, 231-232
        specific pathology and, 232-233
        for temporomandibular joint disorders, 233
    precautions and contraindications to mobilization
        and manipulation interventions for, 220
    upper, 230*f*, 231, 233-236
        capsular pattern of restriction of, 233
        concave joint surface of, 233
        distraction of, 234, 234*f*
        forward-bending glide of, 235, 235*f*
        ligaments of, 233
        orientation of, 233
        rotation glide of, 236, 236*f*
Chiropractic medicine, 3
Clavicle
    on sternum, anterior glide of, 54, 54*f*
Close-packed position, 21
Compression, 11, 12*f*
    of humeroradial joint, 72, 72*f*
Convex-concave rules, 15-18, 15*f*-18*f*, 19*t*
Costochondral joint, 260*f*
Costotransverse joint, 260*f*
Costovertebral joint, 260*f*
Counternutation, of sacroiliac joint, 315
Coupled motion, spinal, 219-220
Cracking noise, 23
Cross-linking, 6
Cuboid
    dorsal glide of, 199, 199*f*
    plantar glide of, 200, 200*f*
    whip/manipulation of, 201, 201*f*
Cuneiform articulations, 171
Cyriax, 4

D

Degrees of freedom, osteokinematic, 6
Distal fibula
    anterior glide of, 177, 177*f*
    posterior glide of, 176, 176*f*

Distal interphalangeal joints, of hand, convex-concave rules for, 19*t*

Distal radioulnar joint, 60*f*, 61, 78-80, 82*f*
  capsular pattern of restriction of, 78
  close-packed position of, 78
  concave surface of, 78
  convex-concave rules for, 19*t*
  ligaments of, 78
  orientation of, 78
  osteokinematic motion of, 78
  resting position of, 78

Distal radius
  anterior glide of, 80, 80*f*
  posterior glide of, 79, 79*f*

Distal row carpal joints
  anterior glide of, 112, 112*f*
  posterior glide of, 110, 111*f*

Distal tibiofibular joint, 170*f*, 171, 175-179
  in ankle sprain, 172
  capsular pattern of restriction of, 175
  close-packed position of, 175
  concave surface of, 175
  convex-concave rules for, 19*t*
  distal fibula in
    anterior glide of, 177, 177*f*
    posterior glide of, 176*f*
  fibula in
    inferior glide of, 179, 179*f*
    superior glide of, 178, 178*f*
  ligaments of, 175
  orientation of, 175
  resting position of, 175

Distraction, 11
  of cervical joints
    lower, 238, 239*f*
    upper, 234, 234*f*
  of glenohumeral joint, 30, 31*f*
  of hip joint, 141, 141*f*
  of humeroradial joint, 70, 71*f*
  of humeroulnar joint, 62, 63*f*
  of interphalangeal joints
    of fingers, 133, 133*f*
    of toes, 212, 212*f*
  of metacarpophalangeal joints
    first, 123, 123*f*
    two through five, 127, 127*f*
  of metatarsophalangeal joints, 206, 206*f*
  of midcarpal joints, 101, 101*f*
  of radiocarpal joint, 85, 85*f*
  of sacroiliac joint, 317, 317*f*
  of scapulothoracic joint, 43, 43*f*
  of subtalar joint, 191, 191*f*
  of symphysis pubis, 325, 325*f*
  of talocrural joint, 181, 181*f*
  of temporomandibular joint, 225, 225*f*
  of thoracic joints, grade V manipulation, 278
  of tibiofemoral joint, 153, 153*f*

Distraction *(Continued)*
  of trapeziometacarpal joint, 114, 114*f*
  of ulnocarpal joints, 85, 85*f*

Dorsal glide
  of cuboid, 199, 199*f*
  of intermetatarsal joints, 203, 203*f*
  of interphalangeal joints, of toes, 213, 213*f*
  of metatarsophalangeal joints, 207, 207*f*
  of navicular, 197, 197*f*

E
Elastic phase, of stress-strain curve, 13, 13*f*

Elbow joint(s), 60-81
  distal radioulnar, 60*f*, 61, 78-80
  humeroradial, 60*f*, 61, 69-74
    anterior glide of, 74, 74*f*
    distraction of, 70, 71*f*
    posterior glide of, 73, 73*f*
  humeroulnar, 60*f*, 61-68
    distraction of, 62, 63*f*
    lateral glide of, 66, 66*f*
      mobilization with movement for, 68, 68*f*
    medial glide of, 64, 65*f*
      mobilization with movement, 67, 67*f*
  lateral epicondylalgia of, 61
  mobilization/manipulation of, 61
  proximal radioulnar, 60*f*, 61
  specific pathology of, 61

End feel, examination and evaluation of, 14-15

Epicondylalgia, lateral, 61
  cervical spine joint mobilization/manipulation for, 233
  thoracic spine and rib joint mobilization/ manipulation for, 262

Evaluation. *see* Examination and evaluation

Evidence-based practice, 5-6

Evidence-informed practice, 5-6

Examination and evaluation, 11-15
  of accessory movements, 11
    compression in, 11, 12*f*
    end feel in, 14-15
    excursion in, 13-14, 13*f*
    with glides, 11, 12*f*
    with oscillation motion, 11
    pain in, 14
    resting position in, 11
    traction or distraction in, 11, 12*f*
    treatment plane in, 11
  of capsular patterns, 18-20
  convex-concave rules in, 15-18, 15*f*-18*f*, 19*t*
  of positional faults, 20
  precautions and contraindications for, 20

Excursion, examination and evaluation of, 13-14, 13*f*

Expiration glide, of rib joints
  five through eleven, 285, 285*f*
  two through seven, 284, 284*f*

Extensibility, increasing, 6
Extension, sacral, 315

F
Facet joints
    cervical, 230*f*
        anterior glide using
            first technique, 248, 249*f*
            second technique, 250, 251*f*
        lumbar, 290*f*, 291
        thoracic, 260*f*, 261
Failure point, on stress-strain curve, 13, 13*f*
Femur, 150*f*
    on pelvis, posterolateral glide of, 146, 146*f*
    tibia on, anterior glide of, 155-157, 155*f*-157*f*
Fibula, 150*f*
    distal
        anterior glide of, 177, 177*f*
        posterior glide of, 176, 176*f*
    inferior glide of, 179, 179*f*
    proximal
        anterior glide of, 174, 174*f*
        posterior glide of, 173, 173*f*
    superior glide of, 178, 178*f*
    talus on, anterior glide of, 183-184, 183*f*,
        185*f*
Finger joint(s), 82*f*, 83
    interphalangeal, 82*f*, 132-135
        anterior glide of, 135, 135*f*
        distraction of, 133, 133*f*
        posterior glide of, 134, 134*f*
    metacarpophalangeal, 82*f*, 83
        decreased range of motion of, 83
        first, 122-125
            distraction of, 123, 123*f*
            lateral (radial) glide of, 124*f*, 125
            medial (ulnar) glide of, 124, 125*f*
        two through five, 126-131
            anterior glide of, 129, 129*f*
            distraction of, 127, 127*f*
            lateral (radial) glide of, 130*f*, 131
            medial (ulnar) glide of, 130, 131*f*
            posterior glide of, 128, 128*f*
    trapeziometacarpal, 113-118
        anterior glide of, 116, 116*f*
        distraction of, 114, 114*f*
        lateral (radial) glide of, 117*f*, 118
        medial (ulnar) glide of, 117, 118*f*
        posterior glide of, 115, 115*f*
Firm end feels, 14-15
First metacarpophalangeal joint, 122-125
    distraction of, 123, 123*f*
    lateral (radial) glide of, 124*f*, 125
    medial (ulnar) glide of, 124, 125*f*
First rib, inferior glide of, 283, 283*f*
Flexion, sacral, 315

Foot joints, 170-215, 170*f*
    anatomic terminology for, 171
    intermetatarsal, 171, 202-204
        dorsal glide of, 203, 203*f*
        plantar glide of, 204, 204*f*
    interphalangeal, 170*f*, 171, 211-214
        distraction of, 212, 212*f*
        dorsal glide of, 213, 213*f*
        plantar glide of, 214, 214*f*
    metatarsophalangeal, 170*f*, 171, 205-210
        distraction of, 206, 206*f*
        dorsal glide of, 207, 207*f*
        lateral glide of, 210, 210*f*
        medial glide of, 209, 209*f*
        plantar glide of, 208, 208*f*
    midtarsal, 170*f*, 171, 196-201
        cuboid in
            dorsal glide of, 199, 199*f*
            plantar glide of, 200, 200*f*
            whip/manipulation of, 201, 201*f*
        navicular in
            dorsal glide of, 197, 197*f*
            plantar glide of, 198, 198*f*
    pronation and supination of, 171
    triplanar motion of, 171
Force
    amount and speed of, 21
    direction of, 21
Forearm joint, 60-81, 60*f*
Forward-bending glide
    of lumbar spine, mobilization with movement, 308,
        308*f*
    of upper cervical spine, 235, 235*f*

G
Glenohumeral joint, 28*f*, 29
    anterior glide of
        first technique, 36, 37*f*
        second technique, 38, 39*f*
    capsular pattern of restriction of, 30
    close-packed position of, 30
    concave surface of, 30
    convex-concave rules for, 17, 19*t*
    distraction of, 30, 31*f*
    inferior glide of, 32, 33*f*
    ligaments of, 30
    orientation of, 30
    osteokinematic motions of, 30
    posterior glide of, 34, 35*f*
    resting position of, 30
Glide(s), 11, 12*f*
    anterior
        of acromioclavicular joint, 57, 57*f*
        of clavicle on sternum, 54, 54*f*
        of distal fibula, 177, 177*f*
        of distal radius, 80, 80*f*

Glide(s) *(Continued)*
    of distal row carpal joints, 112, 112*f*
    of glenohumeral joint
        first technique, 36
        second technique, 38, 39*f*
    of hip joint, 144-145, 144*f*-145*f*
    of humeroradial joint, 74, 74*f*
    of iliac crest, 320, 320*f*
    of intermetacarpal joints two through five, 121,
        121*f*
    of interphalangeal joints, 135, 135*f*
    of lower cervical joint
        using facet joints of, 248, 249*f*, 250, 251*f*
        using spinous processes of, 240, 241*f*
    of lumbar joints
        using spinous processes, 294, 295*f*
        using transverse processes, 302, 303*f*, 304, 305*f*
    of metacarpophalangeal two through five, 129,
        129*f*
    of midcarpal joints, 103, 103*f*
        specific mobilizations/manipulations for, 108,
        109*f*
    of proximal fibula, 174, 174*f*
    of proximal radius, 77, 77*f*
    of proximal row carpal, 96, 97*f*
    of radiocarpal joint, 87, 87*f*
        specific mobilizations/manipulations for, 90, 91*f*
    of ribs, 288, 288*f*
    sacral, 322, 322*f*
    of sacroiliac joints, 321, 321*f*
    of talus mobilization with movement, 186, 187*f*
    of talus on tibia and fibula, 183-184, 183*f*, 185*f*
    of temporomandibular joint, 226, 226*f*
    of thoracic joints
        grade V manipulation, 280-282, 281*f*
        using spinous processes/passive accessory
            vertebral motion, 264, 265*f*, 266, 267*f*, 268,
            269*f*
        using transverse processes, 272, 274, 275*f*
    of tibia on femur, 155-157, 155*f*-157*f*
    of trapeziometacarpal joint, 116, 116*f*
    of ulnocarpal joint, 87, 87*f*
  anterior/superior glide, of lower cervical joint, using
      spinous processes of
    first technique, 242, 243*f*
    second technique, 244, 245*f*
  backward-bending
    of lower cervical joint
        mobilization of, 254, 254*f*
        self mobilization of, 255, 255*f*
    of lumbar joints, 309, 309*f*
    of thoracic joints, 276
  convex-concave rules in, 15-16, 16*f*
  dorsal
    of cuboid, 199, 199*f*
    of intermetatarsal joints, 203, 203*f*

Glide(s) *(Continued)*
    of interphalangeal joints of toes, 213, 213*f*
    of metatarsophalangeal joints, 207, 207*f*
    of navicular, 197, 197*f*
  expiration, of ribs
    five through eleven, 285, 285*f*
    two through seven, 284, 284*f*
  forward-bending
    of lumbar joints, 308, 308*f*
    of upper cervical joint, 235, 235*f*
  inferior
    of fibula, 179, 179*f*
    of first rib, 283, 283*f*
    of glenohumeral joint, 32, 33*f*
    of hip joint, 142, 142*f*
    of patellofemoral joint, 164, 164*f*
    of scapulothoracic joint, 46, 47*f*
    of sternoclavicular joint, 52, 52*f*
  inspiration, of ribs
    five through eleven, 287, 287*f*
    two through seven, 286, 286*f*
  lateral
    of hip joint, 147, 147*f*
    of humeroulnar joint, 66, 66*f*
    of lumbar joints, using spinous processes, 300,
      301*f*
    of metacarpophalangeal joint, 130*f*, 131
        first, 124*f*, 125
        two through five, 130*f*, 131
    of metatarsophalangeal joints, 210, 210*f*
    of midcarpal joints, 104*f*, 105
    of patellofemoral joint, 166, 166*f*
    of radiocarpal joint, 88*f*, 89
    of scapulothoracic joint, 49, 49*f*
    of subtalar joint, 193, 193*f*
    of thoracic joints, using spinous processes/passive
      accessory vertebral motion, 270, 271*f*
    of tibiofemoral joint, 159, 159*f*
    of trapeziometacarpal joint, 117*f*, 118
    of triquetrum-pisiform joint, 98, 99*f*
    of ulnocarpal joint, 88*f*, 89
  medial
    of humeroulnar joint, 64
    of metacarpophalangeal joint
        first, 124, 125*f*
        two through five, 130, 131*f*
    of metatarsophalangeal joints, 209, 209*f*
    of midcarpal joints, 104, 105*f*
    of patellofemoral joint, 165, 165*f*
    of radiocarpal joint, 88, 89*f*
    of scapulothoracic joint, 48, 48*f*
    of subtalar joint, 192, 192*f*
    of temporomandibular joint, 227, 227*f*
    of tibiofemoral joint, 158*f*
    of trapeziometacarpal joint, 117, 118*f*
    of triquetrum-pisiform joint, 98, 99*f*

Glide(s) *(Continued)*
    plantar
        of cuboid, 200, 200*f*
        of intermetatarsal joints, 204, 204*f*
        of interphalangeal joints of toes, 214, 214*f*
        of metatarsophalangeal joints, 208, 208*f*
        of navicular, 198, 198*f*
    posterior
        of acromioclavicular joint, 56, 56*f*
        of distal fibula, 176, 176*f*
        of distal radius, 79, 79*f*
        of distal row carpal joints, 110, 111*f*
        of glenohumeral joint, 34, 35*f*
        of hip joint, 143, 143*f*
        of humeroradial joint, 73, 73*f*
        of iliac crest, 318, 318*f*
        of intermetacarpal joints two through five, 120, 120*f*
        of interphalangeal joints, 134, 134*f*
        of metacarpophalangeal joints two through five, 128, 128*f*
        of midcarpal joints, 102, 102*f*
        of proximal fibula, 173, 173*f*
        of proximal radius, 76, 76*f*
        of radiocarpal joint, 86, 86*f*
            specific mobilizations/manipulations for, 90, 91*f*
        sacral, 323, 323*f*
        of sacroiliac joints, 319, 319*f*
        specific mobilizations/manipulations for, 102, 107*f*
        of sternoclavicular joint, 53, 53*f*
        of talocrural joint, 182, 182*f*
            for ankle sprains, 172
        of talus mobilization with movement, 188, 189*f*
        of tibiofemoral joint, 154, 154*f*
        of trapeziometacarpal, 115, 115*f*
        of ulnocarpal joint, 86, 86*f*
            specific mobilizations/manipulations for, 90, 91*f*
    posterior/superior, of more superior on more inferior thoracic vertebra, 281*f*
    posterolateral
        of femur on pelvis, 146, 146*f*
        of humerus mobilization with movement, 40-41, 40*f*
    proximal, of proximal row carpal joint, 94, 95*f*
    radial
        of metacarpophalangeal joint, 130*f*, 131
            first, 124*f*, 125
        of midcarpal joints, 104*f*, 105
        of radiocarpal joint, 88*f*, 89
        of trapeziometacarpal joint, 117*f*, 118
        of triquetrum-pisiform joint, 98, 99*f*
        of ulnocarpal joint, 88*f*, 89
    rotation
        of cervical joints
            lower, 256-257, 256*f*-257*f*
            upper, 236, 236*f*
        of lumbar joints, 306, 307*f*
    side, of lower cervical spine, 252, 252*f*

Glide(s) *(Continued)*
    side-bending, mobilization with movement, 258, 258*f*
    superior
        of fibula, 178, 178*f*
        of lumbar joints, using spinous processes, 296, 297*f*, 298, 299*f*
        of patellofemoral joint, 163, 163*f*
        of scapulothoracic joint, 44, 45*f*
        of sternoclavicular joint, 51, 51*f*
    ulnar
        of metacarpophalangeal joint
            first, 124, 125*f*
            two through five, 130, 131*f*
        of midcarpal joints, 104, 105*f*
        of radiocarpal joint, 88, 89*f*
        of trapeziometacarpal joint, 117, 118*f*
        of triquetrum-pisiform joint, 98, 99*f*
Grade V manipulation, of thoracic joints
    anterior glide, 280-282, 281*f*
    distraction, 278

H
Hand joints, 82*f*
    carpometacarpal, 82*f*
    intermetacarpal two through five, 119-121
        anterior glide of, 121, 121*f*
        posterior glide of, 120, 120*f*
    interphalangeal, 82*f*, 132-135
        anterior glide of, 135, 135*f*
        distraction of, 133, 133*f*
        posterior glide of, 134, 134*f*
    metacarpophalangeal, 82*f*
        decreased range of motion of, 83
        first, 122-125
            distraction of, 123, 123*f*
            lateral (radial) glide of, 124*f*, 125
            medial (ulnar) glide of, 124, 125*f*
        two through five, 126-131
            anterior glide of, 129, 129*f*
            distraction of, 127, 127*f*
            lateral (radial) glide of, 130*f*, 131
            medial (ulnar) glide of, 130, 131*f*
            posterior glide of, 128, 128*f*
    trapeziometacarpal, 113-118
        anterior glide of, 116, 116*f*
        distraction of, 114, 114*f*
        lateral (radial) glide of, 117*f*, 118
        medial (ulnar) glide of, 117, 118*f*
        posterior glide of, 115, 115*f*
Headache, cervical spine joint mobilization/manipulation for, 232
Hip joint, 138-148, 138*f*
    anterior glide of, 144-145, 144*f*-145*f*
    capsular pattern of restriction of, 140
    close-packed position of, 140
    concave surface of, 140

Hip joint *(Continued)*
  convex-concave rules for, 19*t*
  distraction of, 141, 141*f*
  inferior glide of, 142, 142*f*
  lateral glide of, 147, 147*f*
  ligaments of, 140
  mobilization/manipulation of, 139
  nonarthritic pain in, 139
  orientation of, 140
  osteoarthritis of, 139
  osteokinematic motions of, 140
  pathology of, 139
  posterior glide of, 143, 143*f*
    of femur on pelvis, 146, 146*f*
  resting position for, 11, 140
Hip pain, of sacroiliac joint, 315-316
Hippocrates, 3
Humeroradial joint, 60*f*, 61, 69-74
  anterior glide of, 74, 74*f*
  capsular pattern of restriction, 69
  close-packed position of, 69
  concave surface of, 69
  convex-concave rules for, 19*t*
  distraction of, 70, 71*f*
  ligaments of, 69
  orientation of, 69
  osteokinematic motions of, 69
  posterior glide of, 73, 73*f*
  resting position of, 69
Humeroulnar joint, 60*f*, 61-68
  capsular pattern of restriction in, 62
  close-packed position of, 62
  concave surface of, 62
  convex-concave rules for, 19*t*
  distraction of, 62, 63*f*
  lateral glide of, 66, 66*f*
    mobilization with movement, 68, 68*f*
  ligaments of, 62
  medial glide of, 64, 65*f*
    mobilization with movement, 67, 67*f*
  orientation of, 62
  osteokinematic motion of, 62
  resting position of, 62
  traction mobilizations/manipulations of, 11-12, 12*f*
Humerus, mobilization with movement of, posterolateral glide of, 40-41, 40*f*
Hypermobility, with or without pain, 14
Hypomobility
  evaluation for, 219
  identifying, 8
  with or without pain, 14

I
Iliac crest
  anterior glide of, 320, 320*f*
  posterior glide of, 318, 318*f*
Immobilization, on joint capsules, 6

Impingement syndrome, of shoulder joint, 29
Inferior glide
  of fibula, 179, 179*f*
  of first rib, 283, 283*f*
  of glenohumeral joint, 32, 33*f*
  of hip joint, 142, 142*f*
  of patellofemoral joint, 164, 164*f*
  of scapulothoracic joint, 46, 47*f*
  of sternoclavicular joint, 52, 52*f*
Inspiration glide, of ribs
  five through eleven, 287, 287*f*
  two through seven, 286, 286*f*
Intercarpal joints, convex-concave rules for, 19*t*
Intermetacarpal joints
  convex-concave rules for, 19*t*
  two through five, 119-121
    anterior glide of, 121, 121*f*
    posterior glide of, 120, 120*f*
Intermetatarsal joints, 171, 202-204
  convex-concave rules for, 19*t*
  dorsal glide of, 203, 203*f*
  ligaments of, 202
  orientation of, 202
  osteokinematic motion of, 202
  plantar glide of, 204, 204*f*
Interphalangeal joints
  of fingers, 82*f*
    anterior glide of, 135, 135*f*
    capsular pattern of restriction of, 132
    close-packed position of, 132
    concave surface of, 132
    distraction of, 133, 133*f*
    ligaments of, 132
    orientation of, 132
    osteokinematic motion of, 132
    posterior glide of, 134, 134*f*
    resting position of, 132
  of toes, 170*f*, 171, 211-214
    close-packed position of, 211
    concave joint surface of, 211
    convex-concave rules for, 19*t*
    distraction of, 212, 212*f*
    dorsal glide of, 213, 213*f*
    ligaments of, 211
    orientation of, 211
    osteokinematic motion of, 211
    plantar glide of, 214, 214*f*
    resting position of, 211
Intervention, 20-22
  amount and speed of force for, 21
  direction of force for, 21
  joint position for, 21
  mobilization with movement as, 23
  muscle energy as, 23-24
  in plan of care, 24
  timing of, 22
Intraarticular disc, 223

J

Jaw opening, 223
Joint capsule, adhesions of, 6
Joint cavitation, 23
Joint cracking, 23
Joint extensibility, increasing, 6
Joint manipulation, cracking noise during, 23
Joint mobility, examination and evaluation of, 13
Joint mobilization/manipulation
    definition of, 3
    effects of, 6-8
        mechanical, 6-7
        neurophysiological, 7-8
    evidence-based/evidence-informed practice of, 5-6
    general concepts of, 3-9
    history of, 3
    intervention strategies for, 8
    practitioners contributing to knowledge base of, 3-4
    regional interdependence and, 8
    technique for, 22-23
    variations in, 23-24
Joint motion, types of, 15-16
Joint position, during treatment, 21

K

Kaltenborn, 4
Knee joints, 150-169, 150f
    mobilization/manipulation of, 151
    osteoarthritis of, 151
    patellofemoral, 151, 162-168
        inferior glide of, 164, 164f
        lateral glide of, 166, 166f
        lateral tilt of, 168, 168f
        medial glide of, 165, 165f
        medial tilt of, 167, 167f
        superior glide of, 163, 163f
    specific pathology of, 151
    tibiofemoral, 151-161
        anterior glide of tibia on femur of, 155-157, 155f-157f
        distraction of, 153, 153f
        lateral glide of, 159, 159f
        medial glide of, 158, 158f
        posterior glide of, 154, 154f

L

Lateral epicondylalgia, 61
    cervical spine joint mobilization/manipulation for, 233
    thoracic spine and rib joint mobilization/manipulation for, 262
Lateral glide
    of hip joint, 147, 147f
    of humeroulnar joint, 66, 66f
        mobilization with movement, 68, 68f
    of metacarpophalangeal joint
        first, 124f, 125
        two through five, 130f, 131

Lateral glide (Continued)
    of metatarsophalangeal joints, 210, 210f
    of midcarpal joints, 104f, 105
    of patellofemoral joint, 166, 166f
    of radiocarpal joint, 88f, 89
    of scapulothoracic joint, 49, 49f
    of subtalar joint, 193, 193f
    of thoracic joints, using spinous processes/passive accessory vertebral motion, 270, 271f
    of trapeziometacarpal joint, 117f, 118
    of triquetrum-pisiform joint, 98, 99f
    using spinous processes, 300, 301f
Lateral tilt
    of patellofemoral joint, 168, 168f
    of subtalar joint, 195, 195f
Load deformation, 13, 13f
Long-axis tractions, 11-12
Loose-packed position, 11
Low back pain, nonspecific, lumbar spine mobilization/manipulation for, 291-292
Lower leg joint, 170-215
    distal tibiofibular, 170f, 171, 175-179
        distal fibula in
            anterior glide of, 177, 177f
            posterior glide of, 176, 176f
        fibula in
            inferior glide of, 179, 179f
            superior glide of, 178, 178f
    proximal tibiofibular, 170f, 171-174
        anterior glide of proximal fibula of, 174, 174f
        posterior glide of proximal fibula of, 173, 173f
Lumbar joints, 290f, 291, 293-311
    coupled motion of, 219-220
    facet, 290f, 291
    ligaments of, 293
    mobilization/manipulation of
        for lumbar radiculopathy, 292
        for nonspecific low back pain, 291-292
        risks of, 291
        specific pathology of, 291-292
    mobilization with movement
        backward-bending glide, 309, 309f
        forward-bending glide, 308, 308f
    orientation of, 293
    osteokinematic motions of, 293
    precautions and contraindications to mobilization and manipulation interventions for, 220
    rotation glide of, 306, 307f
    rotation manipulation of, 310, 310f
        lumbosacral, 311, 311f
    spinous processes of
        anterior glide using, 294, 295f
        lateral glide using, 300, 301f
        superior glide using, 296, 297f, 298, 299f
    superior glide using spinous processes/passive accessory vertebral motion of, 296, 297f, 298, 299f

Lumbar joints *(Continued)*
    transverse processes of, anterior glide using, 302, 303*f*, 304, 305*f*
    vertebral body joint in, 290*f*
Lumbar radiculopathy, 292
Lumbar rotation manipulation, 310, 310*f*
Lumbosacral rotation manipulation, 311, 311*f*

M
Maitland, 4
Maitland mobilization/manipulation, 21, 22*f*
Mechanical effects, of joint mobilization/manipulation, 6-7
Medial glide
    of humeroulnar joint, 64, 65*f*
        mobilization with movement, 67, 67*f*
    of metacarpophalangeal joint
        first, 124, 125*f*
        two through five, 130, 131*f*
    of metatarsophalangeal joints, 209, 209*f*
    of midcarpal joints, 104, 105*f*
    of patellofemoral joint, 165, 165*f*
    of radiocarpal joint, 88, 89*f*
    of scapulothoracic joint, 48, 48*f*
    of subtalar joint, 192, 192*f*
    of temporomandibular joint, 227, 227*f*
    of tibiofemoral joint, 158, 158*f*
    of trapeziometacarpal joint, 117, 118*f*
    of triquetrum-pisiform joint, 98, 99*f*
Medial tilt
    of patellofemoral joint, 167, 167*f*
    of subtalar joint, 194, 194*f*
Mennell, 4
Metacarpal joints, 82*f*, 83
Metacarpophalangeal joint(s), 82*f*, 83
    convex-concave rules for, 19*t*
    decreased range of motion of, 83
    first, 122-125
        capsular pattern of restriction of, 122
        close-packed position of, 122
        concave surface of, 122
        distraction of, 123, 123*f*
        lateral (radial) glide of, 124*f*, 125
        ligaments of, 122
        medial (ulnar) glide of, 124, 125*f*
        orientation of, 122
        osteokinematic motion of, 122
        resting position of, 122
    two through five, 126-131
        anterior glide of, 129, 129*f*
        capsular pattern of restriction of, 126
        close-packed position of, 126
        concave surface of, 126
        convex-concave rules for, 19*t*
        distraction of, 127, 127*f*
        lateral (radial) glide of, 130*f*, 131
        ligaments of, 126

Metacarpophalangeal joint(s) *(Continued)*
        medial (ulnar) glide of, 130, 131*f*
        orientation of, 126
        osteokinematic motions of, 126
        posterior glide of, 128, 128*f*
        resting position of, 126
Metatarsophalangeal joint(s), 170*f*, 171, 205-210
    capsular pattern of restriction of, 205
    close-packed position of, 205
    concave joint surface of, 205
    convex-concave rules for, 19*t*
    distraction of, 206, 206*f*
    dorsal glide of, 207, 207*f*
    lateral glide of, 210, 210*f*
    ligaments of, 205
    medial glide of, 209, 209*f*
    orientation of, 205
    osteokinematic motions of, 205
    plantar glide of, 208, 208*f*
    range of motion of, 171
    resting position of, 205
Midback pain, thoracic spine and rib joint mobilization/manipulation for, 261
Midcarpal joints, 82*f*, 83, 100-112
    anterior glide of, 103, 103*f*
        specific mobilizations/manipulations for, 108, 109*f*
    capsular pattern of restriction of, 100
    close-packed position of, 100
    concave surface of, 100
    distraction of, 101, 101*f*
    lateral (radial) glide of, 104*f*, 105
    ligaments of, 100
    medial (ulnar) glide of, 104, 105*f*
    orientation of, 100
    osteokinematic motions of, 100
    posterior glide of, 102, 102*f*
        specific mobilizations/manipulations for, 106, 107*f*
    resting position of, 100
Midtarsal joints, 170*f*, 171, 196-201
    capsular pattern of restriction of, 196
    close-packed position of, 196
    cuboid in
        dorsal glide of, 199, 199*f*
        plantar glide of, 200, 200*f*
        whip/manipulation of, 201, 201*f*
    ligaments of, 196
    navicular in
        dorsal glide of, 197, 197*f*
        plantar glide of, 198, 198*f*
    orientation of, 196
    osteokinematic motions of, 196
    resting position of, 196
Mobilization
    grades of, 21
        with oscillations, 21, 22*f*
    with movement, 3-4, 23

Mobilization/manipulation. *see* Joint mobilization/
    manipulation
Motion
    accessory, 6
    arthrokinematic, 6
    coupled, 219-220
    oscillation, 11
    osteokinematic, 6, 23
        convex-concave rules for, 19*t*
Motion segment, 219
Movement
    mobilization with, 3-4, 23
    osteokinematic, 6
Mulligan, 4
Muscle energy, 3, 23-24
    for sacroiliac joint
        with anterior glide, 321, 321*f*
        with distraction, 317, 317*f*
        with posterior glide, 319, 319*f*
    for symphysis pubis, 325, 325*f*

N
Navicular
    dorsal glide of, 197, 197*f*
    plantar glide of, 198, 198*f*
Neck pain
    nonspecific, cervical spine joint mobilization/
        manipulation of, 232
    thoracic spine and rib joint mobilization/
        manipulation for, 261-262
Neuromusculoskeletal examination, osteopathic, 3
Neurophysiological effects, of joint mobilization/
        manipulation, 7-8
Normal mobility, with or without pain, 14
Nutation, of sacroiliac joint, 315

O
Occipitoatlantal joint, 230*f*
    osteokinematic motions of, 233
Oscillation(s), grades of mobilization/manipulation
        with, 21, 22*f*
Oscillation motion, 11
Osteoarthritis
    of hip joint, 139
    of knee, 151
Osteokinematic degrees of freedom, 6
Osteokinematic motion, 6, 23
    convex-concave rules for, 19*t*
Osteopathic neuromusculoskeletal examination, 3
Osteopathy, 3
Ovoid joints, 17, 18*f*

P
Pain
    and accessory motion testing, 22
    examination and evaluation of, 14
    reduction of, 7

Passive accessory vertebral motion
    of iliac crest
        with anterior glide, 320, 320*f*
        with posterior glide, 318, 318*f*
    lower cervical
        with anterior glide
            using facet joints, 250, 251*f*
            using spinous processes, 240, 241*f*
        with anterior/superior glide, using spinous
            processes
            first technique of, 242, 243*f*
            second technique of, 244, 245*f*
        with distraction, 238, 239*f*
        with lateral glide using spinous processes, 246, 247*f*
    lumbar
        with anterior glide
            using spinous processes, 294, 295*f*
            using transverse processes, 304, 305*f*
        with lateral glide, using spinous processes, 300,
            301*f*
        with superior glide, using spinous processes, 296,
            297*f*, 299*f*
    sacral anterior glide with, 322, 322*f*
    sacral posterior glide with, 323, 323*f*
    thoracic
        with anterior glide, using spinous processes, 264,
            265*f*, 266, 267*f*, 268, 269*f*
        with lateral glide using spinous processes, 270, 271*f*
        with posterior/superior glide of more superior on
            more inferior vertebra, 281*f*
    upper cervical, with distraction, 234, 234*f*
Passive physiologic motion, of rib joints
    five through eleven
        with expiration glide, 285, 285*f*
        with inspiration glide, 287, 287*f*
    two through seven
        with expiration glide, 284, 284*f*
        with inspiration glide, 286, 286*f*
Passive physiologic vertebral motion
    lumbar, with rotation glide, 306, 307*f*
    upper cervical
        with forward-bending glide, 235, 235*f*
        with rotation glide, 236, 236*f*
Patella, 150*f*
Patellofemoral joint, 150*f*, 151, 162-168, 170*f*
    capsular pattern of restriction of, 162
    close-packed position of, 162
    concave surface of, 162
    convex-concave rules for, 17, 19*t*
    inferior glide of, 164, 164*f*
    lateral glide of, 166, 166*f*
    lateral tilt of, 168, 168*f*
    ligament of, 162
    medial glide of, 165, 165*f*
    medial tilt of, 167, 167*f*
    orientation of, 162
    osteokinematic motion of, 162

Patellofemoral joint (Continued)
  resting position of, 162
  superior glide of, 163, 163f
Pelvic joint(s), 314-326, 314f
  precautions and contraindications to mobilization
      and manipulation interventions for, 220
  sacroiliac, 314f, 315-323
    anterior glide/muscle energy for, 321, 321f
    capsular pattern of restriction of, 316
    distraction/muscle energy for, 317, 317f
    iliac crest of
      anterior glide/passive accessory motion of, 320,
          320f
      posterior glide/passive accessory vertebral
          motion of, 318, 318f
    impairment of, 315
      hip pain and, 315-316
    ligaments of, 316
    motion at, 315
    orientation of, 316
    osteokinematic motions of, 316
    pain in, 315-316
    posterior glide/muscle energy for, 319, 319f
    sacral anterior glide/passive accessory motion for,
        322, 322f
    sacral posterior glide/passive accessory motion for,
        323, 323f
    types of, 316
  symphysis pubis as, 315, 324-325
    distraction/muscle energy for, 325, 325f
Pelvis, posterolateral glide of femur on, 146, 146f
Plan of care, mobilization/manipulation in, 24
Plantar glide
  of cuboid, 200, 200f
  of intermetatarsal joints, 204, 204f
  of interphalangeal joints of toes, 214, 214f
  of metatarsophalangeal joints, 208, 208f
  of navicular, 198, 198f
Plastic phase, of stress-strain curve, 13, 13f
Positional faults
  defined, 7
  examination and evaluation of, 20
  of sacroiliac joints, 315
Posterior glide
  of acromioclavicular joint, 56, 56f
  of distal fibula, 176, 176f
  of distal radius, 79, 79f
  of distal row carpal joints, 110, 111f
  of glenohumeral joint, 34, 35f
  of hip joint, 143, 143f
  of humeroradial joint, 73, 73f
  of iliac crest, 318, 318f
  of intermetacarpal joints two through five, 120, 120f
  of interphalangeal joints, 134, 134f
  of metacarpophalangeal joints two through five, 128, 128f
  of midcarpal joints, 102, 102f
    specific mobilizations/manipulations for, 106, 107f

Posterior glide (Continued)
  of proximal fibula, 173, 173f
  of proximal radius, 76, 76f
  of proximal row carpal joint, 94, 95f
  of radiocarpal joint, 86, 86f
    specific mobilizations/manipulations for, 90, 91f
  sacral, 323, 323f
  of sacroiliac joints, 319, 319f
  of sternoclavicular joint, 53, 53f
  of talocrural joint, 182, 182f
    for ankle sprains, 172
  of talus mobilization with movement, 188, 189f
  of tibiofemoral joint, 154, 154f
  of trapeziometacarpal joint, 115, 115f
  of ulnocarpal joint, 86, 86f
    specific mobilizations/manipulations for, 90, 91f
Posterior/superior glide, of more superior on more
    inferior thoracic vertebra, 281f
Posterolateral glide, of femur on pelvis, 146, 146f
Pronation, 171
Proximal fibula
  anterior glide of, 174, 174f
  posterior glide of, 173, 173f
Proximal interphalangeal joints, of hand, convex-
    concave rules for, 19t
Proximal radioulnar joint, 60f, 61
  capsular pattern of restriction of, 75
  close-packed position of, 75
  concave surface of, 75
  convex-concave rules for, 19t
  ligaments of, 75
  orientation of, 75
  osteokinematic motion of, 75
  resting position of, 75
Proximal radius
  anterior glide of, 77, 77f
  posterior glide of, 76, 76f
Proximal row carpal joint
  anterior glide of, 96, 97f
  posterior glide of, 94, 95f
Proximal tibiofibular joint, 150f, 170f, 171-174
  capsular pattern of, 172
  close-packed position of, 172
  concave joint surface of, 172
  convex-concave rules for, 19t
  ligaments of, 172
  orientation of, 172
  proximal fibula in
    anterior glide of, 174, 174f
    posterior glide of, 173, 173f
  resting position of, 172

R
Radial glide
  of metacarpophalangeal joints
    first, 124f, 125
    two through five, 130f, 131

Radial glide (Continued)
   of midcarpal joints, 104f, 105
   of radiocarpal joint, 88f, 89
   of trapeziometacarpal joint, 117f, 118
   of triquetrum-pisiform joint, 98, 99f
   of ulnocarpal joint, 88f, 89
Radiculopathy, lumbar, 292
Radiocarpal joint(s), 82f, 83-98
   anterior glide of, 87, 87f
     specific mobilizations/manipulations for, 92, 93f
   capsular pattern of restriction of, 84
   close-packed position of, 84
   concave surface of, 84
   convex-concave rules for, 19t
   distraction of, 85, 85f
   lateral (radial) glide, 88f, 89
   ligaments of, 84
   medial (ulnar) glide of, 88, 89f
   orientation of, 84
   osteokinematic motions of, 84
   posterior glide of, 86, 86f
     specific mobilizations/manipulations for, 90, 91f
   resting position of, 84
   specific pathology of, 84-98
Radioulnar joint
   convex-concave rules for, 19t
   distal, 60f, 61, 78-80, 82f
     convex-concave rules for, 19t
   proximal, 60f, 61
     convex-concave rules for, 19t
Range-of-motion exercises, joint mobility and, 7
Regional interdependence, 8
Resting position, 11
   during treatment, 21
Rib joint(s), 260f, 261, 282-288
   anterior glide of, 288, 288f
   first, inferior glide of, 283, 283f
   five through eleven
     expiration glide of, 285, 285f
     inspiration glide of, 287, 287f
   ligaments of, 282
   mobilization/manipulation of, 261-262
   orientation of, 282
   osteokinematic motions of, 282
   two through seven
     expiration glide of, 284, 284f
     inspiration glide of, 286, 286f
Rolling, 15-16, 15f
Rotation glide
   of cervical joints
     lower, 256-257, 256f-257f
     upper, 236, 236f
   of lumbar spine joint, 306, 307f
Rotation manipulation, of lumbar spine joint, 310, 310f
   lumbosacral, 311, 311f

S
Sacral anterior glide, 322, 322f
Sacral extension, 315
Sacral flexion, 315
Sacral posterior glide, 323, 323f
Sacroiliac joint(s), 314f, 315
   anterior glide/muscle energy for, 321, 321f
   capsular pattern of restriction of, 316
   distraction of/ muscle energy for, 317, 317f
   iliac crest of
     anterior glide/passive accessory motion of, 320, 320f
     posterior glide/passive accessory vertebral motion of, 318, 318f
   impairment of, 315
     hip pain and, 315-316
   ligaments of, 316
   mobilization/manipulation of, 315-316
     for hip pain, 315-316
   motion at, 315
   orientation of, 316
   osteokinematic motions of, 316
   pain in, 315-316
   posterior glide/muscle energy for, 319, 319f
   sacral anterior glide/passive accessory motion of, 322, 322f
   sacral posterior glide/passive accessory motion of, 323, 323f
   specific pathology of, 315-316
   types of, 316
Scapulothoracic joint, 29, 42-49
   capsular pattern of restriction of, 42
   close-packed position of, 42
   concave surface of, 42
   distraction of, 43, 43f
   inferior glide of, 46, 47f
   lateral glide of, 49, 49f
   ligaments of, 42
   medial glide of, 48, 48f
   orientation of, 42
   osteokinematic motions of, 42
   resting position of, 42
   superior glide of, 44, 45f
Selective tissue tension testing, 4
Sellar joints, 17, 18f
Shoulder joint(s), 28-58, 28f
   acromioclavicular, 28f, 29, 55-57
     anterior glide of, 57, 57f
     posterior glide of, 56, 56f
   adhesive capsulitis of, 29
   glenohumeral, 28f, 29
     anterior glide of, 36, 37f
     distraction of, 30, 31f
     inferior glide of, 32, 33f
     posterior glide of, 34, 35f
     posterolateral glide of humerus mobilization with movement in, 40-41, 40f

Shoulder joint(s) (*Continued*)
    impingement syndrome of, 29
    nonspecific pain in, 29
    rotator cuff injuries in, 29
    scapulothoracic joint in, 29, 42-49
        distraction of, 43, 43*f*
        inferior glide of, 47*f*
        lateral glide of, 49, 49*f*
        medial glide of, 48, 48*f*
        superior glide of, 44, 45*f*
    specific pathology of, 29
    sternoclavicular joint in, 28*f*, 29, 50-54
        anterior glide of clavicle on sternum of, 54, 54*f*
        inferior glide of, 52, 52*f*
        posterior glide of, 53, 53*f*
        superior glide of, 51, 51*f*
Side-bending glide mobilization, of lower cervical joints, 258, 258*f*
Side glide, of lower cervical joints, 252, 252*f*
Somatic dysfunction, 3
Spinal joint
    coupled motion of, 219-220
    precautions and contraindications to mobilization and manipulation interventions for, 220
Spinning, 15-16, 15*f*
Spinous processes
    cervical
        anterior glide using, 240, 241*f*
        anterior/superior glide using
            first technique, 242, 243*f*
            second technique, 244, 245*f*
        lateral glide using, 246, 247*f*
    lumbar
        anterior glide using, 294, 295*f*
        lateral glide using, 300, 301*f*
        superior glide using, 296, 297*f*, 298, 299*f*
    thoracic
        anterior glide using passive accessory vertebral motion and, 264, 265*f*, 266, 267*f*, 268, 269*f*
        lateral glide using passive accessory vertebral motion and, 270, 271*f*
Sternoclavicular joint, 28*f*, 29, 50-54
    anterior glide of clavicle on sternum of, 54, 54*f*
    capsular pattern of restriction of, 50
    close-packed position of, 50
    concave surface of, 50
    convex-concave rules for, 19*t*
    inferior glide of, 52, 52*f*
    ligaments of, 50
    orientation of, 50
    osteokinematic motions of, 50
    posterior glide of, 53, 53*f*
    resting position of, 50
    superior glide of, 51, 51*f*
Sternum, anterior glide of clavicle on, 54, 54*f*
Strengthening exercises, joint mobility and, 7

Stress-strain curve, 13, 13*f*
Subluxations, 7
Subtalar joint, 170*f*, 171, 190-195
    capsular pattern of restriction of, 190
    close-packed position of, 190
    convex-concave rules for, 19*t*
    distraction of, 191, 191*f*
    lateral glide of, 193, 193*f*
    lateral tilt of, 195, 195*f*
    ligaments of, 190
    medial glide of, 192, 192*f*
    medial tilt of, 194, 194*f*
    orientation of, 190
    osteokinematic motion of, 190
    range of motion of, 171
    resting position of, 190
Superior glide
    of fibula, 178, 178*f*
    of lumbar joint, using spinous processes, 296, 297*f*, 298, 299*f*
    of patellofemoral joint, 163, 163*f*
    of scapulothoracic joint, 44, 45*f*
    of sternoclavicular joint, 51, 51*f*
Supination, 171
Symphysis pubis, 315, 324-325
    distraction/muscle energy for, 325, 325*f*

T
Talocrural joint, 170*f*, 171, 180-188
    anterior glide of talus on tibia and fibula of, 183-184, 183*f*, 185*f*
    capsular pattern of restriction of, 180
    close-packed position of, 180
    concave joint surface of, 180
    convex-concave rules for, 19*t*
    distraction of, 181, 181*f*
    ligaments of, 180
    orientation of, 180
    osteokinematic motions of, 180
    posterior glide of, 182, 182*f*
        for ankle sprains, 172
    range of motion of, 171
    resting position of, 180
Talonavicular joint, 170*f*, 171, 196
    convex-concave rules for, 19*t*
    dorsal glide of navicular of, 197, 197*f*
    plantar glide of navicular of, 198, 198*f*
Talus, on tibia and fibula, anterior glide of, 183-184, 183*f*, 185*f*
Tarsometatarsal joints, 170*f*
Temporomandibular joint, 222-228, 222*f*
    anterior glide of, 226, 226*f*
    basics, 223
    capsular pattern of restriction of, 224
    close-packed position of, 224
    concave surface of, 224

Temporomandibular joint *(Continued)*
    convex-concave rules for, 19*t*
    disorders of, 223
        cervical spine joint mobilization/manipulation for, 233
    distraction of, 225, 225*f*
    ligaments of, 224
    medial glide of, 227, 227*f*
    mobilization/manipulation of, 223
    orientation of, 224
    osteokinematic motions of, 224
    resting position of, 224
    specific pathology of, 223
Thoracic joint(s), 260-289, 260*f*
    anterior glide of
        grade V manipulation, 280-282, 281*f*
        using spinous processes/passive accessory vertebral motion, 264, 265*f*, 266, 267*f*, 268, 269*f*
        using transverse processes, 272, 274, 275*f*
    coupled motion of, 219-220
    distraction grade V manipulation of, 278
    lateral glide of, using spinous processes/passive accessory vertebral motion, 270, 271*f*
    ligaments of, 263
    mobilization/manipulation of, 261-262
        for lateral epicondylalgia, 262
        for midback pain, 261
        for neck pain, 261-262
    orientation of, 263
    osteokinematic motions of, 263
    posterior/superior glide of more superior on more inferior vertebra/manipulation/passive accessory vertebral motions of, 281*f*
    type of, 263
    upper, 231
Thrust joint manipulation, 21
Thumb joints, 82*f*, 83
    interphalangeal, 82*f*, 132-135
        anterior glide of, 135, 135*f*
        distraction of, 133, 133*f*
        posterior glide of, 134, 134*f*
    metacarpophalangeal, 82*f*, 122-125
        decreased range of motion of, 83
        distraction of, 123, 123*f*
        first
            lateral (radial) glide of, 124*f*, 125
            medial (ulnar) glide of, 124, 125*f*
    trapeziometacarpal, 113-118
        anterior glide of, 116, 116*f*
        distraction of, 114, 114*f*
        lateral (radial) glide of, 117*f*, 118
        medial (ulnar) glide of, 117, 118*f*
        posterior glide of, 115, 115*f*
Tibia, 150*f*
    on femur, anterior glide of, 155-157, 155*f*-157*f*
    talus on, anterior glide of, 183-184, 183*f*, 185*f*

Tibiofemoral joint, 150*f*, 151-161, 170*f*
    anterior glide of tibia on femur of, 155-157, 155*f*-157*f*
    capsular pattern of restriction of, 152
    close-packed position of, 152
    concave surface of, 152
    convex-concave rules for, 17*f*, 19*t*
    distraction of, 153, 153*f*
    lateral glide of, 159, 159*f*
        mobilization with movement, 161, 161*f*
    ligaments of, 152
    medial glide of, 158, 158*f*
        mobilization with movement, 160, 160*f*
    orientation of, 152
    osteokinematic motions of, 152
    posterior glide of, 154, 154*f*
    proximal, 150*f*
    resting position of, 152
Tibiofibular joint
    in ankle sprain, 172
    convex-concave rules for, 19*t*
    distal, 170*f*, 171, 175-179
        in ankle sprain, 172
        capsular pattern of restriction of, 175
        close-packed position of, 175
        concave joint surface of, 175
        distal fibula in
            anterior glide of, 177, 177*f*
            posterior glide of, 176, 176*f*
        fibula in
            inferior glide of, 179, 179*f*
            superior glide of, 178, 178*f*
        ligaments of, 175
        orientation of, 175
        resting position of, 175
    proximal, 170*f*, 171-174
        capsular pattern of, 172
        close-packed position of, 172
        concave joint surface of, 172
        ligaments of, 172
        orientation of, 172
        proximal fibula in
            anterior glide of, 174, 174*f*
            posterior glide of, 173, 173*f*
        resting position of, 172
Tilt
    lateral
        of patellofemoral joint, 168, 168*f*
        of subtalar joint, 195, 195*f*
    medial
        of patellofemoral joint, 167, 167*f*
        of subtalar joint, 194, 194*f*
Toe joints, 171
    interphalangeal, 170*f*, 171, 211-214
        distraction of, 212, 212*f*
        dorsal glide of, 213, 213*f*
        plantar glide of, 214, 214*f*

Toe joints (Continued)
  metatarsophalangeal, 170f, 171, 205-210
    distraction of, 206, 206f
    dorsal glide of, 207, 207f
    lateral glide of, 210, 210f
    medial glide of, 209, 209f
    plantar glide of, 208, 208f
Traction, 11, 12f
  long-axis, 11-12
Transverse processes
  anterior glide using, 272, 274, 275f
  of lumbar spine, anterior glide using, 302, 303f, 304,
    305f
Trapeziometacarpal joint, 83
  anterior glide of, 116, 116f
  capsular pattern of restriction of, 113
  close-packed position of, 113
  concave surface of, 113
  distraction of, 114, 114f
  lateral (radial) glide of, 117f, 118
  ligaments of, 113
  medial (ulnar) glide of, 117, 118f
  orientation of, 113
  osteokinematic motions of, 113
  posterior glide of, 115, 115f
  resting position of, 113
Treatment plane, 11
Triquetrum-pisiform articulation, 83
  lateral (radial) and medial (ulnar) glide of, 98, 99f

U
Ulnar glide
  of metacarpophalangeal joint
    first, 124, 125f
    two through five, 130, 131f
  of midcarpal joints, 104, 105f
  of radiocarpal joint, 88, 89f
  of trapeziometacarpal joint, 117, 118f
  of triquetrum-pisiform joint, 98, 99f
Ulnocarpal joints, 82f, 83
  anterior glide of, 87, 87f
    specific mobilizations/manipulations for, 92, 93f
  capsular pattern of restriction of, 84
  close-packed position of, 84
  concave surface of, 84
  distraction of, 85, 85f
  lateral (radial) glide of, 88f, 89
  ligaments of, 84

Ulnocarpal joints (Continued)
  medial (ulnar) glide, 88, 89f
  orientation of, 84
  osteokinematic motions of, 84
  posterior glide of, 86, 86f
    specific mobilizations/manipulations for, 90, 91f
  resting position of, 84
  specific pathology of, 83-98

V
Validity, of studies, 5
Vertebral body joint
  cervical, 230f
  lumbar, 290f
  thoracic, 260f
Vertebral motion, 219

W
Whip/manipulation, of cuboid, 201, 201f
Wrist joint(s), 82f, 83
  distal row carpal
    anterior glide of, 112, 112f
    posterior glide of, 110, 111f
  midcarpal, 82f
    anterior glide of, 103, 103f
      specific mobilizations/manipulations for, 108,
        109f
    distraction of, 101, 101f
    lateral (radial) glide of, 104f, 105
    medial (ulnar) glide of, 104, 105f
    posterior glide of, 102, 102f
      specific mobilizations/manipulations for, 106,
        107f
    resting position of, 100
  proximal row carpal
    anterior glide of, 96, 97f
    posterior glide of, 94, 95f
  radiocarpal and ulnocarpal, 82f, 84-98
    anterior glide of, 87, 87f
      specific mobilizations/manipulations for, 92, 93f
    distraction of, 85, 85f
    lateral (radial) glide, 88f, 89
    medial (ulnar) glide, 88, 89f
    posterior glide of, 86, 86f
      specific mobilizations/manipulations for, 90, 91f
  specific pathology of, 83
  triquetrum-pisiform, lateral (medial) and radial
    (ulnar) glide of, 98, 99f